Gastrointestinal Emergencies

Guest Editors

ANGELA M. MILLS, MD
ANTHONY J. DEAN, MD

EMERGENCY MEDICINE CLINICS OF NORTH AMERICA

www.emed.theclinics.com

Consulting Editor
AMAL MATTU, MD

May 2011 • Volume 29 • Number 2

SAUNDERS an imprint of ELSEVIER, Inc.

W.B. SAUNDERS COMPANY

A Division of Elsevier Inc.

1600 John F. Kennedy Boulevard • Suite 1800 • Philadelphia, Pennsylvania 19103-2899

http://www.theclinics.com

EMERGENCY MEDICINE CLINICS OF NORTH AMERICA Volume 29, Number 2
May 2011 ISSN 0733-8627, ISBN-13: 978-1-4557-0439-2

Editor: Patrick Manley
Developmental Editor: Donald Mumford

Emergency Medicine Clinics of North America (ISSN 0733-8627) is published quarterly by Elsevier Inc., 360 Park Avenue South, New York, NY, 10010-1710. Months of issue are February, May, August, and November. Business and Editorial Offices: 1600 John F. Kennedy Boulevard, Suite 1800, Philadelphia, PA 19103-2899. Customer Service Office: 6277 Sea Harbor Drive, Orlando, FL 32887-4800. Periodicals postage paid at New York, NY, and additional mailing offices. Subscription prices are $133.00 per year (US students), $264.00 per year (US individuals), $455.00 per year (US institutions), $189.00 per year (international students), $379.00 per year (international individuals), $549.00 per year (international institutions), $189.00 per year (Canadian students), $326.00 per year (Canadian individuals), and $549.00 per year (Canadian institutions). International air speed delivery is included in all *Clinics'* subscription prices. All prices are subject to change without notice. **POSTMASTER:** Send address changes to *Emergency Medicine Clinics of North America*, Elsevier Periodicals Customer Service, 11830 Westline Industrial Drive, St. Louis, MO 63146. Customer Service (orders, claims, online, change of address): Elsevier Periodicals Customer Service, 11830 Westline Industrial Drive, St. Louis, MO 63146. Tel: 1-800-654-2452 (U.S. and Canada); 314-453-7041 (outside U.S. and Canada). Fax: 314-453-5170. E-mail: journalscustomerservice-usa@elsevier.com (for print support); journalsonline support-usa@elsevier.com (for online support).

Reprints. For copies of 100 or more of articles in this publication, please contact the Commercial Reprints Department, Elsevier Inc., 360 Park Avenue South, New York, NY 10010-1710. Tel.: 212-633-3812; Fax: 212-462-1935; E-mail: reprints@elsevier.com.

Emergency Medicine Clinics of North America is covered in *MEDLINE/PubMed (Index Medicus), Current Contents/Clinical Medicine, EMBASE/Excerpta Medica, BIOSIS, SciSearch, CINAHL, ISI/BIOMED,* and *Research Alert.*

Printed and bound by CPI Group (UK) Ltd, Croydon, CR0 4YY

Transferred to Digital Print 2011

Contributors

CONSULTING EDITOR

AMAL MATTU, MD, FAAEM, FACEP
Program Director, Emergency Medicine Residency; Professor, Department of Emergency Medicine, University of Maryland School of Medicine, Baltimore, Maryland

GUEST EDITORS

ANGELA M. MILLS, MD
Assistant Professor of Emergency Medicine, Department of Emergency Medicine, University of Pennsylvania School of Medicine, Philadelphia, Pennsylvania

ANTHONY J. DEAN, MD, FAAEM, FACEP
Associate Professor of Emergency Medicine, Associate Professor of Emergency Medicine in Radiology; Director, Division of Emergency Ultrasonography, Department of Emergency Medicine, University of Pennsylvania Medical Center, Philadelphia, Pennsylvania

AUTHORS

ELIZABETH R. ALPERN, MD, MSCE
Associate Professor of Pediatrics, Division of Emergency Medicine, Department of Pediatrics, The Children's Hospital of Philadelphia, Philadelphia, Pennsylvania

CPT KENTON L. ANDERSON, MD, USAF, MC
Director of Emergency Ultrasound, Department of Emergency Medicine, Wilford Hall Medical Center, Lackland Air Force Base, San Antonio, Texas

MICHAEL BREYER, MD
Associate Program Director, Residency in Emergency Medicine, Denver Health and Hospital Authority; Assistant Professor, University of Colorado School of Medicine, Denver, Colorado

MATTHEW C. CARLISLE, MD
Chief Resident, Emergency Medicine Residency, Department of Emergency Medicine, Palmetto Health Richland, Columbia, South Carolina

ESTHER H. CHEN, MD
Associate Professor of Emergency Medicine, Department of Emergency Medicine, University of San Francisco, San Francisco, California

ANTHONY J. DEAN, MD, FAAEM, FACEP
Associate Professor of Emergency Medicine; Associate Professor of Emergency Medicine in Radiology; Director, Division of Emergency Ultrasonography, Department of Emergency Medicine, University of Pennsylvania Medical Center, Philadelphia, Pennsylvania

DANIEL J. EGAN, MD
Department of Emergency Medicine, St Luke's Roosevelt Hospital Center, New York, New York

J. MATTHEW FIELDS, MD
Assistant Professor of Emergency Medicine, Department of Emergency Medicine, Thomas Jefferson University Hospital, Philadelphia, Pennsylvania

LEILA GETTO, MD
Academic Faculty, Department of Emergency Medicine, Christiana Care Health System, Newark, Delaware

GEOFFREY E. HAYDEN, MD
Adjunct Faculty Member, Department of Emergency Medicine, Vanderbilt University Medical Center, Nashville, Tennessee

AMANDA E. HORN, MD
Assistant Professor of Emergency Medicine, Department of Emergency Medicine, Temple University School of Medicine, Philadelphia, Pennsylvania

KATHERINE JAHNES, MD
Department of Emergency Medicine, New York Methodist Hospital, Brooklyn, New York

RITU KUMAR, MD
Resident Physician in Emergency Medicine, Department of Emergency Medicine, University of Pennsylvania School of Medicine, Philadelphia, Pennsylvania

RESA E. LEWISS, MD
Department of Emergency Medicine, St Luke's Roosevelt Hospital Center, New York, New York

ALESSANDRO MANGILI, MD
Assistant Professor, Department of Emergency Medicine, Oregon Health and Science University, Portland, Oregon

JENNIFER R. MARIN, MD, MSc
Assistant Professor of Pediatrics, Division of Emergency Medicine, Department of Pediatrics, Children's Hospital of Pittsburgh, Pittsburgh, Pennsylvania

ROBERT MCNAMARA, MD, FAAEM
Professor and Chairman, Department Emergency Medicine, Temple University School of Medicine, Philadelphia, Pennsylvania

ANGELA M. MILLS, MD
Assistant Professor of Emergency Medicine, Department of Emergency Medicine, University of Pennsylvania School of Medicine, Philadelphia, Pennsylvania

JAMES K. PALMA, MD, MPH
Emergency Ultrasound Fellow, Department of Emergency Medicine, Palmetto Health Richland, Columbia, South Carolina

NOVA L. PANEBIANCO, MD, MPH
Assistant Professor of Emergency Medicine, Department of Emergency Medicine, University of Pennsylvania School of Medicine, Philadelphia, Pennsylvania

TROY W. PRIVETTE Jr, MD
Associate Program Director, Emergency Medicine Residency; Academic Attending, Department of Emergency Medicine, Palmetto Health Richland; Medical Director, Chest Pain Unit, Palmetto Health Richland ED, Columbia, South Carolina

LUNA RAGSDALE, MD, MPH
Assistant Professor of Surgery, Division of Emergency Medicine, Duke University Medical Center, Durham, North Carolina

ASHLEY SHREVES, MD
Department of Emergency Medicine, St Luke's Roosevelt Hospital Center, New York, New York

LAUREN SOUTHERLAND, MD
Emergency Medicine Resident, Division of Emergency Medicine, Duke University Medical Center, Durham, North Carolina

KEVIN L. SPROUSE, DO
Chief Resident, Department of Emergency Medicine, New York Methodist Hospital, Brooklyn, New York

JACOB W. UFBERG, MD
Associate Professor of Emergency Medicine, Department of Emergency Medicine, Temple University School of Medicine, Philadelphia, Pennsylvania

ELI ZESERSON, MD
Academic Faculty, Department of Emergency Medicine, Christiana Care Health System, Newark, Delaware

Contents

> Evaluation of the emergency department patient with acute abdominal pain may be challenging. Many factors can obscure the clinical findings leading to incorrect diagnosis and subsequent adverse outcomes. Clinicians must consider multiple diagnoses with limited time and information, giving priority to life-threatening conditions that require expeditious management to avoid morbidity and mortality. This article seeks to provide the clinician with the clinical tools to achieve these goals by reviewing the anatomic and physiological basis of abdominal pain and key components of the history and the physical examination. In addition, this article discusses the approach to unstable patients with abdominal pain.

> When discussing which laboratory tests or imaging to order in the setting of acute abdominal pain, it is practical to organize information by disease process (eg, acute appendicitis, cholecystitis). Because studies on the accuracy of diagnostic tests are of necessity related to the presence or absence of specific diagnoses, and because clinicians frequently look to tests to help them rule in or rule out specific conditions, this article is organized by region of pain and common abdominal diagnoses. It focuses on the contributions that laboratory testing and imaging make in the emergency management of abdominal complaints.

> A variety of systemic and extra-abdominal diseases can cause symptoms within the abdominal cavity. Systemic and extra-abdominal diseases may include abdominal symptoms caused by several mechanisms. This article discusses the most important and common of these causes, namely the metabolic/endocrine causes, hematologic causes, inflammatory causes, infectious causes, functional causes, and the neurogenic causes.

> Diseases that cause vomiting, diarrhea, constipation, and gastroenteritis are major problems for populations worldwide. Patients, particularly

infants, elderly, and immunocompromised individuals, may present at any point in a wide spectrum of disease states, underscoring the need for the clinician to treat these ailments aggressively. Several promising new treatment modalities, from oral rehydration solutions to antiemetic therapies, have been introduced over the past decade. Future directions include the use of probiotic agents and better tolerated rehydration solutions. Gastrointestinal disease will continue to be a focus worldwide in the search for better ways to cure illnesses associated with vomiting and diarrhea.

Gastrointestinal bleeding is a common complaint encountered in the emergency department and frequent cause of hospitalization. Important diagnostic factors that increase morbidity and mortality include advanced age, serious comorbid conditions, hemodynamic instability, esophageal varices, significant hematemesis or melena, and marked anemia. Because gastrointestinal bleeding carries a 10% overall mortality rate, emergency physicians must perform timely diagnosis, aggressive resuscitation, risk stratification, and early consultation for these patients.

Patients with nonspecific abdominal pain can have any one of many disease processes. The physical examination may not reveal clear abnormalities, making the diagnosis more difficult. Vascular abdominal emergencies are not common but, when present, may be catastrophic, with significant morbidity and, frequently, mortality. Most of the conditions are time sensitive, leaving the integrity of organ blood flow at risk. Thromboembolic disease leads to ischemia and eventual infarction of the intraabdominal organs. Aneurismal dilation of the aorta with rupture leads to rapid hypovolemic shock and death if not diagnosed. A high index of suspicion is critical to the successful diagnosis.

The pathophysiology of esophageal and gastric disorders is complicated and broad and includes iatrogenic, structural, inflammatory, neuromuscular, neoplastic, and infectious causes. Symptoms can be nonspecific and are often initially attributed to cardiac or respiratory causes. These disorders have both acute and chronic presentations that require different approaches to diagnosis and management. A thorough history and physical examination enable emergency physicians to initiate evaluation of gastroesophageal disorders. Complete evaluation often requires a combination of emergent screening to rule out life-threatening problems as well as coordinated outpatient testing.

Abdominal pain is a common presenting complaint in today's emergency department (ED). Disorders related to the liver, gallbladder, and pancreas are responsible for many of these presentations. With the increasing prevalence of gallstones, as well as alcohol use and abuse, the numbers of cases are likely to increase. This article examines hepatic emergencies including alcoholic hepatitis, spontaneous bacterial peritonitis, hepatorenal syndrome, and hepatic encephalopathy. In addition, the authors review the presentation, evaluation, and management of acute biliary tract disorders with some emphasis on bedside ultrasonography. Evaluation and treatment of pancreatitis and its complications in the ED are discussed.

distinguish diagnoses requiring immediate attention from self-limiting processes. Pediatric patients can be challenging, particularly those who are preverbal, and therefore, the clinician must rely on a detailed history from a parent or caregiver as well as a careful physical examination in order to narrow the differential diagnosis. This article highlights several pediatric diagnoses presenting as abdominal pain, including surgical emergencies, nonsurgical diagnoses, and extraabdominal processes, and reviews the clinical presentation, diagnostic evaluation, and management of each.

Abdominal pain in older adults is a concerning symptom common to a variety of diagnoses with high morbidity and mortality. Organizing the differential into categories based on pathology (inflammatory, obstructive, vascular, or other causes) provides a framework for the history, physical, and diagnostic studies. An organized approach and treatment and considerations specific to the geriatric population are discussed.

Evaluation and management of acute abdominal pain in special populations can be challenging for the emergency physician. This article focuses on two specific populations: patients with altered immunologic function and postprocedural patients. Recognition of life-threatening abdominal diseases may be delayed in immunosuppressed patients because of the atypical presentations of these conditions. In postprocedural patients, evaluation of acute abdominal symptoms requires an understanding of the complications of procedures often performed by others. The unique characteristics of abdominal pain in these two populations and, more specifically, which diseases to consider and how to use appropriate testing to detect life-threatening conditions, are discussed.

RELATED INTEREST

Ultrasound Clinics, January 2008, Vol. 3, No. 1 (pages 1–178)
Emergency Ultrasound
Vikram S. Dogra, MD and Shweta Bhatt, MD, *Guest Editors*

THE CLINICS ARE NOW AVAILABLE ONLINE!

Access your subscription at:
www.theclinics.com

GOAL STATEMENT

The goal of *Emergency Medicine Clinics of North America* is to keep practicing physicians up to date with current clinical practice in emergency medicine by providing timely articles reviewing the state of the art in patient care.

ACCREDITATION

The *Emergency Medical Clinics of North America* is planned and implemented in accordance with the Essential Areas and Policies of the Accreditation Council for Continuing Medical Education (ACCME) through the joint sponsorship of the University of Virginia School of Medicine and Elsevier. The University of Virginia School of Medicine is accredited by the ACCME to provide continuing medical education for physicians.

The University of Virginia School of Medicine designates this educational activity for a maximum of 15 *AMA PRA Category 1 Credits*™ for each issue, 60 credits per year. Physicians should only claim credit commensurate with the extent of their participation in the activity.

The American Medical Association has determined that physicians not licensed in the US who participate in this CME activity are eligible for a maximum of 15 *AMA PRA Category 1 Credits*™ for each issue, 60 credits per year.

The Emergency Medicine Clinics of North America CME program is approved by the American College of Emergency Physicians for 60 hours of ACEP Category I Credit per year.

Credit can be earned by reading the text material, taking the CME examination online at http://www.theclinics.com/home/cme, and completing the evaluation. After taking the test, you will be required to review any and all incorrect answers. Following completion of the test and evaluation, your credit will be awarded and you may print your certificate.

FACULTY DISCLOSURE/CONFLICT OF INTEREST

The University of Virginia School of Medicine, as an ACCME accredited provider, endorses and strives to comply with the Accreditation Council for Continuing Medical Education (ACCME) Standards of Commercial Support, Commonwealth of Virginia statutes, University of Virginia policies and procedures, and associated federal and private regulations and guidelines on the need for disclosure and monitoring of proprietary and financial interests that may affect the scientific integrity and balance of content delivered in continuing medical education activities under our auspices.

The University of Virginia School of Medicine requires that all CME activities accredited through this institution be developed independently and be scientifically rigorous, balanced and objective in the presentation/discussion of its content, theories and practices.

All authors/editors participating in an accredited CME activity are expected to disclose to the readers relevant financial relationships with commercial entities occurring within the past 12 months (such as grants or research support, employee, consultant, stock holder, member of speakers bureau, etc.). The University of Virginia School of Medicine will employ appropriate mechanisms to resolve potential conflicts of interest to maintain the standards of fair and balanced education to the reader. Questions about specific strategies can be directed to the Office of Continuing Medical Education, University of Virginia School of Medicine, Charlottesville, Virginia.

The faculty and staff of the University of Virginia Office of Continuing Medical Education have no financial affiliations to disclose.

The authors/editors listed below have identified no professional or financial affiliations for themselves or their spouse/partner:
Elizabeth R. Alpern, MD, MSCE; Kenton L Anderson, MD; Michael Breyer, MD; Matthew C. Carlisle, MD; Esther H. Chen, MD; Anthony J. Dean, MD (Guest Editor); Daniel J. Egan, MD; J. Matthew Fields, MD; Leila Getto, MD; Geoffrey E. Hayden, MD; Amanda E. Horn, MD; Ritu Kumar, MD; Resa E. Lewiss, MD; Alessandro Mangili, MD; Patrick Manley, (Acquisitions Editor); Jennifer R. Marin, MD, MSc; Amal Mattu, MD (Consulting Editor); Robert McNamara, MD; James K. Palma, MD, MPH; Nova L. Panebianco, MD, MPH; Troy W. Privette, Jr, MD; Luna Ragsdale, MD, MPH; Ashley Shreves, MD; Lauren Southerland, MD; Kevin L. Sprouse, DO; Bill Woods, MD (Test Author) and Eli Zeserson, MD.

The authors/editors listed below have identified the following professional or financial affiliations for themselves or their spouse/partner:
Katherine Jahnes, MD's spouse is employed by General Electric; owns stock in General Electric.
Angela M. Mills, MD (Guest Editor) is an industry funded research/investigator for AspenBio Pharma, Inc. and Siemens, and is a consultant for Becker & Associates Consulting, Inc.
Jacob W. Ufberg, MD is an industry funded research/investigator for Vapotherm, Inc.

Disclosure of Discussion of Non-FDA Approved Uses for Pharmaceutical Products and/or Medical Devices.
The University of Virginia School of Medicine, as an ACCME provider, requires that all faculty presenters identify and disclose any off-label uses for pharmaceutical and medical device products. The University of Virginia School of Medicine recommends that each physician fully review all the available data on new products or procedures prior to clinical use.

TO ENROLL

To enroll in the Emergency Medicine Clinics of North America Continuing Medical Education program, call customer service at 1-800-654-2452 or visit us online at www.theclinics.com/home/cme. The CME program is available to subscribers for an additional fee of $190.00.

Foreword

Gastrointestinal Emergencies

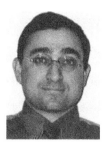

Amal Mattu, MD
Consulting Editor

Many physicians consider the brain to be the "black box" of the human body … that area of the body that may be difficult to understand and diagnose, one that harbors often occult but deadly pathologies. Personally, however, I consider the abdomen and gastrointestinal (GI) system to be the true "black box." Within the abdomen lies myriad organs and vessels, each with multiple functions, and any one of which can produce death without fair warning symptoms or signs. Complicating matters further, abdominal pain and other GI symptoms are among the most common reasons that patients seek medical attention. Abdominal pain, nausea, vomiting, and diarrhea are presentations for an enormous number of diseases, from relatively mundane conditions to deadly conditions. These "typical" symptoms are often present in young patients with benign conditions such as mild stomach flu; yet on the other hand are often lacking in elderly patients with the most deadly conditions such as mesenteric ischemia. Furthermore, GI symptoms are frequently produced by extra-abdominal *conditions*, both benign and deadly, such as viral syndromes and myocardial infarctions. Conversely, GI conditions may present with extra-abdominal *complaints*, such as chest pain or back pain. In fact, my own personal "worst cases" during my career were patients that died of intra-abdominal maladies several hours after their admission. In both cases, the patients presented to the emergency department (ED) for chest pain, and in both cases they were admitted for suspected acute coronary syndromes based on their presenting complaints and examinations.

Some might suggest that the advent and accessibility of advanced imaging modalities have made the diagnosis of abdominal and GI conditions much easier. While this might be partially true, numerous challenges still remain. Computerized tomography (CT) has certainly revolutionized the diagnosis of many conditions within this black box. However, debate regarding overuse of the CT has reached a fever-pitch as recent awareness of radiation-induced cancer risks has increased; there are also concerns about the effect of overuse of CT on ED overcrowding as well as concerns about

Emerg Med Clin N Am 29 (2011) xiii–xiv
doi:10.1016/j.emc.2011.03.002
0733-8627/11/$ – see front matter © 2011 Elsevier Inc. All rights reserved.

contrast-induced nephrotoxicity. Bedside ultrasound offers some solutions to the concerns of CT-induced radiation risk and nephrotoxicity, and it is certainly a much quicker test. However, ultrasound is able to diagnose fewer conditions and is very user-dependent. Despite the technological advances, the abdomen remains a black box.

In this issue of *Emergency Medicine Clinics of North America*, guest editors Drs Angela Mills and Anthony Dean have assembled an outstanding team to try to shed some light on the black box of the abdomen. The authors address the spectrum of GI diseases, from top (esophagus) to bottom (rectum). Detailed but clinically pertinent information regarding pathophysiology, presentations, workup and diagnosis, and treatment is provided. Patient groups that are at especially high risk of misdiagnosis such as the extremes of age are discussed, and other special groups including immunocompromised patients and postprocedure patients are addressed as well.

Because GI symptoms and signs are so common in many fields of medicine, I must say that this issue of *Emergency Medicine Clinics* is one of the most useful issues for multiple specialties that I've encountered. It will be an invaluable addition to the library of almost all physicians, especially for those of us in emergency medicine. Knowledge and practice of the concepts that are discussed in the following pages are certain to save lives. The guest editors and authors are to be commended for providing this outstanding resource for our specialty.

Amal Mattu, MD
Department of Emergency Medicine
University of Maryland School of Medicine
110 S. Paca Street, 6th Floor, Suite 200
Baltimore, MD 21201, USA

E-mail address:
amattu@smail.umaryland.edu

Preface

Gastrointestinal Emergencies

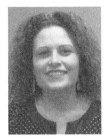 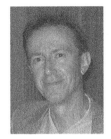

Angela M. Mills, MD   Anthony J. Dean, MD
Guest Editors

The abdomen is like a stage
Enclosed within a fleshy cage,
The symptoms are the actors who
Although they are a motley crew
Act often with consummate art
The major or the minor part;
Nor do they usually say
Who is the author of the play.
That is for you to try and guess,
A problem which, I must confess
Is made less easy from the fact
You seldom see the opening act,
And by the time that you arrive
The victim may be just alive.
(Cope Z. The Acute Abdomen in Rhyme. 5th edition. London: H.K. Lewis & Co
Ltd; 1972.)

Despite our wish to avoid the tendency of editors to make hyperbolic claims regarding the import of their book's subject matter, no less an authority than the Centers for Disease Control and Prevention states that abdominal symptoms (pain, nausea, vomiting) are the commonest presenting complaint among those seeking emergency care in the United States. They account for 10.8 million or 9.2% of annual emergency department (ED) visits.[1] As such, accurate and efficient management of undifferentiated abdominal complaints is an important skill for the emergency physician. Management of a patient with abdominal pain calls upon three mutually interdependent tiers of knowledge. The fundamental level requires an understanding of the epidemiology, prevalence, and presentation of abdominal complaints encountered in ED practice. It is essentially an intimate familiarity with differential diagnosis. With the exception

Emerg Med Clin N Am 29 (2011) xv–xvii
doi:10.1016/j.emc.2011.03.001
0733-8627/11/$ – see front matter © 2011 Elsevier Inc. All rights reserved.

of peptic ulcer disease, this has only changed modestly in the fifteen years since *Emergency Medicine Clinics* last devoted a volume to this topic. The next level is specific diagnosis of the particular disease(s) causing the patient's complaints. In this area the past two decades have brought advances that have resulted in important changes in emergency practice. These will be discussed in further detail below. The final tier is that of treatment, which has also seen significant advances, but because treatment of many gastrointestinal complaints occurs after admission, many of these changes are of less immediate consequence during a patient's ED stay.

In 1921 when Dr Cope published the first edition of his book, the evaluation of the abdomen was almost exclusively a clinical undertaking based on the history and physical examination. Since then, laboratory testing and imaging have supplemented the clinical exam and steadily increased the likelihood of accurate diagnosis. Despite this, until recently, the diagnosis of gastrointestinal illness continued to be somewhat uncertain and anxiety-provoking due to the intrinsic limitations of the available diagnostic tools. In the past 15 years, diagnostic accuracy has been radically improved by widely available computed tomography (CT) and increasing availability of ultrasonography (and a concomitant decrease in reliance on plain radiography). However, these advances have not obviated the importance of clinical skill in the evaluation of gastrointestinal illness because the increase in CT utilization has had some unintended consequences. First, it has caused increased levels of radiation exposure (often repeated in patients with chronic conditions). Second, while unloading the hospital of many unnecessary admissions and in-patient workups, CT has increased the financial, logistical, and manpower burdens of the ED. As a result, the need for sound clinical skills for accurate diagnosis has to some extent been replaced by the need for sound clinical skills to avoid profligate use of diagnostic tests.

In this volume most of the articles discuss gastrointestinal illnesses using the three tiers discussed above, with an emphasis on the key issues involved in their accurate diagnosis. Several articles review the management of select populations, such as children, older adults, the immunosuppressed, and postprocedure patients. It should be noted that while gastrointestinal conditions underlie the majority of cases of abdominal pain, the primary focus of this volume is on gastrointestinal emergencies, not "abdominal pain" per se. Thus, this volume does not address abdominal trauma, urologic disorders, obstetrics, or gynecology.

We would like to express our deep gratitude to the extraordinary effort put in by the authors who have contributed to this volume. We are confident that if the reader can take just a fraction of what we have learned from reviewing their work, then the study of this issue will be highly rewarding.

Angela M. Mills, MD
Department of Emergency Medicine
University of Pennsylvania School of Medicine
3400 Spruce Street, Ground Ravdin
Philadelphia, PA 19104, USA

Anthony J. Dean, MD
Division of Emergency Ultrasonography
Department of Emergency Medicine
University of Pennsylvania Medical Center
3400 Spruce Street, Philadelphia, PA 19104, USA

E-mail addresses:
Angela.Mills@uphs.upenn.edu (A.M. Mills)
Anthony.Dean@uphs.upenn.edu (A.J. Dean)

REFERENCE

1. Niska R, Bhuiya F, Xu J. National Hospital Ambulatory Medical Care Survey: 2007 Emergency Department Summary. National Health Statistics Reports Number 26; 2010. Available at: http://www.cdc.gov/nchs/data/nhsr/nhsr026.pdf. Accessed March 16, 2011.

Approach to Acute Abdominal Pain

Robert McNamara, MD[a],*, Anthony J. Dean, MD[b]

KEYWORDS

• Acute abdomen • Abdominal pain • Peritonitis

Abdominal pain is the most common reason for a visit to the emergency department accounting for 8 million (7%) of the 119 million emergency department (ED) visits in 2006.[1] Skill in the assessment of abdominal pain is an essential requirement of emergency medicine (EM). Although a common presentation, abdominal pain is often a symptom of serious disease and may be difficult to diagnose, resulting in a high percentage of medicolegal actions against both general and pediatric EM physicians.[2,3] The modern physician should know that despite diagnostic and therapeutic advances (computed tomography [CT], ultrasonography, laparoscopy), the misdiagnosis rate of acute appendicitis has changed little over time.[4]

HISTORY

The clinician should try to obtain as complete a history as possible because this is generally the cornerstone of an accurate diagnosis. As with other undifferentiated symptoms, the history should include a complete description of the patient's pain and associated symptoms. The medical, surgical, and social history may provide important additional information.

Assessment of the Patient's Pain

The classic PQRST mnemonic for a complete pain history is as follows:

P3: positional, palliating, and provoking factors
Q: quality
R3: region, radiation, referral
S: severity
T3: temporal factors (time and mode of onset, progression, previous episodes).

[a] Department of Emergency Medicine, Temple University School of Medicine, 3500 North Broad Street, Philadelphia, PA 19140, USA
[b] Division of Emergency Ultrasonography, Department of Emergency Medicine, University of Pennsylvania Medical Center, 3400 Spruce Street, Philadelphia, PA 19104, USA
* Corresponding author.
E-mail address: MCNAMAR@tuhs.temple.edu

Emerg Med Clin N Am 29 (2011) 159–173
doi:10.1016/j.emc.2011.01.013
0733-8627/11/$ – see front matter © 2011 Elsevier Inc. All rights reserved.

Although this mnemonic helps to ensure a thorough history, the above-mentioned sequence may result in a choppy interview, so it is preferable to ask the patient where they feel the pain (location), what kind of pain it is (character), when and how it began (onset), how bad it is (intensity), where else do they feel it, what makes it worse or better, how has it changed over time, and whether they ever had it before.

Location

Embryology determines where a patient feels visceral pain, which is generally perceived in the midline because afferent impulses from visceral organs are poorly localized. Pain fibers travel to the central nervous system via both autonomic nerves and spinal afferents. The latter fibers tend to synapse with second-order neurons in the posterior horns that are shared with afferent fibers from other visceral structures as well as somatic afferents (convergence). This arrangement with projections extending over several spinal cord levels results in poorly localized pain that may be referred to musculoskeletal structures as well as other visceral organs.[5,6] To further complicate the situation, numerous studies have indicated that patients with chronic painful or inflammatory conditions have heightened sensitivity to pain in anatomically remote visceral and somatic structures.[7,8]

Visceral nociceptors can be stimulated by distention, stretching, vigorous contraction, and ischemia. Pain from foregut structures, which include the stomach, pancreas, liver, biliary system, and the proximal duodenum, is typically localized to the epigastric region. The rest of the small bowel and the proximal third of colon, including the appendix, are midgut structures, and visceral pain associated with these organs is perceived in the periumbilical region. Hindgut structures, such as the bladder, distal two-thirds of the colon, and pelvic genitourinary (GU) organs, usually cause pain in the suprapubic region. Pain is often reported in the back for retroperitoneal structures, such as the aorta and kidneys.[9,10] The implications of the visceral innervation of the gallbladder are frequently overlooked by clinicians who exclude gallstone disease if patients do not have localized right upper quadrant pain. The gallbladder is innervated by visceral fibers, and studies consistently show that biliary colic is extremely poorly localized, with pain being perceived almost anywhere in the epigastrium or lower chest, and several investigators finding that it is less likely to be perceived in the right upper quadrant than in the epigastrium.[11,12] In summary, with afferent sensory pathways under active scientific investigation, the prudent clinician will be cautious in ascribing a patient's symptoms to a specific organ or location based solely on a patient's localization of his or her symptoms.

Character

Clinicians should seek to distinguish between the dull, poorly localized, aching or gnawing pain generated by viscerally innervated organs, compared with the characteristically sharp, more defined, and localized somatic pain caused by irritation of the parietal peritoneum or other somatically innervated structures. Somatic pain is transmitted via the spinal nerves from the parietal peritoneum or mesodermal structures of the abdominal wall. Noxious stimuli to the parietal peritoneum may be inflammatory or chemical in nature (eg, blood, infected peritoneal fluid, gastric contents).[9,13]

Onset

Acute onset pain, especially if severe, should prompt immediate concern about an intra-abdominal complication. The foremost consideration would be a vascular emergency, such as a ruptured abdominal aortic aneurysm (AAA) or aortic dissection. Other considerations for pain of acute onset include a perforated ulcer, volvulus, mesenteric ischemia, and torsion; however, these conditions may also occur without an acute onset. For example, only 47% of elderly patients with a proven perforated ulcer report the acute onset of pain.[14] Likewise, volvulus, particularly of the sigmoid colon, can present with a gradual onset of pain.[15] Other serious vascular issues, such as mesenteric ischemia, may present with a gradual onset of pain. Conversely, a gradual onset in the setting of an infectious or inflammatory process may be expected. Pain that awakens the patient from sleep should be considered serious until proven otherwise.[16] The time of onset establishes the duration of pain and allows the physician to interpret the current findings in relation to the expected temporal progression of the various causes of abdominal pain.

Intensity
Pain that is severe should heighten the concern for a serious underlying cause; however descriptions of milder pain cannot be relied on to exclude serious illness, especially in older patients who may underreport symptoms.

Patterns of radiation and referral of pain
The previous discussion of afferent neural pathways and convergence gives rise to predictable patterns of referred pain and radiation. Kehr sign is a classic example in which diaphragmatic irritation, usually from free intraperitoneal blood, causes shoulder pain.[17] Any other inflammatory process or organ contiguous to the diaphragm can also cause referred shoulder pain. Another well-described example is ipsilateral scapular pain caused by biliary disease. Radiation may also reflect progression of disease such as with continued aortic dissection or ongoing passage of a ureteral stone. While considering referred pain, it is important to remember that deep musculoskeletal structures (especially of the back) are innervated by visceral sensory fibers with similar qualities to those arising from intra-abdominal organs. These fibers converge in the spinal cord, giving rise to scleratomes, which are regions of referral in the abdomen and flanks. Thus, in cases in which the patients' perceived location of symptoms seems to be completely unrevealing on physical examination, a careful assessment of musculoskeletal structures should be made.[18]

Duration and progression
Persistent worsening pain is worrisome, whereas pain that is improving is typically favorable. Serious causes of abdominal pain may present early in their course, allowing opportunity for intervention if promptly diagnosed. However, delays in onset of symptoms or in presentation frequently occur, especially in the elderly. Certain patterns of progression can be diagnostic, such as the migration of pain in appendicitis where the initial distention of the appendix causes a periumbilical visceral pain that shifts to the right lower quadrant once the inflammatory process is detected by the somatic sensors of the parietal peritoneum. It should be noted that in contrast to other forms of colic, gallbladder pain caused by an affected stone is not waxing and waning in quality. It is steady, almost never lasts less than 1 hour, and with an average of 5 to 16 hours duration, ranges up to 24 hours.[11,19] Small bowel obstruction typically progresses from an intermittent (colicky) pain to more constant pain when distention occurs. One would only expect somatic pain (arising from transmural ischemia or perforation contiguous to the parietal peritoneum) very late in the course.

Provocative and palliating factors
The clinician needs to ask what, if anything, worsens and improves the pain. It is important to establish whether jarring motions, such as coughing or walking, exacerbate the pain, suggesting peritoneal irritation.[13] Patients with peritonitis often remark on increased pain with jolts or bumps in the road. With upper abdominal pain, the

clinician should specifically determine if it is pleuritic because this may signify chest disease. Peptic ulcer disease may be exacerbated (gastric) or relieved (duodenal) by eating. Mesenteric ischemia may be precipitated by eating, as can the pain of inter-mittently symptomatic gallstones, often associated with fatty meals. The patient should be questioned about any self-treatment, particularly analgesics and antacids, and the response to these measures.

Previous episodes
Recurrent episodes generally point to a medical cause with the exceptions of mesen-teric ischemia (intestinal angina), gallstones, ureterolithiasis, diverticulitis, or partial bowel obstruction.

Assessment of the Associated Symptoms

Gastrointestinal (GI) and urinary symptoms are the primary focus; however, it is impor-tant to ask about fever and cardiopulmonary symptoms. Associated symptoms should be placed in the clinical context, including the patient's age and the current status in the course of the illness.

Anorexia
With appendicitis most physicians expect the patient to report anorexia. However, pooling of the literature indicates that, although anorexia is a discriminatory symptom, it is only present in 68% of patients with appendicitis.[20] The report of this symptom decreases to 20% to 44% in elderly patients with appendicitis.[21]

Vomiting
Vomiting may occur in almost any abdominal disease. Pain generally precedes vomit-ing in surgical conditions, with the important exception of esophageal rupture from forceful emesis.[16,22] It is usually present in small bowel obstruction unless the obstruc-tion is partial or the patient is presenting early in the course. Many other serious enti-ties, including large bowel obstruction, frequently present without vomiting. The nature of the vomiting may be diagnostically helpful. With small bowel obstruction, a progression from gastric contents to bilious to feculent emesis is anticipated as the duration of the illness increases. Frequent nonproductive retching can point to gastric volvulus,[23] whereas repetitive nonbilious vomiting may indicate gastric outlet obstruction. The presence of blood or bile should be noted. Bilious vomiting in an infant is always considered a harbinger of serious abdominal illness such as malrotation.[24] Blood or coffee-ground emeses is usually caused by gastric diseases or complications of liver disease. Hematemesis caused by aortoenteric fistula is bright red, massive, and usually catastrophic and should be suspected with a history of a prior AAA repair.[25] The key feature of vomiting from more benign causes, such as viral or food-borne illness, is that it is self-limited.

Bowel symptoms
Although diarrhea is a frequent accompaniment of more benign abdominal conditions, its presence alone should never rule out serious disease. For example, diarrhea is common with mesenteric ischemia and is frequently reported in conditions such as appendicitis.[20,26] In one series of 1000 ED patients presenting with abdominal pain, 18% presented with diarrhea. No patient younger than 40 years with diarrhea and continuous pain was found to have a surgical cause for their symptoms.[27] Conversely, diarrhea can occur in up to one-fifth of patients with colonic obstruction.[28] Diarrhea also occurs in early small bowel obstruction as the reflexively hyperactive bowel distal

to the obstruction clears itself, and with partial obstruction, diarrhea may be ongoing. Absence of flatus is a more reliable sign than constipation in bowel obstruction because the bowel clears gas more rapidly than fluid. In addition, gas, in contrast to fluid, cannot be replaced by intestinal secretory mechanisms distal to an obstruction. Bloody stool in the presence of significant abdominal pain should raise the suspicion for mucosal compromise from ischemia. Melena suggests an upper source of bleeding, whereas frank blood can indicate a lower source or a massive upper bleed with rapid transit time. In a patient with acute abdominal pain, the urge to defecate has been described as a harbinger of serious disease, including a ruptured aneurysm in the older patient or ruptured ectopic pregnancy in the young.[29]

Other symptoms

Many GU tract diseases can present with abdominal pain. Conversely, any inflammatory process contiguous to the GU tract (including appendicitis, cholecystitis, pancreatitis, or any inflammatory process involving bowel) may result in both pyuria and dysuria. This condition can lead to misdiagnosis of both GI and GU conditions. In men, testicular torsion may present as abdominal pain with nausea and vomiting, and chronic prostatitis may cause nonspecific symptoms. In women, pelvic inflammatory disease, endometriosis, and ovarian pathologic condition frequently cause abdominal or GI symptoms.[6] The enlarging uterus of pregnancy can itself cause discomfort and displace abdominal organs in such a way as to further complicate the diagnosis of many abdominal conditions, especially appendicitis. For these reasons a menstrual (where applicable), sexual, and GU history should be obtained in most patients with abdominal pain. The report of normal regular menses should not preclude consideration of current pregnancy.[30] Cardiopulmonary symptoms, such as cough and dyspnea, can point to a nonabdominal cause of abdominal pain. Syncope may indicate disease originating in the chest (pulmonary embolism, dissection) or abdomen (acute aortic aneurysm, ectopic pregnancy).

Medical and Surgical History, Current Medications

A history of abdominal surgery can rule out a condition or raise the suspicion for a complication such as obstruction from adhesions. Although many chronic medical conditions cause acute abdominal pain (diabetic ketoacidosis, hypercalcemia, Addison disease, sickle cell crisis), the emergency physician first considers those that can precipitate an abdominal crisis, such as atrial fibrillation or chronic low-output heart failure (leading to mesenteric ischemia), or a history of pelvic inflammatory disease (a risk factor for ectopic pregnancy). Other less common metabolic causes of acute abdominal pain include uremia, lead poisoning, hereditary angioedema, and porphyria. The patient's current medications should be reviewed with attention to those affecting the integrity of the gastric mucosa (nonsteroidal antiinflammatory drugs [NSAIDs] and steroids), immunosuppressive agents (impair host defenses and the generation of painful stimuli), and any medication that can impair nociception (narcotics may also be a cause of pain due to constipation).

Social History

The patient's use of drugs and alcohol may have important diagnostic implications. Cocaine use may cause intestinal as well as cardiac ischemia. GI complications of alcohol abuse are extensive and well known. Direct questions regarding domestic violence may reveal a traumatic source of pain.

PHYSICAL EXAMINATION

The general appearance of the patient is always important. The clinician should take note of the patient's position, spontaneous movements, respiratory pattern, and facial expression. An ill-appearing patient with abdominal pain is always of great concern, given the variety of potentially lethal underlying causes. On the other hand, especially in the elderly, the clinician must not be misled by the well-appearing patient who may still have serious underlying disease.[31]

Vital Signs

Vital sign abnormalities should alert the clinician to a serious cause of the abdominal pain. However, the presence of normal vital signs does not exclude a serious diagnosis. Although fever certainly points to an infectious cause or complication, it is frequently absent with infectious causes of abdominal pain. For example, fever is absent in more than 30% of patients with appendicitis and in most of those with acute cholecystitis.[20,32] Tachypnea may be a nonspecific finding but it should prompt consideration of chest disease and metabolic acidosis from entities such as ischemic bowel or diabetic ketoacidosis.

The Abdominal Examination

The emergency physician should know the key elements of the abdominal examination while understanding their limitations. In particular, all techniques for the detection of peritonitis yields both false-negative and false-positive results.

Inspection, auscultation, and percussion

Inspection is important for the detection of surgical scars, skin changes including signs of herpes zoster, liver disease (caput medusa), and hemorrhage (Grey Turner sign of flank ecchymosis with a retroperitoneal source, Cullen sign of a bluish umbilicus with intraperitoneal bleeding).[17] With distention, percussion allows the differentiation between large bowel obstruction (drum-like tympany) and advanced ascites (shifting dullness). Auscultation is of very limited diagnostic utility, and prolonged listening for bowel sounds is ineffective use of time, although it may reveal high-pitched sounds in early small bowel obstruction or the silence encountered with ileus or late in the course of any abdominal catastrophe. Bruits have been described with aortic, renal, or mesenteric stenosis but are rarely appreciated in a busy emergency department.[33]

Palpation

The ED abdominal examination is directed primarily to the localization of tenderness, the detection of abdominal guarding, and the identification of peritonitis. For this reason, it should generally be limited to light and sensitive palpation. In contrast, the deep palpation traditionally conducted at the culmination of the abdominal examination was directed to the detection of abnormal masses and organomegaly. Deep palpation is extremely painful for a patient with a serious intra-abdominal condition, has limited diagnostic accuracy, and may interfere with the ability of any subsequent examiner to obtain an accurate examination due to the patient's apprehension. Furthermore, its purpose of identifying abdominal masses and organomegaly is anachronistic if modern tools of diagnostic imaging are available. Various strategies have been advocated to improve the palpation phase of the examination, including progression from nonpainful areas to the location of pain. It may be useful to palpate the abdomen of anxious or less cooperative children with the stethoscope to define areas of tenderness.[34] Meyerowitz[35] advocates following up the initial examination with a secondary palpation with a stethoscope while telling the patient that one is listening to uncover exaggerated symptoms. It is preferable to have the patient flex the knees and hips to allow for relaxation of the abdominal musculature (see later discussion of guarding).

Localized tenderness is generally a reliable guide to the underlying cause of the pain. More generalized tenderness presents a greater diagnostic challenge. Unless the patient has had an appendectomy, the authors recommend, given its frequency as a serious cause of abdominal pain, continued consideration of appendicitis in any patient with right lower quadrant tenderness. Despite the known issues with diagnosing appendicitis in the elderly, virtually all of them have right lower quadrant tenderness.[14] If tolerated by the patient, palpation or percussion may include assessment of the liver and spleen size, a search for pulsatile or other masses, and an assessment of the quality of femoral pulses. A tender pulsatile and expansile mass is the key distinguishing feature of an acute AAA, although this and most other masses are much more accurately diagnosed with the aid of a bedside ultrasound machine, if available.[36] The femoral pulses may be unequal with aortic dissection.[37] Inspection and palpation of the patient while they are standing may reveal the presence of hernias undetected in the supine position.

Tests for peritoneal irritation

Determining the presence or absence of peritonitis is a primary objective of the abdominal examination; however, the methods for detecting it are often inaccurate. Traditional rebound testing is performed by gentle depression of the abdominal wall for approximately 15 to 30 seconds with sudden release. The patient is asked whether the pain was greater with downward pressure or with release. Despite limitations, the test was one of the most useful in a metanalysis of articles investigating the diagnosis of appendicitis in children.[34] *Cope's Early Diagnosis of the Acute Abdomen* recommends against this test because it is unnecessarily painful; it suggests gentle percussion as more accurate and humane.[33] The literature demonstrates traditional rebound testing has sensitivity for the presence of peritonitis near 80%, yet its specificity is only 40% to 50%, and it is entirely nondiscriminatory in the identification of cholecystitis.[32,38,39] The use of indirect tests, such as the cough test, in which one looks for signs of pain such as flinching, grimacing, or moving the hands to the abdomen on coughing, has a similar sensitivity but a specificity of 79%.[40] In children, indirect tests would include the "heel drop jarring" test (child rises on toes and drops weight on heels) or asking the child to jump up and down while looking for signs of abdominal pain.[34,41]

Guarding is defined as increased abdominal wall muscular tone and is only of significance as an involuntary reflex when it reflects a physiologic attempt to minimize movement of the intraperitoneal structures. In contrast, voluntary guarding can be induced by any person with conscious control of their abdominal wall musculature and is frequently seen in completely normal patients with apprehension about the abdominal examination. Rigidity is the extreme example of true guarding. To identify true guarding, the examiner gently assesses muscle tone through the respiratory cycle, preferably with the knees and hips flexed to further relax the abdomen. With voluntary guarding, the tone decreases with inspiration, whereas with true guarding, the examiner is able to detect continued abdominal wall tension throughout the respiratory cycle. With delicate palpation it may also be possible to detect asymmetry of the abdominal muscular tension with a localized unilateral inflammatory process, such as appendicitis or diverticulitis. The clinician should also be aware that true guarding may also occur with a thoracic inflammatory process adjacent to the diaphragm.

Guarding and rigidity may be lacking in the elderly because of laxity of the abdominal wall musculature. However, only 21% of patients older than 70 years with a perforated ulcer presented with epigastric rigidity.[14]

The Rectal Examination

The diagnostic value of a rectal examination in the evaluation of acute abdominal pain is limited; however, it may be of use in detecting intestinal ischemia, late intussusception, or colon cancer. The routine performance of a rectal examination in suspected appendicitis is not supported by the available literature.[42] It is recommended that, as a general rule, one should not perform this examination in children because it adds little to the diagnostic process at the cost of significant discomfort.[43] On the other hand, the examination's utility may increase with the patient's age, and one study found that within 1 year, nearly 11% of patients older than 50 years diagnosed with nonspecific abdominal pain in an ED were found to have cancer, principally of the colon.[44] The use of the rectal examination in other age groups should be targeted to diagnoses in which it may yield important information.[42]

Special Abdominal Examination Techniques

There are several examination techniques that may be useful to the emergency physician in helping to establish a diagnosis. Some of these tests have not been well studied, but documentation of their presence or absence on the chart indicates a consideration of a specific disease process such as appendicitis.

Carnett sign

Abdominal wall tenderness can be caused by trauma and, with increasing numbers of patients on therapeutic anticoagulation, abdominal wall hematoma. The following technique, described by Carnett in 1926, may confirm the abdominal wall as the source of the patient's pain. The point of maximal pain is identified and palpated, with the abdomen wall relaxed and then tensed through the performance of a half sit-up with the arms crossed. Increased pain with the wall tensed is a positive sign of abdominal wall pathologic condition; a decrease in pain is considered a negative test result. When prospectively applied in 120 patients, the test result was positive in 24, with only 1 having intra-abdominal pathologic condition.[45] Other investigators have found it less accurate but still useful.[46] This test should not be routinely applied but is considered when there is a supportive history and absence of indicators of other illness.[47]

Cough test

Originally described by Rostovzev in 1909, this test seeks evidence of peritoneal irritation by having the patient cough.[48] Jeddy and colleagues[49] described a positive test result as a cough causing a sharp localized pain. They applied this description prospectively to patients with right lower quadrant pain and found it to have near perfect sensitivity with a 95% specificity for the detection of appendicitis or peritonitis (1 patient with perforated diverticulitis). Bennett and colleagues[40] consider signs of pain on coughing such as flinching, grimacing, or moving ones hands to the abdomen as a positive test result and reported a sensitivity of 78% with a specificity of 79% for the detection of peritonitis in a prospective study of 150 consecutive patients with abdominal pain.

Closed eyes sign

Based on the assumption that the patient with an acute abdominal condition carefully watches the examiner's hands to avoid unnecessary pain, this test is considered an indicator of nonorganic cause of abdominal pain. The test result is considered positive if the patients keep their eyes closed when abdominal tenderness is elicited. In a prospective study of 158 patients, Gray and colleagues[50] found that 79% of the 28 patients who closed their eyes did not have identifiable organic pathologic condition.

Murphy sign

Murphy described cessation of inspiration in cholecystitis when the examiner curled their fingers below the anterior right costal margin from above the patient.[51] Now most commonly performed from the patient's side, inspiratory arrest while deeply palpating the right upper quadrant is the most reliable clinical indicator of cholecystitis, although it only has a sensitivity of 65%.[32] The sonographic Murphy sign is actually gallbladder palpation under direct sonographic visualization. It is performed by bringing the ultrasound probe as close to the gallbladder as possible below the costal margin and asking the patient whether pressure, applied with the probe directly in the direction of the gallbladder, reproduces the symptoms. If the answer is affirmative, the same question is asked when similar pressure is applied in the epigastrium at a location remote from the gallbladder. The same procedure is repeated again directly on the gallbladder and in the midaxillary line, lateral to the gallbladder. If the patient can consistently discriminate between probe pressure applied to the gallbladder from that applied elsewhere, the test result is deemed positive. In the hands of emergency physicians, the sensitivity of the sonographic Murphy sign is remarkably consistent at around 75%, whereas specificity ranges from 55% to 80%.[52–54] The test appears to be more sensitive in the hands of emergency physicians than when performed in radiology imaging suites (without loss of specificity).[52,55] This difference may be because of the clinical experience that practicing physicians bring to the test compared with ultrasound technologists.

The psoas sign

The psoas sign is provoked by having the supine patient lift the thigh against hand resistance or with the patient laying on their contralateral side the hip joint is passively extended. Increased pain suggests irritation of the psoas muscle by an inflammatory process contiguous to the muscle. When positive on the right, this is a classic sign suggestive of appendicitis. Other inflammatory conditions involving the retroperitoneum, including pyelonephritis, pancreatitis, and psoas abscess, also elicit this sign.

The obturator sign

The obturator sign is elicited with the patient supine and the examiner supporting the patient's lower extremity with the hip and knee both flexed to 90°. The sign is positive if passive internal and external rotation of the hip causes reproduction of pain. It suggests the presence of an inflammatory process adjacent to the muscle deep in the lateral walls of the pelvis. Potential diagnoses include a pelvic appendicitis (on the right only), sigmoid diverticulitis, pelvic inflammatory disease, or ectopic pregnancy.

The Rovsing sign

The Rovsing sign is a classic test used in the diagnosis of appendicitis. It is a form of indirect rebound testing in which the examiner applies pressure in the left lower quadrant, remote from the usual area of appendiceal pain and tenderness. The test result is positive if the patient reports rebound pain in the right lower quadrant when the examiner releases pressure.[20]

In limited studies, the psoas, obturator, and Rovsing signs demonstrate a low sensitivity (15%–35%) but a relatively high specificity (85%–95%) for appendicitis.[20,34,56]

Other Examination Elements

Careful examination of adjacent areas is a key part of the assessment of the patient with abdominal pain. In addition to skin inspection, the back should be assessed for tenderness at the costovertebral angle, spinous processes, and paraspinal regions. Because virtually any chest disease can present with abdominal pain, particular attention should be paid to the cardiopulmonary examination. The groin is assessed for hernias. If this diagnosis is under serious consideration, this examination should be performed with the patient standing. The male patient must be inspected for testicular pathologic condition, including torsion and infection. In female patients with lower abdominal pain, a pelvic examination is almost always necessary. Even if all potentially offending structures have been surgically removed, the examination may reveal a rectovaginal fistula or abscess, an unanticipated mass, or acute cystitis. The pelvic examination presents an opportunity to assess the pelvic peritoneum directly for signs of inflammation through the assessment of cervical motion tenderness and for evidence of cystitis by palpation of the bladder through the anterior wall of the vagina. If Fitzhugh-Curtis syndrome is a consideration, a pelvic examination may be indicated with upper abdominal pain.[13]

Analgesia and the Abdominal Examination

The emergency physician should not hesitate to administer adequate analgesic medication to the patient with acute abdominal pain. When studied, the administration of narcotic analgesics does not obscure the diagnosis or interfere with the treatment of the patient, and multiple well-designed randomized trials have demonstrated that the use of analgesia in acute abdominal pain does not lead to adverse outcomes.[57–63] The United States Agency for Health care Research and Quality issues reports regarding making health care safer and recommended this practice after a review of the literature.[64] Previously, *Cope's Early Diagnosis of the Acute Abdomen* was against the physician for administering morphine, but this stance has been reversed in more recent editions.[64,65] The current editor of this book, William Silen, was a co-author on a prospective study where the administration of up to 15 mg of morphine did not affect diagnostic accuracy in patients with acute abdominal pain. Thomas and colleagues[57] recommend its use in that it fulfills the physician's "imperative to relieve suffering."

APPROACH TO THE UNSTABLE PATIENT

On occasion, a patient with acute abdominal pain presents in extremis. The ill-appearing patient with abdominal pain requires immediate attention. This requirement is particularly so in the elderly because the overall mortality rate for all older patients with acute abdominal pain ranges from 11% to 14%, and those presenting in an unstable fashion have an even poorer prognosis.[31]

The usual sequence of resuscitation is applied to the patient with unstable abdominal pain, with airway control achieved as necessary. Hypotension requires the parallel process of treatment and an early assessment for life threatening conditions requiring emergent surgical intervention. Hypotension from blood and fluid loss from the GI tract is usually apparent from the history coupled with a digital rectal examination. If this evidence is lacking in the patient with abdominal pain, there needs to be early consideration of third spacing, which can cause enormous fluid shifts into the bowel lumen or peritoneal space in bowel obstruction or other intestinal catastrophes. Bedside ultrasonography is an extremely useful diagnostic adjunct in such patients. In the older patients, hypotension should prompt an immediate search for an AAA, immediately followed by sonographic evaluation of the inferior vena cava for intravascular volume status, and sonography of the heart, pleural, and peritoneal spaces to exclude massive effusions or evidence of massive pulmonary embolus. Bedside echocardiography also identifies severe global myocardial depression as a cardiogenic cause of shock. In the younger patient, a large amount of free fluid detected by ultrasonography in an unstable patient is most commonly because of rupture of an ectopic pregnancy, spleen, or hemorrhagic ovarian cyst. An immediate urine pregnancy test is the first step in distinguishing these.

The proper place for the unstable patient with an acute AAA is the operating room or, in some centers, the interventional suite for emergency aortic stent placement. Attempts to obtain CT imaging may cause fatal delays in definitive treatment. With a high clinical index of suspicion (if possible supported by emergency bedside ultrasonography [EMBU]), most patients sent directly to surgery is found to have an acute AAA, and nearly all others have an alternative diagnosis that still needs operative intervention.[66]

DIAGNOSTIC STUDIES AND DISPOSITION

Appropriate diagnostic testing is covered in the respective articles for specific entities; however, it must be emphasized that there are significant limitations of imaging and laboratory studies in the evaluation of acute abdominal pain, and all diagnostic tests have a false-negative rate. If the history and physical examination lead to a high pretest probability of a disease, a negative test result cannot exclude the diagnosis. For example, the total leukocyte count can be normal in the face of serious infection such as appendicitis or cholecystitis.[34,67] CT is frequently used in evaluation of the patient with abdominal pain. Clinicians are assisted by the recent advances in the technology that have allowed for improved image resolution and shorter acquisition times along with coronal and 3-dimensional reconstruction. However, it remains an imperfect test for conditions such as appendicitis and may add little to the clinical assessment.[68,69]

As noted, EMBU is particularly useful in the unstable patient with abdominal pain because of the immediate information it can provide regarding intravascular volume status and cardiac function. EMBU is also helpful in narrowing the range of diagnostic possibilities in stable patients with undifferentiated abdominal complaints. EMBU assessment of the abdominal aorta is extremely accurate and obviates the transfer of a potentially unstable patient to the CT suite.[70] Ultrasonography in the hands of emergency physicians attains extremely high sensitivity for identification of gallstones (similar to that attained by imaging specialists: around 95%), although studies of its specificity (65%-95%) are more varied.[52–54] The accuracy of EMBU in the identification of acute cholecystitis also seems to have a high sensitivity around 90% with lower specificity.[54] In early pregnancy, the goal of bedside ultrasonography is to exclude ectopic pregnancy by the demonstration of definitive evidence of an intrauterine pregnancy (yolk sac or better). If the pretest index of suspicion is high (particularly in patients on progestational agents), it may be prudent to perform a formal complete radiology study to search for adnexal evidence of a heterotopic pregnancy. Smaller studies suggest that EMBU may also provide useful information beyond that obtained from the physical examination in nonpregnant patients with pelvic and right lower quadrant complaints.[71,72]

Plain abdominal radiographs are of limited utility in the evaluation of acute abdominal pain.[73] Although they may identify free intraperitoneal air, calcified aortic aneurysm, or air-fluid levels in obstruction, other diagnostic studies are almost always indicated or perform better as the initial testing. If plain radiographs are used, the limitations must be appreciated. For example, a standard upright film does not demonstrate free air in up to 40% of patients with a perforated ulcer.[74]

The oft-repeated axiom of "treat the patient, not the test" certainly applies to the patient with acute abdominal pain. An unexpected negative test result should prompt a reassessment of the patient and consideration for observation and repeat examination for disease progression. Whenever the diagnosis is doubtful, serial examination as an inpatient or in an observation unit is a sound strategy. When a patient is discharged home after an evaluation for abdominal pain, the authors recommend instructions to return if the pain worsens, new vomiting or fever occurs, or if the pain persists beyond 8 to 12 hours. Such instructions are targeted at ensuring the return of a patient who has progressed from an early appendicitis or small bowel obstruction, the 2 most common surgical entities erroneously discharged from an emergency department.[17,22]

SUMMARY

The assessment of abdominal complaints calls on the traditional clinical method of a careful history and physical examination followed by targeted laboratory tests and imaging studies. There is no clinical finding or test result that is unfailingly accurate or diagnostic, so that each data point should be interpreted as a part of the overall clinical picture. Older or very young patients or those with conditions that interfere with the perception of pain require special caution. With serious abdominal conditions, ongoing monitoring, supportive care, pain relief, and empiric treatment are concurrent with the diagnostic workup.

REFERENCES

1. Pitts SR, Niska RW, Xu J, et al. National hospital ambulatory medical care survey: 2006 emergency department summary. National health statistics report; no. 7. Hyattsville (MD): National Center for Health Statistics; 2008.
2. Selbst SM, Friedman MJ, Singh SB. Epidemiology and etiology of malpractice lawsuits involving children in US emergency departments and urgent care centers. Pediatr Emerg Care 2005;21:165–9.
3. Kachalia A, Gandhi TK, Puopolo AL, et al. Missed and delayed diagnoses in the emergency department: a study of closed malpractice claims from 4 liability insurers. Acad Emerg Med 2007;49:196–205.
4. Flum DR, Morris A, Koepsell T, et al. Has misdiagnosis of appendicitis decreased over time? JAMA 2001;286:1748–53.
5. Bielefeldt K, Christianson JA, Davis BM. Basic and clinical aspects of visceral sensation: transmission in the CNS. Neurogastroenterol Motil 2005;17(4):488–99.
6. Brinkert W, Dimcevski G, Arendt-Nielsen L, et al. Dysmenorrhoea is associated with hypersensitivity in the sigmoid colon and rectum. Pain 2007;132(Suppl 1): S46–51.
7. Giamberardino MA, De Laurentis S, Affaitati G, et al. Modulation of pain and hyperalgesia from the urinary tract by algogenic conditions of the reproductive organs in women. Neurosci Lett 2001;304(1–2):61–4.
8. Sarkar S, Aziz Q, Woolf CJ, et al. Contribution of central sensitisation to the development of non-cardiac chest pain. Lancet 2000;356:1154–9.
9. Jung PJ, Merrell RC. Acute abdomen. Gastroenterol Clin North Am 1988;17: 227–44.

10. Jones RS, Claridge JA. Acute abdomen. In: Townsend CM, Beauchamp RD, Evers BM, et al, editors. Sabiston textbook of surgery: the biologic basis of modern surgical practice. 17th edition. Philadelphia: Elsevier; 2004. p. 1219–38. Chapter: 43.
11. Traverso LW. Clinical manifestations and impact of gallstone disease. Am J Surg 1993;165:405–9.
12. Berger MY, van der Velden JJ, Lijmer JG, et al. Abdominal symptoms: do they predict gallstones? A systematic review. Scand J Gastroenterol 2000;35:70–6.
13. Abbott J. Pelvic pain: lessons from anatomy and physiology. J Emerg Med 1990; 8:441–7.
14. Fenyo G. Acute abdominal disease in the elderly: experience from two series in Stockholm. Am J Surg 1982;143:751–4.
15. Anderson JR, Lee D. The management of acute sigmoid volvulus. Br J Surg 1981; 68:117–20.
16. Silen W. Method of diagnosis: the history. In: Cope's early diagnosis of the acute abdomen. New York: Oxford; 2010. p. 18–27.
17. Hickey MS, Kiernan GJ, Weaver KE. Evaluation of abdominal pain. Emerg Med Clin North Am 1989;7:437–52.
18. Feinstein B, Langton JNK, Jameson RM, et al. Experiments on pain referred from deep somatic tissues. J Bone Joint Surg Am 1954;36:981–97.
19. Silen W. Cholecystitis and other causes of acute pain in the right upper quadrant of the abdomen. In: Cope's early diagnosis of the acute abdomen. New York: Oxford; 2010. p. 131–40.
20. Wagner JM, McKinney WP, Carpenter JL. Does this patient have appendicitis? JAMA 1996;2786:1589–94.
21. Kraemer M, Franke C, Ohmann C, et al. Acute appendicitis in late adulthood: incidence, presentation, and outcome. Results of a prospective multicenter acute abdominal pain study and a review for the literature. Arch Surg 2000;3835: 470–81.
22. Brewer RJ, Golden GT, Hitch DC, et al. Abdominal pain: an analysis of 1,000 consecutive cases in a university hospital emergency room. Am J Surg 1976; 131:219–24.
23. Godshall D, Mossallam W, Rosenbaum R. Gastric volvulus: case report and review of the literature. J Emerg Med 1999;17:837–40.
24. Schafermeyer Robert W. Pediatric abdominal emergencies. In: Tintinalli JE, Kelen GD, Stapczynski S, et al, editors. Emergency medicine: a comprehensive study guide. 6th edition. New York: McGraw-Hill; 2004. p. 844–51. Chapter: 123.
25. Busuttil SJ, Goldstone J. Diagnosis and management of aortoenteric fistulas. Semin Vasc Surg 2001;14:302–11.
26. Inderbitzi R, Wagner HE, Seiler C, et al. Acute mesenteric ischaemia. Eur J Surg 1992;158:123–6.
27. Chen EH, Shofer FS, Dean AJ, et al. Derivation of a clinical prediction rule for evaluating patients with abdominal pain and diarrhea. Am J Emerg Med 2008; 26(4):450–3.
28. Greenlee HB, Pienkos EJ, Vamderbilt PC, et al. Acute large bowel obstruction. Comparison of county, Veterans Administration, and community hospital populations. Arch Surg 1974;108:470–6.
29. Hadjis NS, McAuley G, Ruo L, et al. Acute abdominal pain and the urge to defecate in the young and old: a useful symptom complex? J Emerg Med 1999;17: 239–42.
30. Ramoska EA, Sacchetti AD, Nepp M. Reliability of patient history in determining the possibility of pregnancy. Ann Emerg Med 1989;18:48–50.

31. McNamara R. Abdominal pain in the elderly. In: Tintinalli JE, Kelen GD, Stapczynski S, et al, editors. Emergency medicine: a comprehensive study guide. 6th edition. New York: McGraw-Hill; 2004. p. 515–9. Chapter: 69.

32. Trowbridge RL, Ruttconski NK, Shojania KG. Does this patient have acute cholecystitis? JAMA 2003;289:80–6.

33. Silen W. Method of diagnosis: the examination of the patient. In: Cope's early diagnosis of the acute abdomen. New York: Oxford; 2010. p. 28–40.

34. Bundy DG, Byerley JS, Liles EA, et al. Does this child have appendicitis? JAMA 2007;298:438–51.

35. Meyerowitz BR. Abdominal palpation by stethoscope [letter]. Arch Surg 1976; 111:831.

36. Marston WA, Ahlquist R, Johnson G, et al. Misdiagnosis of ruptured abdominal aortic aneurysms. J Vasc Surg 1992;16:17–22.

37. Klompas M. Does this patient have an acute thoracic aortic dissection? JAMA 2002;287:2262–72.

38. Prout WG. The significance of rebound tenderness in the acute abdomen. Br J Surg 1970;57:508–10.

39. Liddington MI, Thomson WHF. Rebound tenderness test. Br J Surg 1991;78: 795–6.

40. Bennett DH, Tambeur LJ, Campbell WB. Use of coughing test to diagnose peritonitis. BMJ 1994;308:1336.

41. Markle GB. Heel-drop jarring test for appendicitis. Arch Surg 1985;120:243.

42. Brewster GS, Herbert ME. Medical myth: a digital rectal examination should be performed on all individuals with suspected appendicitis. West J Med 2000; 173:207–8.

43. Jesudason EC, Walker J. Rectal examination in paediatric surgical practice. Br J Surg 1999;86:376–8.

44. DeDombal FT, Matharu SS, Staniland JR, et al. Presentation of cancer to a hospital as 'acute abdominal pain'. Br J Surg 1980;67:413–6.

45. Thomson H, Francis DMA. Abdominal-wall tenderness: a useful sign in the acute abdomen. Lancet 1977;2:1053–4.

46. Gray DW, Seabrook G, Dixon JM, et al. Is abdominal wall tenderness a useful sign in the diagnosis of non-specific abdominal pain? Ann R Coll Surg Engl 1988;70:233–4.

47. Thomson WH, Dawes RF, Carter SS. Abdominal wall tenderness: a useful sign in chronic abdominal pain. Br J Surg 1991;78:223–5.

48. Kovachev LS. 'Cough sign': a reliable test in the diagnosis of intra-abdominal inflammation [letter]. Br J Surg 1994;81:1541.

49. Jeddy TA, Vowles RH, Southam JA. 'Cough sign': a reliable test in the diagnosis of intra-abdominal inflammation. Br J Surg 1994;81:279.

50. Gray DW, Dixon JM, Collin J. The closed eyes sign: an aid to diagnosing non-specific abdominal pain. BMJ 1988;297:837.

51. Aldea PA, Meehan JP, Sternbach G. The acute abdomen and Murphy's signs. J Emerg Med 1986;4:57–63.

52. Kendall JL, Shimp RJ. Performance and interpretation of focused right upper quadrant ultrasound by emergency physicians. J Emerg Med 2001;21:7–13.

53. Miller AH, Pepe PE, Brockman CR, et al. ED ultrasound in hepatobiliary disease. J Emerg Med 2006;30:69–74.

54. Rosen CL, Brown DF, Chang Y, et al. Ultrasonography by emergency physicians in patients with suspected cholecystitis. Am J Emerg Med 2001;19: 32–6.

55. Ralls PW, Halls J, Lapin SA, et al. Prospective evaluation of the sonographic Murphy sign in suspected acute cholecystitis. J Clin Ultrasound 1982;10(3): 113–5.
56. Kharbanda AB, Taylor GA, Fishman SJ, et al. A clinical decision rule to identify children at low risk for appendicitis. Pediatrics 2005;116:709–16.
57. Thomas SH, Silen WH, Cheema F, et al. Effects of morphine analgesia on diagnostic accuracy in emergency department patients with abdominal pain: a prospective, randomized trial. J Am Coll Surg 2003;196:18–31.
58. Attard AR, Corlett MJ, Kidner NJ, et al. Safety of early pain relief for acute abdominal pain. BMJ 1992;305(6853):554–6.
59. LoVecchio F, Oster N, Sturmann K, et al. The use of analgesics in patients with acute abdominal pain. J Emerg Med 1997;15(6):775–9.
60. Ranji SR, Goldman LE, Simel DL, et al. Do opiates affect the clinical evaluation of patients with acute abdominal pain? JAMA 2006;296(14):1764–74.
61. Zoltie N, Cust MP. Analgesia in the acute abdomen. Ann R Coll Surg Engl 1986; 68(4):209–10.
62. Gallagher EJ, Esses D, Lee C, et al. Randomized clinical trial of morphine in acute abdominal pain. Ann Emerg Med 2006;48(2):150–60, 160.e1–4.
63. Manterola C, Astudillo P, Losada H, et al. Analgesia in patients with acute abdominal pain. Cochrane Database Syst Rev 2007;3:CD005660.
64. Brownfield E. Pain management. Use of analgesics in the acute abdomen. In: Making health care safer: a critical analysis of patient safety practices. Evidence Report/Technology Assessment, No. 43. AHRQ Publication No. 01-E058. Rockville (MD): Agency for Healthcare Research and Quality; 2001. p. 396–400. Available at: http://www.ahrq.gove/clinic/ptsafety/. Accessed February 26, 2011.
65. Silen W. Principles of diagnosis in acute abdominal disease. In: Cope's early diagnosis of the acute abdomen. New York: Oxford; 2010. p. 3–17.
66. Valentine RJ, Barth M, Myers S, et al. Nonvascular emergencies presenting as ruptured abdominal aortic aneurysms. Surgery 1993;113:286–9.
67. Kessler N, Cyteval C, Gallix B, et al. Appendicitis: evaluation of sensitivity, specificity, and predictive value of US, Doppler US, and laboratory findings. Radiology 2004;230:472–8.
68. Gwynn LK. The diagnosis of acute appendicitis: clinical assessment versus computed tomography evaluation. J Emerg Med 2001;21:119–23.
69. Lee SL, Walsh AJ, Ho HS. Computed tomography and ultrasonography do not improve and may delay the diagnosis and treatment of acute appendicitis. Arch Surg 2001;136:556–62.
70. Kuhn M, Bonnin RL, Davey MJ, et al. Emergency department ultrasound scanning for abdominal aortic aneurysm: accessible, accurate, and advantageous. Ann Emerg Med 2000;36:219–23.
71. Tayal VS, Bullard M, Swanson DR, et al. ED endovaginal pelvic ultrasound in nonpregnant women with right lower quadrant pain. Am J Emerg Med 2008; 26(1):81–5.
72. Tayal VS, Crean CA, Norton HJ, et al. Prospective comparative trial of endovaginal sonographic bimanual examination versus traditional digital bimanual examination in nonpregnant women with lower abdominal pain with regard to body mass index classification. J Ultrasound Med 2008;27(8):1171–7.
73. Smith JE, Hall EJ. The use of plain abdominal x rays in the emergency department. Emerg Med J 2009;26:160–3.
74. Maull KI, Reath DB. Pneumogastrography in the diagnosis of perforated peptic ulcer. Am J Surg 1984;148:340–5.

Imaging and Laboratory Testing in Acute Abdominal Pain

Nova L. Panebianco, MD, MPH[a],*, Katherine Jahnes, MD[b],
Angela M. Mills, MD[a]

KEYWORDS

• Abdominal pain • Computed tomography • Ultrasonography

As noted by almost every author in this issue, the diagnosis of emergency abdominal conditions involves the integration of information from the history, physical examination, laboratory testing, and imaging studies. Only rarely does the history or physical examination provide information that is conclusive or unequivocal, so that in most cases the clinician must resort to laboratory testing or imaging studies, which may themselves be equivocal or inaccurate. To prioritize and weight the information obtained from testing, it is important for the clinician to know the accuracy of the test being used. When discussing which laboratory tests or imaging to order in the setting of acute abdominal pain, it is convenient to organize information by disease process (eg, acute appendicitis, cholecystitis). Because studies on the accuracy of diagnostic tests are of necessity related to the presence or absence of specific diagnoses, and because clinicians frequently look to tests to help them rule in or rule out specific conditions, this article is organized by region of pain and common abdominal diagnoses. It focuses on the contributions that laboratory testing and imaging make in the emergency management of abdominal complaints as well as potential blind-spots and pitfalls that can arise if the tests are misapplied or misinterpreted.

OVERVIEW OF LABORATORY TESTING

Acute abdominal pain was the leading symptom-related cause for visiting an emergency department (ED), at 6.7% or 8 million visits, in 2006.[1] Laboratory work in the

---

The authors have no financial conflict.
[a] Department of Emergency Medicine, University of Pennsylvania School of Medicine, 3400 Spruce Street, Ground Ravdin, Philadelphia, PA 19104, USA
[b] Department of Emergency Medicine, New York Methodist Hospital, 506 Sixth Street, Brooklyn, NY 11215, USA
* Corresponding author.
E-mail address: Nova.panebianco@uphs.upenn.edu

patient with abdominal pain can serve to make a diagnosis, indicate the severity of disease, or direct attention toward coexisting medical problems. However, tests may result in incidental findings that may confound the clinical picture. For this reason, tests should be ordered with a specific clinical question in mind and, when possible, with a clear sense of the pretest probability and likelihood ratios engendered by a positive or negative outcome of the test.

Determining the value of an individual laboratory test for a patient with abdominal pain is difficult. In fact, the 1994 American College of Emergency Physicians (ACEP) policy statement recommends laboratory analysis for very few clinical diagnoses in patients with abdominal pain. However, clinical practice certainly varies significantly from this policy. Some studies have looked at the diagnostic importance of individual laboratory tests in the evaluation of specific conditions or suspected conditions (eg, suspicion of appendicitis). While review of data shows that individual laboratory studies taken in isolation infrequently "make" a diagnosis, results of laboratory studies do frequently affect disposition or treatment in the ED. In addition, many studies investigating laboratory testing in abdominal pain involve protocols in which laboratory tests are ordered for all patients and then tailored to the individual case after history and physical examination.[2–5] Most abdominal labs test general physiology, for example the complete blood count (CBC). Few tests are as specific as the lipase and urinalysis. In addition, even tests that are relatively specific, such as aspartate transaminase (AST) and alanine aminotransferase (ALT), may be abnormal in many different conditions.

The usefulness of a given test is often evaluated by its ability to rule in or out a given disease process. Using that as a starting point, intuitively it is clear that laboratory tests that give a more systemic glimpse at a patient's physiology, for instance a CBC or electrolytes, will be perceived as less "useful" than laboratory tests that more directly measure injury to an organ that is diseased, for example, troponins in myocardial ischemia or lipase in pancreatitis. However, laboratory tests that give an indication of systemic illness are clinically important for patients with abdominal pain. The most common laboratory tests ordered in the ED by percentage of patient visits are CBC (34.0%), blood urea nitrogen (BUN)/creatinine (20.1%), electrolytes (19.1%), cardiac enzymes (19.0%), and liver function tests (11.5%). Urinalysis was ordered in 20.2% of ED visits.[1] A study of abdominal pain patients at an urban academic ED found that laboratory and imaging tests led to a change in diagnosis in 37% of subjects and in disposition in 41%.[4] The investigators reported the two most useful tests to be abdominal computed tomography (CT) and urinalysis.

Summary

1. Laboratory tests can narrow a differential diagnosis, confirm clinical suspicion of a disease process, and, occasionally confound the treating physician.
2. Labs should be obtained to answer a focused clinical question.

OVERVIEW OF DIAGNOSTIC IMAGING

Imaging plays an important role in the evaluation of patients with acute abdominal pain. In 2005, 44% of ED visits included imaging; 35% of visits included plain radiography, 11% had CT, 3% had ultrasonography (US), and 0.5% magnetic resonance imaging (MRI).[6] While these statistics are for all complaints, not just for abdominal pain, it reflects the reliance on ancillary testing in the ED. When evaluating a patient with acute abdominal pain, the decision to order an imaging study, just as with laboratory testing, should come from information gleaned from a comprehensive yet focused history and physical examination. It is important to remember that all diagnostic testing has significant false-positive and false-negative results, and in the setting of a high pretest suspicion for disease, a negative test does not rule out disease. In addition, radiographic imaging may carry risks such as contrast and radiation exposure, and as such it is important to consider risks and benefits of an imaging modality when evaluating a patient with acute abdominal pain.

Plain Abdominal Radiography

Plain radiography has historically been the initial imaging modality used for the evaluation of abdominal pain, due to its ease of acquisition and cost. With the increased availability and technological advances of other imaging modalities such as CT and US, the usefulness of plain radiographs has diminished. With alternative imaging readily available, the usefulness of abdominal radiographs in the nontraumatic patient is controversial. In a recent study of patients whose abdominal radiograph was interpreted as normal or nonspecific, the majority (81%) had positive findings on CT, US, or upper gastrointestinal imaging.[7] The investigators found that plain radiographs led to a change in management in only 4% of patients. In another study, when compared with unenhanced helical CT, 3-view abdominal radiographs yielded only an overall sensitivity of 30%, specificity of 88%, and accuracy of 56% (95% confidence interval 0.46–0.66), with a negative predictive value of 51%.[8] Given the poor performance, added cost, and increased radiation dose, plain radiographs are indicated only in specific, limited settings.

Some have suggested that abdominal radiography be used solely to identify bowel obstruction, perforation, foreign body ingestion, or localization of catheter placement.[9] However, in obstruction, abdominal radiography alone does not provide the exact location or extent of the obstruction (partial, complete, or intermittent) and often requires further imaging such as CT.[10] Thus, a patient may be subjected to multiple tests with ionizing radiation. Pneumoperitoneum can be seen on an abdominal series radiograph; however, is often better visualized on an upright chest radiograph, which subjects the patient to shorter exposure times, less radiographic penetration, and more tangential alignment of the x-ray beam to the diaphragm (**Fig. 1**).[11] Abdominal radiography for the identification and localization of a foreign body or catheter may be the strongest indication for this imaging modality.

Summary

1. Plain abdominal radiography is of limited value and may only increase cost of care and a patient's total exposure to ionizing radiation.
2. Indications for the use of abdominal radiographs include suspicion for pneumoperitoneum or small bowel obstruction in the setting of limited or delayed availability of CT, localization of an ingested foreign body, and the localization of catheters.

Abdominal Computed Tomography

The use of CT for medical imaging is a relatively recent phenomenon, with the first commercially available CT scanner publicly announced in 1972. The benefits of CT include high-contrast resolution of images, multiplanar reformatted imaging, and rapid high-accuracy diagnosis. CT is often the test of choice when multiple diagnoses are being entertained, and greatly increases clinician diagnostic confidence. The disadvantages of CT include exposure to ionizing radiation, increased cost, increased personnel requirements, lack of repeatability, intravenous dye load and contrast allergies, and the risks of removing a patient out of the emergency treatment area.

In the United States the use of CT has increased dramatically in the past few decades, with more than 70 million CT scans performed in 2007.[12,13] Although CT

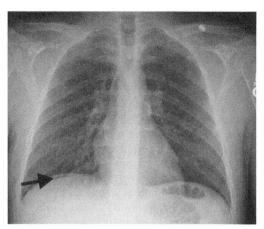

Fig. 1. A small stripe of free air (*arrow*) is seen in this upright chest radiograph. The thin pointy shape of the free air should be contrasted with the "roundy" shape of intraluminal of gas seen under the left hemidiaphragm. (*Courtesy of* Anthony J. Dean, MD, University of Pennsylvania, Philadelphia, PA.)

accounts for only 15% of radiological imaging, it accounts for approximately half of the collective medical radiation performed in the United States.[14,15] The median effective radiation dose for abdomen and pelvis CT ranges from 15 to 31 millisieverts (mSv), in comparison with the chest radiograph, which is 0.1 mSv.[16] In a study by Sodickson and colleagues,[15] cumulative CT radiation exposure added incrementally to baseline cancer risk. Estimated lifetime cancer mortality risks attributable to the radiation exposure from a single abdominal CT in a 1-year-old is 0.18%.[17] Brenner and Hall[18] predicted that 1.5% to 2% of all United States population cancers may be caused by CT radiation exposure. In particular, patients with chronic or recurrent medical conditions have the greatest exposure risk.

There are two groups in whom the cost, delay, and risk of abdominal CT may outweigh the benefits.[19] Those patients with (1) a high index of suspicion for the need for immediate surgical intervention (eg, unstable, obvious peritonitis) and (2) those in whom there is high confidence of a nonsurgical diagnosis based on history, physical examination, and/or other laboratory tests, yielding a low index of suspicion of serious abdominal pathology.[20] For those patients that fall between these two groups, abdominal CT can be invaluable.

An abdominal CT can be performed with or without intravenous (IV) iodinated contrast medium, and with or without oral/rectal contrast. In a prospective study of 100 ED patients with abdominal pain, patients were initially scanned without oral contrast and then again 90 minutes after oral contrast with identical scanning parameters. The investigators concluded that oral contrast takes at least 90 minutes to adequately opacify the bowel, increases length of stay in the ED by almost double that amount of time, but adds little, if anything, to the accuracy of diagnosis in patients with nontraumatic abdominal pain.[21] Similarly, in a study of noncontrast enhanced versus oral-contrast enhanced CTs, there was a 241-minute increase in time until disposition with the use of oral contrast.[22]

Summary

1. CT offers high-contrast resolution of images, multiplanar reformatted imaging, rapid high-accuracy diagnosis, and is often the test of choice when multiple diagnoses are

being considered. However, it may expose the patient to ionizing radiation, contrast dye, higher incurred cost, and removal from the ED treatment area.

2. CT is particularly useful in stable patients without overt surgical pathology but whose differential diagnosis includes significant abdominal pathology.
3. Radiation exposure may have consequences for the patient years to come, and the decision to perform the imaging examination should be taken in context of patients' current complaint and the future of their disease.
4. Oral contrast increases length of stay in the ED and may not add additional information.

Ultrasonography

US of the abdomen can produce anatomic, functional, and dynamic information during a real-time interaction between the examiner and the patient. The examiner may control the image plane, interrogate an area of tenderness, or watch for changes in image over time. US of the abdomen allows for rapid evaluation of an unstable patient, efficient narrowing of the differential diagnosis, repeatability throughout the resuscitation process, and the lack of known adverse biologic effects. The main drawbacks with US are that image acquisition and interpretation is operator dependent, and patient factors including body habitus and bowel gas may limit the examination.

Abdominal ultrasound images are traditionally obtained by technicians, interpreted later by radiologists, and then results are reported to clinicians. With the advent of smaller, more portable, higher-resolution machines, US is currently being used directly by clinicians. For more than a decade emergency physicians (EPs) have been using bedside US, and the ACEP has formally endorsed and supports bedside US by EPs for multiple applications, research, and education.[23] Emergency medicine residents are now required to receive training in point-of-care goal-directed US, and there are currently more than 50 ultrasound fellowships in the United States.

US has proved to be particularly useful in the early evaluation of the unstable patient. Appropriately trained nonradiologist clinician-performed bedside US can reliably detect intraperitoneal free fluid, the presence of an abdominal aortic aneurysm **(Fig. 2)**, and ruptured ectopic pregnancy, and can assess the morphology and collapsibility of the inferior vena cava for volume status.[24–27] In a study by Jones and colleagues,[28] the investigators examined a physician-performed, goal-directed ultrasound protocol for the ED management of patients presenting with nontraumatic, symptomatic, undifferentiated hypotension. It was demonstrated that immediate goal-directed US in the evaluation of patients reduces the number of viable diagnostic possibilities and allows the physician to come to a more accurate final diagnosis.

Summary

1. Clinician-performed US is a repeatable examination that can provide vital diagnostic information at the bedside without exposing a patient to ionizing radiation.
2. In the unstable patient, a goal-directed ultrasound examination may be the most efficient way to narrow a diagnosis.
3. US is limited by patient factors including habitus, wound bandages, abdominal tenderness, and subcutaneous emphysema.

INTEGRATION OF LABORATORY TESTS AND IMAGING STUDIES BASED ON LOCATION OF PAIN AND DISEASE PROCESS
Evaluation of Generalized Abdominal Pain

Generalized abdominal pain can be secondary to infectious, mechanical, vascular, inflammatory, malignant, or traumatic processes ranging from benign to life-threatening

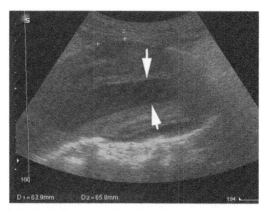

Fig. 2. Longitudinal ultrasound image of an abdominal aortic aneurysm. A thick layer of thrombus has formed within the walls of the aneurysm, creating a "pseudolumen" (*arrows*). Improper gain settings can result in the walls of the pseudolumen being mistaken for the walls of the aorta. (*Courtesy of* Anthony J. Dean, MD, University of Pennsylvania, Philadelphia, PA.)

in etiology. Some causes of generalized abdominal pain include bowel obstruction, abdominal aortic aneurysm (AAA), mesenteric ischemia, peritonitis, narcotic withdrawal, sickle cell crisis, irritable bowel syndrome, and heavy metal poisoning.[29] A workup for generalized abdominal pain will depend on a multitude of clinical factors, including history and physical examination, age, comorbidities, and vital signs, to avoid missing a serious condition. Several studies have shown that CT has an advantage over other imaging modalities in patients with nontraumatic generalized abdominal pain, and can alter disposition decisions in about a quarter of patients.[19,30,31]

A study of 100 young women (age 15–45 years) who presented to the ED with a chief complaint of lower abdominal pain attempted to examine the effects of CBC result on clinical decision making.[32] All patients in this study with appendicitis, as well as the one patient with an ectopic pregnancy, were appropriately diagnosed without the CBC result. In addition, of the 73 patients not admitted or diagnosed with an infectious disease, 17 were found to have an elevated white blood cell (WBC) count. While often ordered, the CBC in this study was found to have limited additional value in the workup of this patient population.

In the critically ill patient, lactate levels, although not specific to abdominal pain, can be a useful adjunct in the evaluation. In a prospective cohort study involving 1278 consecutive patients admitted to the hospital from an urban academic ED with a clinically significant infection (regardless of source), lactate levels were found to be useful as a risk stratification tool for inpatient mortality.[2] Primary end point was 28-day in-hospital mortality with a secondary outcome of "early death" within 3 days of hospitalization. Patients were divided into 3 groups by lactate levels defined as low (<2.5), medium (2.5–3.99), and high (≥4). For the 3 groups, 28-day in-hospital mortality was 4.9%, 9.0%, and 28.4%, respectively, and early mortality was 1.5%, 4.5%, and 22.4%, respectively. Lactate levels greater than 4 were 55% specific and 91% sensitive for early death (positive likelihood ratio [LR+] 1.4, negative likelihood ratio [LR−] 0.22, authors' calculation), and 36% specific and 92% sensitive for 28-day death (LR+ 2.02, LR− 0.16, authors' calculation). The investigators surmise that lactate levels may be helpful in identifying patients who should be targeted for aggressive early therapy.

Mesenteric ischemia is one of the most feared diagnoses for an ED physician with its unfortunate triad of frequent lack of history, unreliable physical examination, and lethality. The identification of laboratory markers to improve the diagnosis has so far proven elusive; however, a few potential markers have been identified. In a systematic review of the literature, 20 articles were identified that investigated serologic markers for intestinal ischemia in a combined 978 patients.[33] The prevalence of intestinal ischemia was 28% and included patients from a variety of settings. Of the multiple serologic markers investigated, 3 offered potential for improved diagnostic accuracy, including D-lactate, glutathione S-transferase (GST), and intestinal fatty acid binding protein (i-FABP). D-Lactate is produced by bacterial organisms and is thought to be a marker for bacterial translocation, as may follow ischemic (or other) mucosal injury. The investigators calculated a pooled positive LR of 2.64 in patients presenting with acute abdomen and a negative LR of 0.23. Physiologically, GST is a less specific marker, as it is released during oxidative stress from both the liver and the intestines; however, the analysis showed a positive LR of 3.28 and a negative LR of 0.23 in patients with acute abdomen. Intestinal fatty acid binding proteins are found in the cytoplasm of enterocytes at the tips of villi, the area most vulnerable to ischemia, thus making i-FABP an interesting candidate for a serologic marker of ischemia. In the analysis, the positive LR was 4.5 and the negative LR was 0.52. All of these markers require further research before becoming routine in the evaluation of ED patients presenting with acute abdominal pain.

As clinical examination and laboratory tests tend to have limited ability to predict the presence of mesenteric ischemia, imaging tests are often needed. Angiography of the mesenteric arteries traditionally has been the gold-standard diagnostic test for mesenteric ischemia. This test is limited by its invasiveness, dye load, and inability to visualize surrounding structures other than the vessel lumen. With the advent of multidetector-row CT and MRI, angiography is no longer a first-choice procedure. CT has many advantages over angiography in that it is minimally invasive, can detect ischemic changes in the affected areas (bowel wall thickening, fat stranding, pneumatosis), and image reformatting can allow for angiographic reconstructions that often eliminate the need for traditional angiography in the case of high clinical suspicion and negative CT (**Fig. 3**).[34] The limitations of CT include high radiation dose and risk of nephrotoxicity secondary to contrast dye. In a review article by Biolato and colleagues,[35] they report that CT with IV contrast has a sensitivity and specificity for acute mesenteric ischemia of 64% and 92%, respectively. Multidetector-row CT with 3-dimensional reformats increases sensitivity and specificity to 96% and 94%, respectively. MR angiography can obtain high-resolution angiograms in 85% to 90% of superior mesenteric arteries, 75% to 90% of celiac arteries, and 25% of inferior mesenteric arteries (lower because of its anatomic location). The superior mesenteric and celiac arteries are clearly visualized using duplex US in more than 90% and 80% of cases, respectively. As with MR, US cannot reliably visualize the inferior mesenteric artery because of its anatomic location.[35]

Summary

1. In the setting of generalized abdominal pain, CT is often the test of choice for evaluating patients with a significant clinical risk of an acute intra-abdominal process.
2. Lactate levels, although not specific to abdominal pain, can be a useful adjunct in the evaluation of patients who may be critically ill.
3. Multidetector-row CT, MRI, and duplex US may replace angiography as the first-line test for mesenteric ischemia.

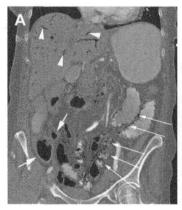
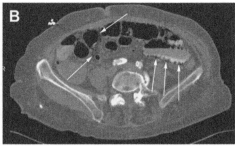

Fig. 3. Coronal (*A*) and axial (*B*) CT images of a patient with mesenteric ischemia demonstrating extensive portal venous gas (*arrowheads*), bowel wall edema (*short arrows*), and marked intestinal pneumatosis (*long arrows*). (*Courtesy of* William W. Boonn, MD, University of Pennsylvania, Philadelphia, PA.)

Right Upper Quadrant

Pain in the right upper quadrant (RUQ) may relate to disorders of the hepatobiliary system, right kidney, pancreas, bowel, pleura/lung, and musculoskeletal system. In a retrospective study of 100 patients with suspected acute cholecystitis who underwent a hepatobiliary scan, Singer and colleagues[36] investigated whether the presence or absence of various clinical or laboratory parameters (including WBC count, total bilirubin, AST, ALT, alkaline phosphatase, and amylase) would identify patients at high risk for having a positive hepatobiliary scan. In fact, none of the laboratory values evaluated in this study were predictive of having a positive hepatobiliary scan. A study of 311 patients admitted with suspected acute cholecystitis described the relationship between elevated liver function tests (LFTs) (specifically bilirubin, ALT, and alkaline phosphatase) and acute cholecystitis.[37] The incidence of confirmed acute cholecystitis was 73.6%, and though LFT abnormalities were statistically more frequent in patients with acute cholecystitis than without acute cholecystitis, these results were not clinically useful because of the broad overlap of values in those with other conditions. Furthermore, normal LFTs did not exclude cholecystitis. Laboratory testing is an adjunct to the workup of patients with suspected acute cholecystitis, but ultimately clinical suspicion and imaging studies are needed for diagnosis.

It is estimated that 20 million persons in the United States have gallstones.[38] Although radionuclide imaging is sensitive for acute cholecystitis, it is expensive, time consuming, and does not assess structures outside of the biliary tract. Thus, RUQ US is considered the test of choice for evaluation of the gallbladder and biliary tree.[39] Multiple studies have shown that EPs can detect cholelithiasis by US, with good sensitivity and specificity.[40,41] Acute cholecystitis is characterized on ultrasound images by the presence of gallstones (particularly if in the neck of the gallbladder), thickened wall, pericholecystic fluid, and the presence of a sonographic Murphy sign (**Fig. 4**). One study of EPs' ability to detect gallstones by bedside US found a sensitivity and specificity of 91% and 66%, respectively.[42] The low specificity may have been secondary to the use of a single criterion in the diagnosis of acute inflammation, a sonographic Murphy sign.

In the setting of acute jaundice, US may be used to detect the presence of biliary stasis, localize the level of ductal obstruction, and identify the cause of obstruction.

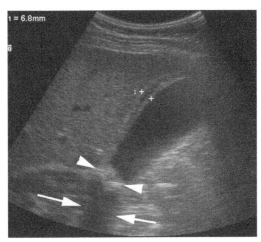

Fig. 4. Longitudinal ultrasound view showing stones (*arrowheads*) impacted in the gall-bladder neck with posterior shadowing (*arrows*). In this case of cholecystitis, the wall is thickened with a dark layer of intramural edema. (*Courtesy of* Anthony J. Dean, MD, University of Pennsylvania, Philadelphia, PA.)

The ability of US to detect common bile duct stones is limited, with some studies reporting a sensitivity of less than 70%; however, the diagnosis of intrahepatic calculi by US may be more accurate than that of CT because these stones lack sufficient calcium to make them radio-opaque.[43,44] US may be useful to rule in disease, but not significantly sensitive to rule it out. In this setting, LFTs including total bilirubin, AST, ALT, and γ-glutamyl transpeptidase (GGT) may be useful.

Other causes of pain in the RUQ include pneumonia, hepatitis, renal colic, musculoskeletal pain, and herpes zoster. RUQ pain secondary to lung infection can often be determined by physical examination and chest radiography. Pain due to renal colic may be identified by the history and physical examination. Urinalysis may contain red blood cells; however, lack of hematuria does not rule out nephrolithiasis. In a study using helical CT as the reference standard for ureterolithiasis, the sensitivity and specificity for a patient with any degree of microscopic hematuria were 89% and 29%, respectively.[45] Imaging may include plain radiography, unenhanced CT, intravenous urography (IVU), and US. A kidney-ureter-bladder (KUB) radiograph can be used to determine the location and size of a kidney stone, and is often used to track the progress of a known stone. The sensitivity and specificity of KUB for nephrolithiasis is 44% to 77% and 80% to 87% respectively.[46] In a study by Wang and colleagues,[47] unenhanced CT was determined to be more effective and efficient than IVU and was recommended to replace IVU as the first-line diagnostic tool for ureteral stone detection in the ED. In a review by Heidenreich and colleagues,[46] the investigators write that "unenhanced helical CT has been demonstrated to be superior (in diagnosing ureteral stones) since (1) it detects ureteral stones with a sensitivity and specificity from 98% to 100% regardless of size, location and chemical composition, (2) it identifies extra-urinary causes of flank pain in about one third of all patients presenting with acute flank pain, (3) it does not need contrast agent, and (4) it is a time saving imaging technique being performed within 5 minutes." Renal US is commonly used in the evaluation of acute flank pain and may reveal hydronephrosis, and occasionally a stone is seen in the ureterovesicular junction. US is appealing, as it is fast, painless, repeatable, does not expose the patient to ionizing radiation, and may be able to rule out obstruction with the presence of ureteral jets. US may be particularly useful in a patient with a history of nephrolithiasis and low risk for alternative diagnosis, in order to avoid a CT scan.

Summary

1. There is no single blood test that predicts the presence or absence of acute cholecystitis.
2. RUQ US is the test of choice in the evaluation of biliary disease.
3. Unenhanced CT of the abdomen has excellent sensitivity and specificity for ureterolithiasis, and can point to an alternative diagnosis if no stones are identified.

Epigastric

Amylase and lipase are the two serologic markers used to diagnose acute pancreatitis. In a retrospective study of 10,931 patients, serum amylase and lipase measurements were compared with discharge diagnosis of acute pancreatitis using radiographic evidence for confirmation of diagnosis.[48] The investigators demonstrated an improved diagnostic accuracy for lipase over amylase, with sensitivity and specificity of 90.3% and 93.0%, respectively for lipase and 78.7% and 92.6%, respectively for amylase. The level of pancreatic enzyme elevation has not been shown to correlate with severity of disease, nor can daily measurement of enzymes be used to assess clinical progress or prognosis.[49]

Enhanced CT of the abdomen is the radiologic test of choice to evaluate for pancreatic necrosis. Abdominal plain radiography typically offers little information in the evaluation of acute pancreatitis. Abdominal US may yield information about the pancreas; however, it may be limited by patient habitus and bowel gas. US may play a role in the assessment of pancreatitis by identifying gallstones as the cause. Patients with necrotizing pancreatitis have been found to have a mortality of 10% to 23% compared with a mortality of less than 1% in those with interstitial pancreatitis.[50] As CT grade of severity increases, so does the rate of complications and mortality. Not all patients with pancreatitis must undergo abdominal CT. For those with a known history of pancreatitis, stable labs, and vital signs, CT may not be of additional value.[51] CT is often used to exclude other sources of pain and to assess the severity of disease, especially in patients with continued symptoms who are not improving.

Summary

1. Elevated lipase is more specific than amylase in the detection of acute pancreatitis.
2. Contrast-enhanced CT can be used to determine the extent of pancreatic injury and identify alternative causes of acute epigastric abdominal pain.

Right Lower Quadrant

Pain in the right lower quadrant (RLQ) may be caused by appendicitis, ovarian pathology, ectopic pregnancy, hernia, intestinal pathology, and renal colic. In the 2009 ACEP clinical policy with regard to the evaluation and management of ED patients with suspected appendicitis, the subcommittee gave a level B recommendation to the use of clinical findings to risk-stratify patients and guide further testing and management. The subcommittee also concluded that WBC alone is not a consistent predictor of appendicitis, as it may frequently be normal especially in the setting of early presentation.[52] A meta-analysis by Andersson[53] of clinical signs and symptoms and laboratory values in suspected appendicitis found individual components to be "of weak discriminatory and predictive capacity." The study reports, however, that a WBC greater than 10 ($\times 10^9$/L) had a positive LR of 2.47 for appendicitis, and

C-reactive protein (CRP) greater than 10 (mg/L) had a positive LR of 1.97. Andersson also calculated LRs for granulocyte counts and proportion of polymorphonuclear neutrophil (PMN) cells, and found appendicitis to be more likely in patients with high granulocyte counts and PMN percentages greater than 75. Appendicitis was unlikely in cases where both WBC and CRP were less than 10. Andersson concluded that "contrary to common opinion, simple and easily performed laboratory tests of the inflammatory response appear to be at least as important as discriminators as the clinical descriptions of peritoneal irritation, especially in advanced appendicitis."

Abdominal radiography has a limited role in the evaluation of the patient with acute RLQ pain. US and CT are often used to evaluate patients for acute appendicitis. CT is more accurate than US in the evaluation of appendicitis (particularly in obese patients), often provides an alternative diagnosis when negative for acute appendicitis, and should be considered in any clinically stable older patient (**Fig. 5**).[54,55] In a study by Balthazar and colleagues,[56] 100 patients had both CT and US evaluation for acute appendicitis. Fifty-four patients had acute appendicitis and 46 did not. Of the 54 patients with appendicitis, analysis of the data for CT versus US revealed sensitivity of 96% versus 76%, respectively, and specificity of 89% versus 91%. In the 46 patients without appendicitis, an alternative diagnosis was made by CT in 22 patients and by US in 15. CT scans showed abscesses and/or phlegmons in 28% of patients with appendicitis versus only 17% using US. Thus, CT was more accurate than US in the diagnosis of acute appendicitis, and offered an alternative diagnosis more often when the patient did not have acute appendicitis.

There are certain populations where CT in the evaluation for acute appendicitis may be contraindicated. Acute appendicitis is the most common cause of surgical abdominal pain in children, and they are most at risk for lifelong effects of ionizing radiation. Children are also less often obese, a common limitation of US for acute appendicitis. Given the risk of ionizing radiation, the advantage of a pediatric physique, and specificities as high as 88% to 99%, it may be best to perform US first in these patients (**Fig. 6**).[55,57] A positive study requires no further testing, and a negative or equivocal study could be followed by CT or observation with serial examinations. A similar argument can be made for pregnant patients in whom ionizing radiation may put the fetus at risk. In these patients, US or MRI may be the initial imaging test of choice. In a small study by Israel and colleagues,[58] when the appendix was visualized on MRI the

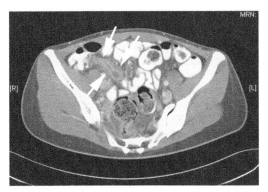

Fig. 5. CT scan showing the appendix (*arrows*) to be very enlarged and unfilled with contrast (compare with bowel). Fat stranding is demonstrated even in this thin patient, where the fat posterior to the appendix is of much higher radiodensity than that on the other side of the abdomen. (*Courtesy of* Nova L. Panebianco, MD, University of Pennsylvania, Philadelphia, PA.)

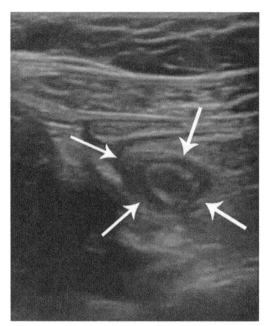

Fig. 6. Ultrasonogram of an inflamed appendix in short-axis plane (outlined by *narrow white arrows*). In real time it is found to be a blind-ending tubular structure that lacks peristalsis and is typically located at the point of maximal tenderness. When viewed in short axis it is often described as a "target" sign. (*Courtesy of* Nova L. Panebianco, MD, University of Pennsylvania, Philadelphia, PA.)

sensitivity, specificity, positive predictive value (PPV), and negative predictive value (NPV) for the diagnosis of appendicitis was 100% for all parameters. When the appendix was visualized by US, the sensitivity, specificity, PPV, and NPV for the diagnosis of appendicitis was 50%, 100%, 100%, and 66%, respectively.

In the female patient with right (or left) lower quadrant pain, ruptured ovarian cysts, ovarian torsion, tubo-ovarian abscess (TOA), and ectopic pregnancy should be considered. Any woman of child-bearing age with acute abdominal pain should have a urine pregnancy test as part of their initial ED evaluation. Urine pregnancy tests can detect human chorionic gonadotropin (hCG) hormone in concentrations as low as 25 mIU/mL. A double decidual sac can be visualized consistently using transabdominal sonography, with a B-hCG of 6500 mIU/mL and 1500 mIU/mL using transvaginal US. Identification of a yolk sac or fetal pole within the uterus effectively rules out ectopic pregnancy in patients who did not undergo assisted reproductive technologies. Although the B-hCG level should not determine whether US should be performed for the evaluation of ectopic pregnancy, it may assist in interpreting the US results.[59]

According to the Centers for Disease Control and Prevention (CDC), the incidence of *Chlamydia*, gonorrhea, and syphilis reported from 1996 to 2008 was 170 in 100,000.[60] Sexually transmitted diseases are associated with pelvic inflammatory disease (PID), TOA, ectopic pregnancy, and decreased fertility. A ruptured TOA has a mortality rate as high as 8.6%.[61] Patients are often tested for *Chlamydia*, gonorrhea, and syphilis while in the ED; however, the results of these tests may not be available for several days. Although the results do not assist the ED physician at the point of care, they are important in public health implications and may be useful in subsequent clinical encounters. There is no single laboratory test to reliably confirm or refute the diagnosis of TOA. An elevated WBC is a nonspecific finding. In a 2007 review article, Blenning and colleagues[62] report that elevated erythrocyte sedimentation rate (ESR) and CRP along with an elevated WBC count may be helpful in diagnosing PID, particularly in mild cases.

The diagnoses of ruptured ovarian cyst, ovarian torsion, TOA, and ectopic pregnancy can be made with US (**Fig. 7**). Pelvic US has a sensitivity of 93% and a specificity of 98% in the diagnosis of TOA.[63] In a study by Lee and colleagues[64] examining ovarian torsion, the twisted vascular pedicle was detected preoperatively by US in 28 of 32 patients with surgically proven torsion, showing a diagnostic accuracy of 87%. In a study by Pascual and colleagues,[65] the sensitivity and specificity of color Doppler transvaginal sonography to detect functional ovarian cysts were 84.6% and 99.2%, respectively, with positive and NPVs of 98% and 93.5%.

Summary

1. CT is more accurate than US in the diagnosis of acute appendicitis; however, in certain populations where the risk of ionizing radiation is great, US or MRI may be the better initial imaging strategy. A positive ultrasonogram rules in the diagnosis, but a negative study does not rule it out.
2. A urine pregnancy test is almost invariably needed in the evaluation of acute abdominal pain in any female patient of child-bearing age.
3. Pelvic US, in most situations, should be the first imaging study in a young woman with acute pelvic pain.

Left Upper Quadrant

Emergent causes of abdominal pain in the left upper quadrant (LUQ) are rare. Diagnoses to consider include disorders of the stomach including gastritis and its related conditions, disorders of the spleen including splenomegaly, splenic infarct or abscess, and pancreatitis, and disorders of the kidney including renal colic and pyelonephritis. Other conditions to consider in the patient with LUQ abdominal pain include herpes

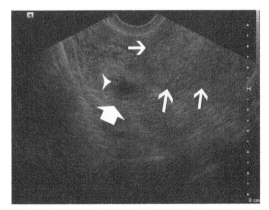

Fig. 7. Ultrasound image shows an empty uterus (outlined by *narrow white arrows*) with a right adnexal ectopic mass (*thick white arrow*). A yolk sac is visualized within the cystic ectopic mass (*arrowhead*). (*Courtesy of* Nova L. Panebianco, MD, University of Pennsylvania, Philadelphia, PA.)

zoster and conditions of the chest such as pneumonia, pleurisy, myocardial infarction, and pericarditis.

Similar to laboratory testing, there is no specific radiologic test for the LUQ. A chest radiograph may reveal pneumonia. If the patient's history and physical examination suggest esophageal or gastric origin, then symptomatic therapy and endoscopy is recommended. If renal colic is suspected then US or CT, as described earlier, may corroborate the diagnosis. CT scan can reveal pancreatitis, splenic infarct or abscess, gastric malignancy, pyelonephritis, and inflammation of the bowel. In the setting of blunt trauma, US may detect free fluid in the abdomen as a surrogate marker for acute splenic trauma (**Fig. 8**). The decision to image, and what imaging modality to use, must be made on a case-by-case basis.

Summary

1. There is limited literature on the usefulness of laboratory and radiologic imaging in the evaluation of acute LUQ abdominal pain, and clinical features should guide testing.
2. US and CT imaging may be used to narrow or make the diagnosis when there is high clinical suspicion for an acute abdominal process, particularly in the elderly, immunosuppressed, or trauma patient.

Left Lower Quadrant

Important diagnoses in patients with acute left lower quadrant (LLQ) pain include diverticulitis and colitis (including Crohn disease, ulcerative colitis, and *Clostridium difficile* colitis) as well as the complications of these conditions. As for patients with RLQ pain, LLQ pain can be secondary to renal colic, ovarian pathology, ectopic pregnancy, and hernia. Laboratory testing and imaging for these conditions is described in the section on RLQ.

Acute diverticulitis is a common cause of LLQ pain. The prevalence of diverticular disease is age dependent, increasing from less than 5% at age 40, to 30% by age 60, to 65% by age 85 years.[66] The patient may have leukocytosis, but in one study 45% of patients had a normal WBC count.[67] LFTs are usually normal. Amylase may be normal or elevated. Urinalysis may reveal sterile pyuria secondary to inflammation adjacent to the bladder. CT with oral and IV contrast is very sensitive for the detection of acute diverticulitis (79%–98%) and can help distinguish this from other causes of

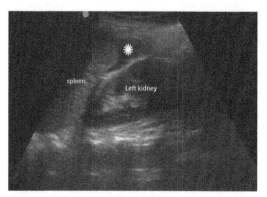

Fig. 8. Longitudinal ultrasound view of the left upper quadrant. Free fluid (*white star*) outlines the lower pole of the spleen and tracts into the splenorenal space. (*Courtesy of* Nova L. Panebianco, MD, University of Pennsylvania, Philadelphia, PA.)

acute LLQ pain (**Fig. 9**).[19] In a study by Rao and colleagues,[68] the sensitivity and specificity of helical CT (with colonic contrast only) was determined to be 97% and 100%, respectively. CT is also useful for identifying complications of acute diverticulitis such as perforation and abscess formation, and allows for an assessment of the severity of the disease. US for the detection of acute diverticulitis has also been studied. In a prospective study of 123 patients with clinical signs of acute intestinal inflammation, the sensitivity of US in comparison with abdominal CT in diagnosing acute colonic diverticulitis was 84.6%, and the specificity 80.3%.[69] US may be less sensitive than CT in detecting abscesses and microperforation.

Summary

1. Acute diverticulitis is a common cause of LLQ pain.
2. CT with oral or rectal, and IV contrast, is very sensitive for this disease.

Suprapubic

Disorders of the bladder and surrounding structures often cause suprapubic abdominal pain. Little and colleagues[70] evaluated the accuracy of urinalysis dipsticks versus a clinical decision rule for diagnosis of urinary tract infection (UTI), and found favorable diagnostic accuracy with dipsticks. In 427 women with suspected UTI, nitrite, leukocyte esterase (+ or greater), and blood (trace hemolyzed or greater) on dipstick analysis were all independently predictive of UTI with adjusted odds ratios of 6.36, 4.52, and 2.23, respectively. The investigators found a PPV of 92% for dipstick-positive nitrite and either blood or leukocyte esterase. In a study by Jou and Powers,[71] urine microscopy prompted a management change in only 9 of 166 patients (5%) after the initial urine dip. Six changes resulted in therapy for UTI, 1 resulted in withholding of therapy for UTI, and 2 resulted in cancellation of plans for diagnostic imaging. It was concluded that primary use of dipstick urinalysis, with microscopy in selected cases, would likely result in considerable cost savings and time saving without compromising patient care. The dipstick-only approach may not be appropriate in elderly patients, children, or any patient in whom urosepsis is suspected, as these patients require adequate sampling for culture.

Acute urinary retention may be secondary to benign prostatic hypertrophy (BPH), a bladder mass, blood clot, medication, or bladder injury. US of the bladder to assess

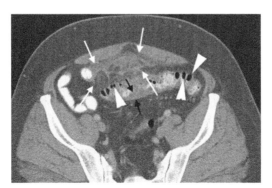

Fig. 9. CT scan of the pelvis showing a loop of bowel with markedly thickened walls (demonstrated by location of intraluminal contrast, *black arrows*), multiple diverticuli (*white arrowheads*), and a large area of intensive stranding anteriorly (*white arrows*). (*Courtesy of* Anthony J. Dean, MD, University of Pennsylvania, Philadelphia, PA.)

for the etiology of acute urinary retention can assist the ED physician. Bladder stones will have a highly reflective surface and a brightly reflective posterior. Clotted blood in the bladder tends to settle down into the most dependent areas and layers out. An enlarged prostate can be seen on transabdominal sonography. US can also be used to confirm Foley placement in a patient who is anuric. If the US is negative for acute pathology then one may consider a CT with or without contrast.

Summary

1. Urine dip is as good as urinary microanalysis at revealing the presence or abscess of a UTI.
2. US can be used to assess bladder volumes. This is important in patients with acute urinary retention whether secondary to bladder pathology (BPH, blood clot), medication induced, or secondary to trauma.

SUMMARY

The evaluation of acute abdominal pain in the ED is challenging. Often laboratory testing and radiologic imaging are needed to supplement the history and physical examination to confirm or exclude a diagnosis. Unfortunately, all diagnostic tests have false-negative and false-positive rates. A negative test does not rule out disease, and in the setting of a high pretest probability of disease, it is prudent to consider reassessment and a short course of observation for serial abdominal examinations for disease progression or resolution. Careful selection of laboratory and imaging studies should be made to efficiently and safely manage patient care.

REFERENCES

1. Pitts SR, Niska RW, Xu J, et al. National Hospital Ambulatory Medical Care Survey: 2006 emergency department summary. Natl Health Stat Report 2008;7: 1–38.
2. Shapiro NI, Howell MD, Talmor D, et al. Serum lactate as a predictor of mortality in emergency department patients with infection. Ann Emerg Med 2005;45:524–8.
3. Sutton P, Humes D, Purcell G, et al. The role of routine assays of serum amylase and lipase for the diagnosis of acute abdominal pain. Ann R Coll Surg Engl 2009; 91(5):381–4.
4. Nagurney JT, Brown DF, Chang Y, et al. Use of diagnostic testing in the emergency department for patients presenting with non traumatic abdominal pain. J Emerg Med 2003;25(4):363–71.
5. Chi CH, Shiesh SC, Chen KW, et al. C-reactive protein for the evaluation of acute abdominal pain. Am J Emerg Med 1996;14(30):254–6.
6. Nawar EW, Niska RW, Xu J. National Hospital Ambulatory Care Survey: 2005 emergency department summary. Vital Health Stat 2007;386:1–32. Available at: http://www.cdc.gov/nchs/data/ad/ad386.pdf. Accessed January 21, 2011.
7. Kellow ZS, MacInnes M, Kurzencwyg D, et al. The role of abdominal radiography in the evaluation of the nontrauma emergency patient. Radiology 2008;248: 887–93.
8. MacKersie AB, Lane MJ, Gerhardt RT, et al. Nontraumatic acute abdominal pain: unenhanced helical CT compared with three-view acute abdominal series. Radiology 2005;237:114–22.
9. Spates M, Schwartz DT, Savitt D. Abdominal imaging. In: Schwartz DT, Reisdorff EJ, editors. Emergency radiology. San Francisco, CA: McGraw-Hill; 2000. p. 509–55.

10. Barker SR. The abdominal plain film: what will be its role in the future? Radiol Clin North Am 1993;31(6):1335–44.
11. Flak B, Rowley A. Acute abdomen: plain film utilization and analysis. Can Assoc Radiol J 1993;44(6):423–8.
12. Amis ES Jr, Butler PF, Applegate KE, et al. American College of Radiology white paper on radiation dose in medicine. J Am Coll Radiol 2007;4:272–84.
13. Smith-Bindman R, Miglioretti DL, Larson EB. Rising use of diagnostic medical imaging in a large integrated health system. Health Aff (Millwood) 2008;27: 1491–502.
14. Mettler FA Jr, Thomadsen BR, Bhargavan M, et al. Medical radiation exposure in the U.S. in 2006: preliminary results. Health Phys 2008;95:502–7.
15. Sodickson A, Baeyens PF, Andriole KP, et al. Recurrent CT, cumulative radiation exposure, and associated radiation-induced cancer risks from CT of adults. Radiology 2009;251(1):175–84.
16. Smith-Bindman R, Lipson J, Marcus R, et al. Radiation dose associated with common computed tomography examinations and the associated lifetime attributable risk of cancer. Arch Intern med 2009;169:2078–86.
17. Brenner D, Elliston C, Hall E, et al. Estimated risks of radiation-induced fatal cancer from pediatric CT. AJR Am J Roentgenol 2001;17(2):289–96.
18. Brenner DJ, Hall EJ. Computed tomography: an increasing source of radiation exposure. N Engl J Med 2007;357:2277–84.
19. Lewis LM. The role of imaging in evaluating emergency patients with abdominal pain. In: Cline DM, Stead LG. Abdominal emergencies. New York: McGraw Hill Medical; 2008.
20. Lewis LM, Klippel AP, Bavolek RA, et al. Quantifying the usefulness of CT in evaluating seniors with abdominal pain. Eur J Radiol 2007;61:290.
21. Lee SY, Coughlin B, Wolfe JM, et al. Prospective comparison of helical ct of the abdomen and pelvis without and with oral contrast in assessing acute abdominal pain in adult Emergency Department patients. Emerg Radiol 2006;12:150–7. Epub 2006 Apr 21.
22. Huynh LN, Coughlin BF, Wolfe J, et al. Patient encounter time intervals in the evaluation of emergency department patients requiring abdominopelvic CT: oral contrast versus no contrast. Emerg Radiol 2004;10:310–3.
23. Emergency ultrasound guidelines. Policy statement. Dallas (TX): American College of Physicians; 2008.
24. Ollerton JE, Sugrue M, Balogh Z, et al. Prospective study to evaluate the influence of FASTon trauma patient management. J Trauma 2006;60(4):785–91.
25. Kuhn M, Bonnin RL, Davey MJ, et al. Emergency department ultrasound scanning for abdominal aortic aneurysm: accessible, accurate and advantageous. Ann Emerg Med 2000;36(3):219–23.
26. Mateer JR, Valley VT, Aiman EJ, et al. Outcome analysis of a protocol including bedside endovaginal sonography in patients at risk for ectopic pregnancy. Ann Emerg Med 1996;27(3):283–93.
27. Stawicki SP, Braslow BM, Panebianco NL, et al. Intensivist use of hand-carried ultrasonography to measure IVC collapsibility in estimating intravascular volume status: correlations with CVP. J Am Coll Surg 2009;209(1):55–61.
28. Jones AE, Tayal VS, Sullivan DM, et al. Controlled trial of immediate versus delayed goal-directed ultrasound to identify the cause of nontraumatic hypotension in emergency department patients. Crit Care Med 2004;32(8):1703–8.
29. Cartwright SL, Knudson MP. Evaluation of acute abdominal pain in adults. Am Fam Physician 2008;77(7):971–8.

30. Tsushima Y, Yamada S, Aoki J, et al. Effect of contrast-enhanced computed tomography on diagnosis and management of acute abdomen in adults. Clin Radiol 2002;57:507.
31. Esses D, Birnbaum A, Bijur P, et al. Ability of CT to alter decision making in elderly patients with acute abdominal pain. Am J Emerg Med 2004;22:270–2.
32. Silver BE, Patterson JW, Kulick M, et al. Effect of CBC results on ED management of women with lower abdominal pain. Am J Emerg Med 1995;13(3):304–6.
33. Evennett NJ, Petrov MS, Mittal A, et al. Systematic review and pooled estimates for the diagnostic accuracy of serologic markers for intestinal ischemia. World J Surg 2009;33:1374–83.
34. Zacho HD, Abrahamsen J. Chronic intestinal ischaemia: diagnosis. Clin Physiol Funct Imaging 2008;28:71–5.
35. Biolato M, Miele L, Gasbarrini G, et al. Abdominal angina. Am J Med Sci 2009; 338(5):389–95.
36. Singer AJ, McCracken G, Henry MC, et al. Correlation among clinical, laboratory, and hepatobiliary scanning findings in patients with acute cholecystitis. Ann Emerg Med 1996;28(3):267–72.
37. Dunlop MG, King PM, Gunn AA. Acute abdominal pain: the value of liver function tests in suspected cholecystitis. J R Coll Surg Edinb 1989;34(3):124–7.
38. Johnston EE, Kaplan MM. Medical progress: pathogenesis and treatment of gallstones. N Engl J Med 1993;328:412–5.
39. Wang HP, Chen SC. Upper abdominal ultrasound in the critically ill. Crit Care Med 2007;35(Suppl 5):S208–15.
40. Lanoix R, Leak LV, Gaeta T, et al. A preliminary evaluation of emergency ultrasound in the setting of an emergency medicine training program. Am J Emerg Med 2000;18:41–5.
41. Schlager D, Lazzareschi G, Whitten D, et al. A prospective study of ultrasonography in the ED by emergency physicians. Am J Emerg Med 1994;12:185–9.
42. Rosen CL, Brown DF, Chang Y, et al. Ultrasonography by emergency physicians in patients with suspected cholecystitis. Am J Emerg Med 2001;19:32–6.
43. Rickes S, Treiber G, Monkemuller K, et al. Impact of the operator's experience on value of high-resolution transabdominal ultrasound in the diagnosis of choledocholithiasis: a prospective comparison using endoscopic retrograde cholangiography as the gold standard. Scand J Gastroenterol 2006;41:838–43.
44. Kim HJ, Kim MH, Lee SK, et al. Characterization of primary pure cholesterol hepatolithiasis: cholangioscopic and selective cholangiographic findings. Gatrointest Endosc 2001;53:324–8.
45. Koeing CJ. Accuracy of hematuria in diagnosing kidney stones. J Fam Pract 1999;48:912–3.
46. Heidenreich A, Desgrandschamps F, Terrier F. Modern approach of diagnosis and management of acute flank pain: review of all imaging modalities. Eur Urol 2002;41:351–62.
47. Wang JH, Shen SH, Huang SS, et al. Prospective comparison of unenhanced spiral computed tomography and intravenous urography in the evaluation of acute renal colic. J Chin Med Assoc 2008;71(1):30–6.
48. Smith RS, Southwell-Keely J, Chesher D. Should serum pancreatic lipase replace serum amylase as a biomarker of acute pancreatitis? ANZ J Surg 2005;75:399–404.
49. Yadav D, Agarwal N, Pitchumoni CS. A critical evaluation of laboratory tests in acute pancreatitis. Am J Gastroenterol 2002;97(6):1309–18.
50. Balthazar EJ. Acute pancreatitis: assessment of severity with clinical and CT evaluation. Radiology 2002;223:603–13.

51. Banks PA, Freeman ML, Practice Parameters Committee of the American College of Gastroenterology. Practice guidelines in acute pancreatitis. Am J Gastroenterol 2006;101:2379–400.

52. Howell JM, Eddy OL, Lukens TW, et al. American College of Emergency Physicians. Clinical policy: critical issues in the evaluation and management of emergency department patients with suspected appendicitis. Ann Emerg Med 2010; 55:71–116.

53. Andersson RE. Meta-analysis of the clinical and laboratory diagnosis of appendicitis. Br J Surg 2004;91:28–37.

54. Keyzer C, Zalcman M, DeMaerteler V, et al. Comparison of US and unenhanced multi-detector row CT in patients suspected of having acute appendicitis. Radiology 2005;236:527.

55. Cline DM, Stead LG. Abdominal emergencies. New York: McGraw Hill Medical; 2008. Chapter 5.

56. Balthazar EJ, Birnabaum BA, Yee J, et al. Acute appendicitis: CT and US correlation in 100 patients. Radiology 1994;190:31–5.

57. Taylor GA. Suspected appendicitis in children: in search of the single best diagnostic test. Radiology 2004;231:293.

58. Israel GM, Malguria N, McCarthy S, et al. MRI vs. ultrasound for suspected appendicitis during pregnancy. J Magn Reson Imaging 2008;28(2):428–33.

59. ACOG practice bulletin no. 3. Medical management of tubal pregnancy. Clinical management guidelines for obstetrician-gynecologists. Washington, DC: American College of Obstetricians and Gynecologists; 1998.

60. Centers for Disease Control and Prevention. Available at: http://wonder.cdc.gov/controller/datarequest/D46. Accessed January 21, 2011.

61. Krivak T, Propst A, Horowitz G. Tubo-ovarian abscess. Principles of contemporary management. Fem Patient 1997;22:27.

62. Blenning CE, Muench J, Zegar Judkins D. Which tests are the most useful for diagnosing PID? J Fam Prac 2007;56(3):216–20.

63. Lambert MJ, Villa M. Gynecologic ultrasound in emergency medicine. Emerg Med Clin North Am 2004;22(3):683–96.

64. Lee EJ, Kwon HC, Joo HJ, et al. Diagnosis of ovarian torsion with color Doppler sonography: depiction of twisted vascular pedicle. J Ultrasound Med 1998;17:83–9.

65. Pascual MA, Hereter L, Tresserra F, et al. Transvaginal sonographic appearance of functional ovarian cysts. Hum Reprod 1997;12(6):1246–9.

66. Parks TG. Natural history of diverticular disease of the colon. Clin Gastroenterol 1975;4:53.

67. Ambrosetti P, Robert JH, Witzig JA, et al. Acute left colonic diverticulitis: a prospective analysis of 226 consecutive cases. Surgery 1994;115(5):546–50.

68. Rao PM, Rhea JT, Novelline RA, et al. Helical CT with only colonic contrast material for diagnosing diverticulitis: prospective evaluation of 150 patients. Am J Roentgenol 1998;170(6):1445–9.

69. Verbanck J, Lambrecht S, Rutgeerts L, et al. Can sonography diagnose acute colonic diverticulitis in patients with acute intestinal inflammation? A prospective study. J Clin Ultrasound 1989;17(9):661–6.

70. Little P, Turner S, Rumsby K, et al. Developing clinical rules to predict urinary tract infection in primary care settings: sensitivity and specificity of near patient tests (dipsticks) and clinical scores. Br J Gen Pract 2006;56(529):606–12.

71. Jou WW, Powers RD. Utility of dipstick urinalysis as a guide to management of adults with suspected infection or hematuria. South Med J 1998;91(3):266–9.

Systemic Causes of Abdominal Pain

J. Matthew Fields, MD[a],*, Anthony J. Dean, MD[b]

KEYWORDS

- Extra-abdominal • Systemic • Intra-abdominal • Abdomen

A variety of systemic and extra-abdominal diseases can cause symptoms within the abdominal cavity (**Box 1**). This article discusses the most important and common of these diseases. Systemic and extra-abdominal diseases may include abdominal symptoms caused by several mechanisms listed in **Table 1**. Mechanisms include direct pathologic effects on intra-abdominal organs (eg, gallstone formation in sickle cell disease); conversely, systemic illnesses (eg, congestive heart failure, diabetic ketoacidosis [DKA], or addisonian crisis) may themselves be precipitated by diseases in the abdomen. Some systemic illnesses have a direct (eg, constipation in hypercalcemia) or indirect (eg, nausea and vomiting in diabetic or alcoholic ketoacidosis [AKA]) effect on the functioning of the gastrointestinal (GI) tract. Abdominal symptoms may be caused by disease in contiguous organs outside the abdomen (eg, diaphragmatic irritation from disease of adjacent structures in the lung and mediastinum).[1–4] Finally, symptoms may be referred to the abdomen from extra-abdominal organs via neural pathways (eg, nausea and vomiting in acute coronary syndrome, glaucoma, ureterolithiasis, or testicular torsion).[5–8] Many diseases cause abdominal symptoms by a combination of these mechanisms. For example, hypercalcemia can cause abdominal symptoms as a result of intestinal dysfunction, ureterolithiasis, pancreatitis, and/or neuropathy. The range of mechanisms gives rise to a similarly wide variety of clinical findings. For example, the painful crisis of sickle cell disease or a widow spider envenomation may cause a rigid abdomen; conversely, the abdominal symptoms of a life-threatening splenic sequestration crisis may be minimal. Careful attention to the patient's history and due consideration of apparently unrelated complaints or findings on the physical examination may guide an astute clinician to consider and perform the appropriate evaluation for an underlying systemic disease.

[a] Department of Emergency Medicine, Thomas Jefferson University Hospital, 1020 Sansom Street, Thompson Building 239, Philadelphia, PA 19107, USA
[b] Division of Emergency Ultrasonography, Department of Emergency Medicine, University of Pennsylvania Medical Center, 3400 Spruce Street, Philadelphia, PA 19104, USA
* Corresponding author.
E-mail address: matthewfields@gmail.com

Emerg Med Clin N Am 29 (2011) 195–210
doi:10.1016/j.emc.2011.01.011
0733-8627/11/$ – see front matter © 2011 Published by Elsevier Inc.

Box 1
Extra-abdominal and systemic causes of abdominal pain

Thoracic

    Acute coronary syndrome

    Pneumonia

    Pulmonary embolism

    Congestive heart failure

    Pericarditis/myocarditis

Metabolic/endocrine

    Metabolic acid syndromes (diabetic ketoacidosis, alcoholic ketoacidosis)

    Uremia

    Thyrotoxicosis

    Adrenal insufficiency

    Porphyria

    C1 inhibitor deficiency

    Hypocalcemia/hypercalcemia

    Pheochromocytoma

Hematologic

    Sickle cell disease

    Ileocecal syndrome

    Acute leukemia

    Lymphoma

Inflammatory

    Familial Mediterranean fever

    Eosinophilic gastroenteritis

    Polyarteritis nodosa

    Henoch-Schönlein purpura

    Systemic lupus erythematosus

    Food allergy

    Chronic angioedema

Infectious

    Tuberculosis

    Epididymitis

    Prostatitis

    Lyme disease

    Pneumonia

    Streptococcal pharyngitis

    Pediatric infections

Toxin/environmental

    Heavy metals

Caustics/corrosives

Lactrodectus mactans (black widow spider) envenomation

Opiates/opioid withdrawal

Alcohol poisoning

Mushroom poisoning

Food allergy

Functional

Cyclic vomiting syndrome

Abdominal migraine

Irritable bowel syndrome

Neurogenic

Herpes zoster

Abdominal epilepsy

Other

Gonadal torsion

Glaucoma

Heat stroke

METABOLIC/ENDOCRINE CAUSES OF ABDOMINAL SYMPTOMS
Metabolic Acidosis Syndromes

Abdominal pain is present in nearly half of patients with DKA and its intensity is associated with worsening metabolic acidosis.[9] The mechanism of abdominal pain in DKA is poorly understood, however gastritis, gastric distension and ileus secondary to metabolic derangement have been suggested.[10] While abdominal pain in DKA is most often non-specific in up to 30% of cases pain is actually secondary to the stressor that precipitated the DKA state.[9-11] Fluid resuscitation and insulin are the mainstays of therapy of DKA, however abdominal pain that persists despite correction of acidosis warrants further investigation.[11,12] While abdominal manifestations are common in DKA they are not commonly seen in hyperosmolar hyperglycemic syndromes.[12]

Alcoholic ketoacidosis also commonly presents with abdominal pain and similarly to DKA gastrointestinal symptoms may be multifactorial in etiology. There is a direct gastritis effect by alcohol and a secondary effect induced by ketoacidosis on gastric functioning leading to nausea, vomiting, and abdominal pain.[13]

Adrenal Insufficiency

Adrenal insufficiency occurs when adrenal gland function is reduced by lack of adrenocorticotropic hormone (ACTH), chronic steroid use, or primary adrenal disease and, as a result, glucocorticoid production is unable to meet physiologic demands. Adrenal (addisonian) crisis generally occurs in patients with underlying adrenal insufficiency in the setting of a physiologic stressor or medical noncompliance; however, it may also occur in normal patients in the settings of blunt trauma, sepsis, meningococcemia, emboli, and other critical illnesses.[14] Symptoms can be acute or insidious at onset but may include weakness, fatigue, prostration, confusion, vomiting, diarrhea, fever,

Table 1
Mechanisms of abdominal symptoms in extra-abdominal and systemic diseases (some diseases cause abdominal symptoms by several mechanisms)

Mechanism	Examples
Systemic disease causes pathologic condition in intra-abdominal organs	Heavy metal toxicity, tuberculosis, CHF, spider envenomation, alcoholic ketoacidosis, sickle cell infarction and biliary disease, neutropenia, hypercalcemia (pancreatitis, ileus, gastritis), C1 inhibitor deficiency, SLE (lupus enteritis)
Systemic disease is precipitated by pathologic condition in intra-abdominal organs	Abdominal disease precipitating DKA, addisonian crisis
Systemic disease causes nausea, vomiting, or other gastrointestinal symptoms	Hypercalcemia and hypocalcemia, sickle cell painful crisis, SLE
Extra-abdominal disease causes abdominal symptoms by neural mechanisms or with functional or poorly understood organic basis	DKA, glaucoma, thyrotoxicosis, porphyria, hypercalcemia (neuropathy, hypomotility), hypocalcemia, adrenal crisis, gonadal torsion, pheochromocytoma
Disease of extra-abdominal organs causes perception of pain in the abdomen because of irritation of contiguous extra-abdominal structures	Lower lobe pneumonia, pulmonary emboli, pleuritis, inferior wall cardiac ischemia, pyelonephritis, spinal and other musculoskeletal diseases, testicular torsion
Abdominal pain due to referred pain from extra-abdominal structures	ACS and other diseases of mediastinal structures, ureterolithiasis, pyelonephritis

Abbreviations: ACS, acute coronary syndrome; CHF, congestive heart failure; DKA, diabetic ketoacidosis; SLE, systemic lupus erethematosus.

hypotension, tachycardia, shock, and abdominal pain.[14] Any of these symptoms in a patient who has been taking steroids for more than a week should prompt consideration of addisonian crisis. The abdominal pain may be severe, causing suspicion of an intra-abdominal catastrophe.[15,16] The basis of the abdominal pain is unknown, although there is evidence to suggest that gastric dysmotility and serositis occur.[17,18] Hypoglycemia (with concomitant mineralocorticoid deficiency), hyponatremia, and hyperkalemia may occur in acute crisis but are more common in chronic deficiency. Recommended treatment is intravenous dexamethasone. Hydrocortisone may also be used but has the drawback of interfering with ACTH stimulation testing.[19]

Thyrotoxicosis

Although abdominal complaints receive scant attention in most texts, they are fairly common in thyrotoxicosis and include nausea, vomiting, loose frequent stools, and weight loss. Perhaps they are overlooked because of the protean and more life-threatening derangements of this disease.[20] In 1 retrospective series, GI symptoms occurred in 36% of cases.[21] Although most patients with abdominal pain and thyrotoxicosis have no demonstrable intra-abdominal pathologic condition, in 1 case series, 16% had an intra-abdominal cause requiring surgery, serving as a reminder that the search for serious medical conditions that have precipitated thyroid storm should not be overlooked.[22]

Porphyria

Acute intermittent porphyria is a rare autosomal dominant condition that presents most commonly with abdominal pain.[23] With variations in penetrance and expressivity, the gene is symptomatic in 1 to 2 persons per 100,000.[24] The mutation leads to a deficiency of porphobilinogen deaminase, a hepatic enzyme involved in heme synthesis. δ-Aminolevulinic acid and porphobilinogen accumulate in tissues, leading to a neuroviseral crisis that results in acute abdominal pain. Attacks can be precipitated by stimulation of the cytochrome P450 system with medications (eg, rifampin, barbiturates, and sulfonamides), estrogens or progesterones, smoking, or alcohol. Attacks may also occur when heme oxygenase is induced by physiologic stressors such as fever, fasting, or infection.[23,24] Pain is thought to be caused by visceral autonomic neuropathy leading to regions of overactive and underactive bowel. Pain may be persistent or colicky and is usually located in the lower part of the abdomen but may also occur in the back or lower limbs.[25] Other symptoms include fever, vomiting, constipation, weakness, muscle cramps, paresthesias, seizures, and neuropsychiatric complaints, including anxiety and depression. Dysautonomias can cause extra-abdominal symptoms with diaphoresis, flushing, tachycardia, and hypertension or hypotension. Seizures are generally because of hyponatremia, which may be secondary to vomiting or to the syndrome of inappropriate antidiuretic hormone hypersecretion. Neuropathy may be rapid and severe, leading to life-threatening respiratory involvement. The abdomen is usually soft, with only mild tenderness. Diagnosis is made by detecting elevated urinary porphobilinogen levels. Short-term management involves pain control, resuscitation, and evaluation for potentially life-threatening complications such as respiratory compromise from phrenic neuropathy or hyponatremia.[26]

C1 Inhibitor Deficiency

C1 inhibitor (C1INH) deficiency may be hereditary or acquired and results in angioedema involving the skin, GI tract, or upper airway. Excess active C1 leads to excessive complement activation and overproduction of bradykinin, resulting in submucosal and subcutaneous vascular permeability.[27] Approximately 25% of patients with C1INH deficiency have predominantly abdominal symptoms.[28] Submucosal edema in the stomach and small bowel leads to episodes of nausea, vomiting, and cramping abdominal pain. Abdominal examination may reveal marked tenderness, guarding, or rigidity, leading to the consideration of intra-abdominal surgical emergencies. Acute attacks may occur without any apparent cause but are more often precipitated by minor trauma (especially dental procedures), menstruation, stress, or use of angiotensin-converting enzyme inhibitors. The diagnosis may be suggested by a history of chronic abdominal complaints with episodic exacerbation. Abdominal symptoms generally precede cutaneous or upper airway symptoms.[29,30] Laryngeal edema, when present, is life threatening. Until recently, management involved airway control and standard supportive care.[31] In October 2009, C1 esterase inhibitor replacement protein was approved by the Food and Drug Administration. Early trials have shown significant improvement of symptoms in acute attacks.[32]

Hypercalcemia

Hypercalcemia is most commonly caused by hyperparathyroidism and malignancy.[33] Elevated calcium levels affect nerve conduction, cardiac rhythm, function of cardiac and skeletal muscles, renal function, and GI motility. Patients may present with isolated abdominal pain that may be multifactorial in etiology.[34] Ileus formation leads to abdominal pain, nausea, and vomiting. Elevated levels of gastrin and lower stomach pH predispose patients to gastritis and peptic ulcer formation. Increased secretion of pancreatic enzymes may lead to acute pancreatitis. In the kidneys, in addition to tubular dysfunction that results in fluid and electrolyte losses, calcium deposition may lead to kidney stone formation and ureterolithiasis.[33] The diagnosis should be considered in patients with diffuse abdominal pain accompanied by weakness, lethargy, and dehydration.

HEMATOLOGIC CAUSES OF ABDOMINAL SYMPTOMS
Sickle Cell Disease

Sickle cell disease is an autosomal recessive hemoglobinopathy characterized by production of hemoglobin S, which causes erythrocyte sickling, leading to chronic hemolytic anemia and recurrent vascular occlusion. Vascular occlusion can cause ischemia or infarction in almost any organ. In the abdomen, this may cause pain by a variety of mechanisms including local ischemia, microinfarction, macroinfarction (eg, of the spleen), cholelithiasis, cholecystitis, pancreatitis, splenic sequestration, hepatic crisis, and intrahepatic cholestasis.[35] Even in the absence of a surgical cause, ischemia and microinfarction can result in an examination that strongly suggests an acute surgical abdomen with peritoneal signs and leukocytosis. The clinician is guided by the patient's description of previous episodes of painful crisis, but in uncertain cases, the increasing availability of bedside ultrasonography and abdominal computed tomography (CT) have made appropriate diagnosis of these patients' condition easier. Crises can be triggered by many factors including infection, dehydration, cold, stress, menses, alcohol consumption, and hypoxemia; however, most of the time, there is no identifiable cause.

Neutropenia

Abdominal pain in patients with neutropenia may be caused by a spectrum of disorders of the ileocecal region that ranges in severity from mild mucosal inflammation to bacterial and fungal invasion of the bowel, leading to transmural ulceration and/ or necrotizing colitis with high mortality rates. The disorder has been variously named neutropenic enterocolitis (NE), typhlitis, and ileocecal syndrome. It is usually seen in patients receiving chemotherapy but occasionally occurs in patients with aplastic anemia, cyclic neutropenia, and AIDS.[36] Presentation is most likely 10 to 14 days after chemotherapy, coincident with the neutrophil nadir. The ileum, cecum, ascending colon, and appendix are the most common sites; however, any portion of the bowel may be affected. Abdominal symptoms in these patients may be masked due to immunosuppression, which inhibits elaboration of the inflammatory mediators that are the primary stimulators of intra-abdominal nociceptors; although focal right lower quadrant pain, abdominal distension, diarrhea, or rebound tenderness may be present.[37] Neutropenia with fever, abdominal pain, and diarrhea should prompt suspicion. *Clostridium difficile* enterocolitis, appendicitis, and diverticulitis are also diagnostic considerations in these patients. CT scan is the preferred diagnostic modality and reveals bowel wall thickening often involving the terminal ileum.[38] *C difficile* colitis is not usually limited to the cecum and rarely involves the ileum in contrast to NE. Ultrasonography has been shown to be useful in the diagnosis and management of critically ill patients in whom CT cannot be obtained. Ultrasonography reveals the affected bowel as a mass with a hyperechoic core and thick hypoechoic walls. In the setting of the abovementioned symptoms, a bowel wall thickness of 4 mm is considered diagnostic and increasing thickness correlates with disease severity.[39] Historically, surgery (right hemicolectomy) was the mainstay of treatment. More recent case series support medical management, including therapy with broad spectrum and antifungal antibiotics, and supportive care. Surgery may still be necessary in some patients, and early consultation is often warranted.[40]

INFLAMMATORY CAUSES OF ABDOMINAL SYMPTOMS
Familial Mediterranean Fever

Familial Mediterranean fever (FMF) is an autosomal recessive disorder characterized by recurrent episodes of fever and serositis resulting in abdominal, chest, joint, or muscular pain. This condition is primarily diagnosed in people of Sephardic Jewish, Arabic, Turkish, Armenian, Egyptian, and Lebanese descents. Because of the involvement of the extensive peritoneal serosa, abdominal pain in FMF causes peritonitis and findings of an acute abdomen. About 95% of patients report abdominal pain as the main symptom of their attacks, and 50% report abdominal pain as their first symptom of disease.[41] Onset is sudden, occurring over 1 to 2 hours, with fever and abdominal pain that may be diffuse or localized. The pain is often worse with movement, and examination reveals distension, rigidity, rebound, and guarding.[42] Laboratory abnormalities include a leukocytosis with left shift and elevated sedimentation rate and C-reactive protein levels. Abdominal radiography may show dilated loops of small bowel and air fluid levels. The most common findings on CT of patients with acute FMF are engorged mesenteric vessels and thickened mesenteric folds. A minority of patients may demonstrate mesenteric and/or retroperitoneal lymphadenopathy, ascites, splenomegaly, and dilated small bowel loops.[43] Less-severe (incomplete) attacks may occur without fever or peritonitis. Symptoms begin to improve within 12 to 24 hours, and complete resolution generally occurs at 96 hours. Colchicine prophylaxis to prevent attacks is the mainstay of therapy; however, it is not effective in an acute attack. Diclofenac has been shown to be effective in addition to standard pain medication regimens.[41] Colchicine has a low therapeutic index, so that in patients on this drug presenting with abdominal pain and diarrhea, the clinician should consider the possibility of colchicine toxicity.

Eosinophilic Gastroenteritis

Eosinophilic gastroenteritis (EG) is a disorder characterized by eosinophilic infiltration of any portion of the GI tract from the esophagus to rectum. The syndrome often presents with abdominal pain. A history of atopy and allergies is present in about 50% of cases. Mucosal EG is the most common subtype and may present with abdominal pain, vomiting, diarrhea, GI bleeding, anemia, or a protein-losing enteropathy.[44,45] Rarely, EG presents with signs of peritoneal inflammation.[46] Eosinophilia may be present but is not necessary for diagnosis. Management includes allergy testing, changes in diet, steroids, mast cell inhibitors, antihistamines, and leukotriene antagonists.[45]

Polyarteritis Nodosa

Polyarteritis nodosa (PAN) is a rare form of systemic vasculitis affecting small- and medium-sized arteries. PAN occurs most commonly in patients aged 40 to 60 years, and 30% to 60% of the cases are associated with hepatitis B, hepatitis C, or human immunodeficiency virus infection.[47,48] Most patients present with subacute symptoms over weeks to months, most commonly with fever, neuropathy, hypertension, weight loss, malaise, and asymmetric arthritis.[49] Approximately half of the patients present with GI symptoms including nausea, vomiting, abdominal pain, and diarrhea. Vasculitis may cause infarction of the GI tract leading to GI bleeding or perforation. Vasculitic cholecystitis, appendicitis, pancreatitis, or even rupture of splenic, hepatic, or renal arteries may occur in severe cases.[50]

Henoch-Schönlein Purpura

Henoch-Schönlein purpura (HSP) is a small-vessel vasculitis caused by deposition of IgA, affecting skin, joints, kidney, and bowel. It is most common in the pediatric age group but may occur in adults. Findings in HSP include palpable purpura, arthralgias, glomerulonephritis, hematuria, and GI symptoms of colicky abdominal pain, nausea, and vomiting.[51] In 1 study, 17% of patients presented with abdominal pain as their only symptom.[52] The most frequent GI complication of HSP is intussusception occurring in approximately 3% to 4% of cases.[53] Other more rare GI complications include bowel ischemia and infarction, fistula formation, ileal stricture, gallbladder hydrops, pancreatitis, and pseudomembranous colitis. Treatment is supportive with detection and treatment of potential complications. Retrospective studies suggest that steroids may decrease the duration of symptoms and complications; however, this has not been demonstrated prospectively.[54]

Systemic Lupus Erythematosus

Systemic lupus erythematosus (SLE) is an autoimmune disorder that in 90% of cases affects women. The disorder can cause nonspecific symptoms of nausea, vomiting and diarrhea, pancreatitis and hepatitis, as well as disease in every part of the GI tract from the mouth to anus. Despite the known pathologic effects, there is no agreement about the prevalence of GI disease in SLE because it is often impossible to determine whether GI pathology is a side effect of medications or the result of intercurrent diseases such as renal failure. Reports of the incidence of GI disease in SLE range widely from 1% to 50%.[55,56] The commonest site of involvement is the oral cavity, where it causes ulcerations, decreased salivation, and a variety of other mucosal lesions.[55] In 1 retrospective review of patients admitted for SLE, 22% presented with abdominal pain, half of who were found to have intestinal vasculitis (referred to as lupus enteritis).[57] In most cases, this condition responds well to supportive care and immunosuppressive therapy, although occasionally, it can progress to infarction. The presence of antiphospholipid antibody increases the risk of thrombosis. In a series of patients with SLE with an acute abdomen, nonvascular causes (mainly cholecystitis, appendicitis, and abscesses) were as frequent as vascular causes. Nearly all patients in this study required surgery either because of a nonvascular source or because of ischemic complications of vasculitis.[58] Medical treatment of lupus flares includes high-dose steroids, increasing the risk of intestinal perforation in the setting of vasculitic ischemia. Abdominal pain in patients with SLE should be approached cautiously with a low threshold to perform abdominal imaging and to obtain surgical consultation.

Food Allergy

Symptoms of food-induced allergy most frequently involve the skin, GI tract, and respiratory system. Urticaria, flushing, angioedema, vomiting, abdominal pain, diarrhea, rhinitis, wheezing, and stridor may be present together or in isolation.[59] Symptoms usually occur soon after ingestion so that identification of the offending allergen is apparent whether or not symptoms are primarily gastrointestinal. Many patients have a history of atopy. Treatments include administration of antihistamines, epinephrine, inhaled β-agonists, and systemic corticosteroids. Referral to an allergist is warranted with avoidance of suspected agents until allergy testing has been undertaken.

INFECTIOUS CAUSES OF ABDOMINAL SYMPTOMS
Tuberculosis

Tuberculosis (TB), caused by *Mycobacterium tuberculosis*, persists as an important diagnostic consideration even in well-developed countries. Extrapulmonary TB may involve the peritoneum in up to 4% of cases, and clinical presentation can vary from insidious onset with fever, weight loss, anorexia, night sweats, and malaise to acute focal abdominal pain.[60,61] Miliary TB less commonly presents with abdominal pain;

however, peritoneal, hepatic, pancreatic, or splenic seeding does occur and may be a focus of pain.[62,63]

Pediatric Infections

Abdominal pain is a frequent manifestation in common pediatric extra-abdominal infections. In a study of more than 1100 children presenting with acute abdominal pain, 59% were diagnosed with extra-abdominal problems including upper respiratory tract infection and/or otitis (18.6%), pharyngitis (16.6%), viral syndrome (16.0%), and acute febrile illness (7.8%). Less than 1% of the group had surgical disease.[64] In regard to pharyngitis, abdominal pain is seen similarly in both streptococcal and non-streptococcal disease.[65]

TOXIN-RELATED OR DRUG-RELATED CAUSES OF ABDOMINAL SYMPTOMS

Toxins and environmental exposures can lead to abdominal pain by a variety of mechanisms including direct corrosive effects (aspirin, iron, mercury, acids, and alkalis), ileus formation (anticholinergics, narcotics), mechanical obstruction (bezoars), systemic effect (black widow spider bite, opioid withdrawal), bowel ischemia secondary to vasoconstriction (amphetamines, ergotamines, cocaine), or damage to intra-abdominal organs (acetaminophen).

Heavy Metals

Acute exposure to heavy metals such as iron, lead, arsenic, cadmium, and thallium may cause abdominal pain and GI symptoms. Anemia may be a clue to chronic heavy metal exposure but is nonspecific. Although abdominal symptoms may be present in chronic toxicity, other systems are more commonly involved. Iron toxicity occurs mainly because of unintentional ingestion in the pediatric population.[60–63,66] Toxicity occurs in 5 phases. Phase 1 begins with acute vomiting due to corrosive effects followed by diarrhea that may be bloody. In phase 2, the acute symptoms resolve after 1 to 2 days. This resolution is followed by phase 3 in which GI symptoms recur with lethargy, anion gap metabolic acidosis, leukocytosis, coagulopathy, renal failure, and arrhythmias. In severe cases, disease may progress to cardiovascular collapse and death. Phase 4, consisting of fulminant hepatic failure, is relatively rare, but when it occurs, it is usually fatal. Phase 5 describes the chronic pyloric or small bowel scarring that may lead to future mechanical obstructions.[67] Emergency management includes supportive care. Deferoxamine should be used in patients with a history or clinical signs of significant exposure.

Lead poisoning is decreasing in incidence because of restrictions on the use of lead in paints and gasoline as well as closer surveillance in work environments.[68] Still, sources of lead exposure persist and include bullets, fishing weights, and contaminated soil or water. Occupational risk is present in industries such as lead smelting, battery manufacturing, radiator repairing, bridge or ship construction or demolition, soldering, or welding.[69,70] Acute lead exposure can lead to crampy abdominal pain, nausea, vomiting, constipation, or diarrhea and has been termed lead colic. Other symptoms include headaches, fatigue, anemia, and peripheral neuropathy. In severe cases, there can be end-organ dysfunction, including renal and hepatic failure, convulsions, and coma.

Arsenic may induce varying degrees of systemic toxicity. Exposures occur at home, in occupational settings, particularly those using and manufacturing arsenic-containing pesticides, and in areas containing high levels of arsenic in rock, which contaminates soil or water. Toxicity may also ensue by exposure to semiconductors, smelting, power plants burning coal, industries involved in glass and microcircuit production, fungicides, insecticides, paint, and tanning agents.[71] Arsenic binds to sulfhydryl groups, inhibiting glycolysis and disrupting oxidative phosphorylation. Acute poisoning is more common in cases of ingestion or inhalation of arsenic fumes in workers. Initial symptoms include nausea, vomiting, abdominal pain, and diarrhea. Patients often complain of a metallic or garlic taste. Massive hemolysis ensues, and severe cases result in encephalopathy, seizures, coma, cardiac arrhythmias, and death. In chronic poisoning, peripheral nerve and skin manifestations are more common than GI disturbances. Emergency department (ED) management includes decontamination of skin, consideration of charcoal and/or nasogastric suctioning in patients who present within 1 hour of ingestion, administration of fluids, monitoring, and chelation therapy with dimercaprol in symptomatic patients.[72]

Caustics

A common pathway for many toxins is initial vomiting and abdominal pain by corrosive properties. Aspirin impairs the gastric mucosal barrier, leading to abdominal pain, vomiting, and hematemesis. Acids and alkalis are known for causing liquefaction and corrosive necrosis, respectively. This process leads to oropharyngeal and esophageal burns, resulting in drooling, stridor, nausea, vomiting, hematemesis, chest pain, odynophagia, dysphagia, abdominal pain, and esophageal or gastric perforation.

Lactrodectus mactans (Black Widow Spider) Envenomation

Spiders of the genus Lactrodectus are found throughout the United States (except Alaska) and are the leading cause of death from arachnid envenomation. The venom acts at the presynapse of the neuromuscular junction, causing release of multiple neurotransmitters and overstimulation of motor end plates. This overstimulation results in pain and cramping of large muscle groups, weakness, hypertension, priapism, and rarely, death. Generalized abdominal or back pain is the most frequent presenting complaint in patients seeking medical attention. The abdomen may be rigid and mimic an acute abdomen.[73] Management includes monitoring, fluid administration, and pain control with opioids. The use of antivenin, which is derived from horse serum, is reserved for severe cases and must be weighed against the risk of potential allergic complications.[74]

Opiates

A known side effect of opiates is the slowing of GI motility and formation of ileus, leading to abdominal pain in many patients. Conversely, in patients who use opioids for long-term, cessation of intake leads to opioid withdrawal, which often presents with nausea, vomiting, abdominal pain, and diarrhea. Symptoms may begin within 6 to 12 hours after the last dose of a short-acting opioid and 24 to 48 hours after cessation of methadone.[75] Physical examination reveals a patient who is often agitated, in acute discomfort, with myalgias, mydriasis, yawning, hyperactive bowel sounds, and piloerection. Vomiting and diarrhea may be severe enough to cause dehydration, tachycardia, and hypotension. Methadone or other narcotics as well as clonidine or benzodiazepines may be used to control symptoms.[76]

FUNCTIONAL CAUSES OF ABDOMINAL SYMPTOMS
Cyclic Vomiting Syndrome

Cyclic vomiting syndrome is characterized by recurrent discrete episodes of vomiting. It occurs in both children and adults. Attacks are severe, generally requiring intravenous hydration and causing patients to miss work or school.[77] Episodes may be stereotypical with identified triggers and are often self-limited. Patients with frequent episodes (>1/month) may require prophylactic therapy including propranolol, cyproheptadine, amitriptyline, phenobarbital, or valproic acid.[78] When attacks occur, parental medications including, ondansetron and ketorolac, are recommended.[79] A change from the patient's wonted symptoms should prompt the clinician to consider other causes.

Abdominal Migraine

Abdominal migraine is similar to cyclic vomiting syndrome, except that the primary complaint is abdominal pain. This term was coined in 1956 by Farquhar, who presumed that these episodes of abdominal pain represented a migraine variant as the source of symptoms.[80] Although this presumption has not been proven, there is an association between migraines, abdominal migraines, and cyclic vomiting syndrome.[81,82]

Irritable Bowel Syndrome

Although primarily a GI disease, irritable bowel syndrome merits mention because of its association with psychological disorders, poor socioeconomic status during childhood, and GI tract infections. Its pathogenesis seems to involve GI motor and sensory dysfunction. Patients often report that specific foods aggravate symptoms.[83] There may be a genetic predisposition in some patients.[83,84] Most patients have had many similar episodes in the past. ED management is directed at ruling out other intra-abdominal diseases. Treatment is supportive.

NEUROGENIC CAUSES OF ABDOMINAL SYMPTOMS
Herpes Zoster

Herpes zoster may involve an abdominal dermatome causing severe pain. Pain often precedes the rash; however, a close physical examination may reveal erythema, small papules, or early vesicles. Pain is often hyperesthetic to light palpation. Rarely, visceral varicella zoster infection occurs, usually in immunocompromised patients in who rash may or may not be present.[85] This entity represents disseminated infection and is life threatening. In immunocompetent patients with localized zoster, oral antiviral therapy with acyclovir or famciclovir has been shown to reduce duration of symptoms and incidence of postherpetic neuralgia if started early (<3 days from onset) in the disease process.[86,87] In disseminated disease, parenteral antiviral therapy and admission are required.

Abdominal Epilepsy

Abdominal epilepsy is an exceedingly rare condition in which seizures manifest as GI symptoms, including vomiting and abdominal pain. The criteria for diagnosis include recurrent paroxysmal GI complaints and findings on electroencephalography suggestinga seizure.[88] Central nervous system involvement with changes in mental status and convulsions may occur but is not always present, and abdominal pain episodes generally improve with anticonvulsant therapy.

SUMMARY

Abdominal pain is a symptom of many extra-abdominal diseases not infrequently seen in patients in the ED. The prudent clinician will consider extra-abdominal causes when patients presenting with abdominal complaints do not have a clear-cut intra-abdominal cause or in patients with repeat visits despite a supposed diagnosis. Familiarity with mechanisms of nociception and systemic diseases that cause abdominal symptoms will facilitate the consideration of alternative causes. In such situations, a careful history including a thorough review of systems combined with careful physical examination will often prompt laboratory tests and/or imaging that leads to an accurate diagnosis.

REFERENCES

1. Potts DE, Sahn SA. Abdominal manifestations of pulmonary embolism. JAMA 1976;235(26):2835–7.
2. Sethuraman U, Siadat M, Lepak-Hitch CA, et al. Pulmonary embolism presenting as acute abdomen in a child and adult. Am J Emerg Med 2009;27(4):514.e1–5.
3. Unluer EE, Denizbasi A. A pulmonary embolism case presenting with upper abdominal and flank pain. Eur J Emerg Med 2003;10(2):135–8.
4. Smith DC. Pulmonary embolism presenting as an acute surgical abdomen. J Emerg Med 1996;14(6):715–7.
5. Constant J. The clinical diagnosis of nonanginal chest pain: the differentiation of angina from nonanginal chest pain by history. Clin Cardiol 1983;6(1):11–6.
6. Gupta M, Tabas JA, Kohn MA. Presenting complaint among patients with myocardial infarction who present to an urban, public hospital emergency department. Ann Emerg Med 2002;40(2):180–6.
7. Watson NJ, Kirkby GR. Acute glaucoma presenting with abdominal symptoms. BMJ 1989;299(6693):254.
8. McCollough M, Sharieff GQ. Abdominal surgical emergencies in infants and young children. Emerg Med Clin North Am 2003;21(4):909–35.
9. Umpierrez G, Freire AX. Abdominal pain in patients with hyperglycemic crises. J Crit Care 2002;17(1):63–7.
10. Kitabchi AE, Umpierrez GE, Miles JM, et al. Hyperglycemic crises in adult patients with diabetes. Diabetes Care 2009;32(7):1335–43.
11. Campbel IW, Duncan LJ, Innes JA, et al. Abdominal pain in diabetic metabolic decompensation: clinical significance. JAMA 1975;233(2):166–8.
12. Kitabchi AE, Umpierrez GE, Fisher JN, et al. Thirty years of personal experience in hyperglycemic crises: diabetic ketoacidosis and hyperglycemic hyperosmolar state. J Clin Endocrinol Metab 2008;93(5):1541–52.
13. McGuire LC, Cruickshank AM, Munro PT. Alcoholic ketoacidosis. Emerg Med J 2006;23(6):417–20.
14. Burke CW. Adrenocortical insufficiency. Clin Endocrinol Metab 1985;14(4):947–76.
15. Laws SA, Cook PR, Rees M. Adrenal insufficiency masquerading as an acute abdomen. Hosp Med 2001;62(2):118–9.
16. Balasubramanian SS, Bose D. Adrenal crisis presenting as an acute abdomen. Anaesthesia 2006;61(4):413–4.
17. Tobin MV, Aldridge SA, Morris AI, et al. Gastrointestinal manifestations of Addison's disease. Am J Gastroenterol 1989;84(10):1302–5.
18. Valenzuela GA, Smalley WE, Schain DC, et al. Reversibility of gastric dysmotility in cortisol deficiency. Am J Gastroenterol 1987;82(10):1066–8.
19. Taylor RL, Grebe SK, Singh RJ. Quantitative, highly sensitive liquid chromatography-tandem mass spectrometry method for detection of synthetic corticosteroids. Clin Chem 2004;50(12):2345–52.
20. Gharahbaghian L, Brosnan DP, Fox JC, et al. New onset thyrotoxicosis presenting as vomiting, abdominal pain and transaminitis in the emergency department. West J Emerg Med 2007;8(3):97–100.
21. Harper MB. Vomiting, nausea, and abdominal pain: unrecognized symptoms of thyrotoxicosis. J Fam Pract 1989;29(4):382–6.
22. Leow MK, Chew DE, Zhu M, et al. Thyrotoxicosis and acute abdomen–still as defying and misunderstood today? Brief observations over the recent decade. QJM 2008;101(12):943–7.

23. Puy H, Deybach JC, Lamoril J, et al. Molecular epidemiology and diagnosis of PBG deaminase gene defects in acute intermittent porphyria. Am J Hum Genet 1997;60(6):1373–83.

24. Herrick AL, McColl KE. Acute intermittent porphyria. Best Pract Res Clin Gastroenterol 2005;19(2):235–49.

25. Ventura P, Cappellini MD, Rocchi E. The acute porphyrias: a diagnostic and therapeutic challenge in internal and emergency medicine. Intern Emerg Med 2009; 4(4):297–308.

26. Badminton MN, Elder GH. Management of acute and cutaneous porphyrias. Int J Clin Pract 2002;56(4):272–8.

27. Bork K, Staubach P, Eckardt AJ, et al. Symptoms, course, and complications of abdominal attacks in hereditary angioedema due to C1 inhibitor deficiency. Am J Gastroenterol 2006;101(3):619–27.

28. Gompels MM, Lock RJ, Abinun M, et al. C1 inhibitor deficiency: consensus document. Clin Exp Immunol 2005;139(3):379–94.

29. Baraza W, Garner JP, Amin SN. Hereditary angioedema-a forgotten cause of the 'medical' acute abdomen. Int J Colorectal Dis 2007;22(11):1415–6.

30. Hong SB, Kim CW, Kim JH, et al. A case of angioedema due to acquired c1 esterase inhibitor deficiency masquerading as suspected peritonitis: a case report. J Emerg Med 2008. [Epub ahead of print].

31. Bowen T, Hebert J, Ritchie B, et al. Management of hereditary angioedema: a Canadian approach. Transfus Apher Sci 2003;29(3):205–14.

32. Waytes AT, Rosen FS, Frank MM. Treatment of hereditary angioedema with a vapor-heated C1 inhibitor concentrate. N Engl J Med 1996;334(25):1630–4.

33. Carroll MF, Schade DS. A practical approach to hypercalcemia. Am Fam Physician 2003;67(9):1959–66.

34. Hsu HC, Chi CH, Tsai MC, et al. An unusual cause of abdominal pain: thiazide-related hypercalcemia in a patient with veiled hyperparathyroidism and thyroid papillary carcinoma. J Emerg Med 2008;34(2):151–3.

35. Ahmed S, Shahid RK, Russo LA. Unusual causes of abdominal pain: sickle cell anemia. Best Pract Res Clin Gastroenterol 2005;19(2):297–310.

36. Bremer CT, Monahan BP. Necrotizing enterocolitis in neutropenia and chemotherapy: a clinical update and old lessons relearned. Curr Gastroenterol Rep 2006;8(4):333–41.

37. Cloutier RL. Neutropenic enterocolitis. Emerg Med Clin North Am 2009;27(3): 415–22.

38. Kirkpatrick ID, Greenberg HM. Gastrointestinal complications in the neutropenic patient: characterization and differentiation with abdominal CT. Radiology 2003; 226(3):668–74.

39. Cartoni C, Dragoni F, Micozzi A, et al. Neutropenic enterocolitis in patients with acute leukemia: prognostic significance of bowel wall thickening detected by ultrasonography. J Clin Oncol 2001;19(3):756–61.

40. Song HK, Kreisel D, Canter R, et al. Changing presentation and management of neutropenic enterocolitis. Arch Surg 1998;133(9):979–82.

41. Simon A, van der Meer JW, Drenth JP. Familial Mediterranean fever-a not so unusual cause of abdominal pain. Best Pract Res Clin Gastroenterol 2005; 19(2):199–213.

42. Drenth JP, van der Meer JW. Hereditary periodic fever. N Engl J Med 2001; 345(24):1748–57.

43. Zissin R, Rathaus V, Gayer G, et al. CT findings in patients with familial Mediterranean fever during an acute abdominal attack. Br J Radiol 2003;76(901):22–5.

44. Chehade M, Sampson HA. Epidemiology and etiology of eosinophilic esophagitis. Gastrointest Endosc Clin N Am 2008;18(1):33–44, viii.
45. Khan S. Eosinophilic gastroenteritis. Best Pract Res Clin Gastroenterol 2005; 19(2):177–98.
46. Sandrasegaran K, Rajesh A, Maglinte DD. Eosinophilic gastroenteritis presenting as acute abdomen. Emerg Radiol 2006;13(3):151–4.
47. Mahr A, Guillevin L, Poissonnet M, et al. Prevalences of polyarteritis nodosa, microscopic polyangiitis, Wegener's granulomatosis, and Churg-Strauss syndrome in a French urban multiethnic population in 2000: a capture-recapture estimate. Arthritis Rheum 2004;51(1):92–9.
48. Mohammad AJ, Jacobsson LT, Mahr AD, et al. Prevalence of Wegener's granulomatosis, microscopic polyangiitis, polyarteritis nodosa and Churg-Strauss syndrome within a defined population in southern Sweden. Rheumatology (Oxford) 2007;46(8):1329–37.
49. Stone JH. Polyarteritis nodosa. JAMA 2002;288(13):1632–9.
50. Levine SM, Hellmann DB, Stone JH. Gastrointestinal involvement in polyarteritis nodosa (1986–2000): presentation and outcomes in 24 patients. Am J Med 2002;112(5):386–91.
51. Chang WL, Yang YH, Lin YT, et al. Gastrointestinal manifestations in Henoch-Schonlein purpura: a review of 261 patients. Acta Paediatr 2004;93(11): 1427–31.
52. Calvino MC, Llorca J, Garcia-Porrua C, et al. Henoch-Schonlein purpura in children from northwestern Spain: a 20-year epidemiologic and clinical study. Medicine (Baltimore) 2001;80(5):279–90.
53. Trapani S, Micheli A, Grisolia F, et al. Henoch Schonlein purpura in childhood: epidemiological and clinical analysis of 150 cases over a 5-year period and review of literature. Semin Arthritis Rheum 2005;35(3):143–53.
54. Weiss PF, Feinstein JA, Luan X, et al. Effects of corticosteroid on Henoch-Schonlein purpura: a systematic review. Pediatrics 2007;120(5):1079–87.
55. Sultan SM, Ioannou Y, Isenberg DA. A review of gastrointestinal manifestations of systemic lupus erythematosus. Rheumatology 1999;38(10):917–32.
56. Hallegua DS, Wallace DJ. Gastrointestinal manifestations of systemic lupus erythematosus. Curr Opin Rheumatol 2000;12(5):379–85.
57. Lee CK, Ahn MS, Lee EY, et al. Acute abdominal pain in systemic lupus erythematosus: focus on lupus enteritis (gastrointestinal vasculitis). Ann Rheum Dis 2002;61(6):547–50.
58. Medina F, Ayala A, Jara LJ, et al. Acute abdomen in systemic lupus erythematosus: the importance of early laparotomy. Am J Med 1997;103(2):100–5.
59. Lack G. Clinical practice. Food allergy. N Engl J Med 2008;359(12):1252–60.
60. Figueiredo AA, Lucon AM, Ikejiri DS, et al. Urogenital tuberculosis in a patient with AIDS: an unusual presentation. Nat Clin Pract Urol 2008; 5(8):455–60.
61. Pandey A, Kumar V, Gangopadhyay AN, et al. Chronic bilious vomiting in children in developing countries due to high bowel obstruction: not always malrotation or tuberculosis. Pediatr Surg Int 2010;26(2):213–7.
62. de Benedictis FM, Nobile S, Lorenzini I. Electronic clinical challenges and images in GI. Abdominal tuberculosis. Gastroenterology 2008;134(3):e3–5.
63. Sikalias N, Alexiou K, Mountzalia L, et al. Acute abdomen in a transplant patient with tuberculous colitis: a case report. Cases J 2009;2:9305.
64. Scholer SJ, Pituch K, Orr DP, et al. Clinical outcomes of children with acute abdominal pain. Pediatrics 1996;98(4 Pt 1):680–5.

65. Kreher NE, Hickner JM, Barry HC, et al. Do gastrointestinal symptoms accompanying sore throat predict streptococcal pharyngitis? An UPRNet study. Upper Peninsula Research Network. J Fam Pract 1998;46(2):159–64.

66. Lai MW, Klein-Schwartz W, Rodgers GC, et al. 2005 Annual Report of the American Association of Poison Control Centers' national poisoning and exposure database. Clin Toxicol (Phila) 2006;44(6–7):803–932.

67. Mills KC, Curry SC. Acute iron poisoning. Emerg Med Clin North Am 1994;12(2): 397–413.

68. Centers for Disease Control and Prevention (CDC). Adult blood lead epidemiology and surveillance–United States, 2005–2007. MMWR Morb Mortal Wkly Rep 2009;58(14):365–9.

69. Centers for Disease Control and Prevention (CDC). Blood lead levels in residents of homes with elevated lead in tap water–District of Columbia, 2004. MMWR Morb Mortal Wkly Rep 2004;53(12):268–70.

70. Centers for Disease Control and Prevention (CDC). Children with elevated blood lead levels related to home renovation, repair, and painting activities–New York State, 2006–2007. MMWR Morb Mortal Wkly Rep 2009;58(3):55–8.

71. Arsenic toxicological profile. Atlanta (GA): ATSDR; 2007. 2010(01/29).

72. Munday SW, Ford MD. Arsenic. In: Lewis SN, Neal AL, Mary AH, et al, editors. Flomenbaum: Goldfrank's toxicologic emergencies. 9th edition. New York (NY): McGraw-Hill Publishing; 2010. Chapter 88.

73. Bush SP. Black widow spider envenomation mimicking cholecystitis. Am J Emerg Med 1999;17(3):315.

74. Clark RF, Wethern-Kestner S, Vance MV, et al. Clinical presentation and treatment of black widow spider envenomation: a review of 163 cases. Ann Emerg Med 1992;21(7):782–7.

75. Doyon S. Opioid. In: Tintinalli JE, Stapczynski JS, Ma OJ, et al, editors. Tintinalli's emergency medicine: a comprehensive study guide. 7th edition. New York (NY): McGraw-Hill Publishing; 2010. Chapter 180.

76. Arnold-Reed DE, Hulse GK. A comparison of rapid (opioid) detoxification with clonidine-assisted detoxification for heroin-dependent persons. J Opioid Manag 2005;1(1):17–23.

77. Li BU, Lefevre F, Chelimsky GG, et al. North American Society for Pediatric Gastroenterology, Hepatology, and Nutrition consensus statement on the diagnosis and management of cyclic vomiting syndrome. J Pediatr Gastroenterol Nutr 2008;47(3):379–93.

78. Pareek N, Fleisher DR, Abell T. Cyclic vomiting syndrome: what a gastroenterologist needs to know. Am J Gastroenterol 2007;102(12):2832–40.

79. Chepyala P, Svoboda RP, Olden KW. Treatment of cyclic vomiting syndrome. Curr Treat Options Gastroenterol 2007;10(4):273–82.

80. Farquhar HG. Abdominal migraine in children. Br Med J 1956;1(4975):1082–5.

81. Symon DN, Russell G. The relationship between cyclic vomiting syndrome and abdominal migraine. J Pediatr Gastroenterol Nutr 1995;21(Suppl 1):S42–3.

82. Stickler GB. Relationship between cyclic vomiting syndrome and migraine. Clin Pediatr (Phila) 2005;44(6):505–8.

83. Cremonini F, Talley NJ. Irritable bowel syndrome: epidemiology, natural history, health care seeking and emerging risk factors. Gastroenterol Clin North Am 2005;34(2):189–204.

84. Agrawal A, Houghton LA, Reilly B, et al. Bloating and distension in irritable bowel syndrome: the role of gastrointestinal transit. Am J Gastroenterol 2009;104(8): 1998–2004.

85. Chan SS. An unusual cause of abdominal pain: implications for infection control in the ED. Am J Emerg Med 2008;26(9):1062–3.

86. Tyring S, Barbarash RA, Nahlik JE, et al. Famciclovir for the treatment of acute herpes zoster: effects on acute disease and postherpetic neuralgia. A randomized, double-blind, placebo-controlled trial. Ann Intern Med 1995;123(2):89–96.

87. Dworkin RH, Johnson RW, Breuer J, et al. Recommendations for the management of herpes zoster. Clin Infect Dis 2007;44(Suppl 1):S1–26.

88. Zinkin NT, Peppercorn MA. Abdominal epilepsy. Best Pract Res Clin Gastroenterol 2005;19(2):263–74.

Vomiting, Diarrhea, Constipation, and Gastroenteritis

Leila Getto, MD[a],*, Eli Zeserson, MD[a], Michael Breyer, MD[b]

KEYWORDS

• Vomiting • Diarrhea • Constipation • Gastroenteritis

VOMITING

Vomiting is a reflex composed of the coordinated series of motor and autonomic responses that results in the forceful expulsion of gastric contents through the mouth activated by humoral or neuronal stimuli.[1] Vomiting should not be confused with regurgitation or retching. Regurgitation is the return of esophageal contents to the hypopharynx with little effort, whereas retching is unsuccessful vomiting due to absence of gastric contents or closure of the upper esophageal sphincter. Vomiting continues to be a major problem throughout the world. An analysis of the 2006 National Hospital Ambulatory Medical Care Survey (NHAMCS) found nausea and vomiting as the chief complaint for 3.7% of Emergency Department (ED) visits.[2] Pregnant women are particularly afflicted, as 56% of women experience vomiting during their pregnancies.[3] The cost of nausea and vomiting to society is high, with a 2002 study estimating a yearly cost of $3.4 billion for food-related and gastrointestinal infections.[4]

Differential Diagnosis and Initial Approach

Nausea and vomiting are symptoms of a wide variety of underlying conditions that may involve almost any organ system. Accordingly, when faced with a patient with vomiting, the differential is broad and includes gastrointestinal, infectious, central nervous system, drug reaction, and cardiac origins (**Table 1**). While the most common causes of nausea and vomiting are acute gastroenteritis, febrile systemic illness, and drug effects,[5] one must also consider certain critical and emergent diagnoses such as Boerhaave syndrome, intracranial bleed or raised intracranial pressure, meningitis, diabetic ketoacidosis, myocardial ischemia, sepsis, gonadal torsion, abdominal inflammatory processes, bowel obstruction, adrenal insufficiency, and toxic ingestions.

[a] Department of Emergency Medicine, Christiana Care Health System, 4755 Ogletown-Stanton Road, Newark, DE 19718, USA
[b] Department of Emergency Medicine, Denver Health and Hospital Authority, 660 Bannock Street, Denver, CO 80204, USA
* Corresponding author.
E-mail address: lgetto@christianacare.org

Emerg Med Clin N Am 29 (2011) 211–237
doi:10.1016/j.emc.2011.01.005
0733-8627/11/$ – see front matter © 2011 Elsevier Inc. All rights reserved.

emed.theclinics.com

Table 1
Differential diagnosis of vomiting

System	Disease
Gastrointestinal	Gastroenteritis (viral or bacterial), gastric outlet obstruction, small bowel obstruction, gastroparesis, cyclic vomiting syndrome, irritable bowel syndrome, neoplasm, peptic ulcer disease, gastritis, gastroesophageal reflux disease, hepatitis, cholecystitis, biliary colic, appendicitis, mesenteric ischemia, Crohn disease, pancreatitis, diverticulitis, volvulus, intussusception, pyloric stenosis, intestinal perforation
Central nervous system	Migraine, tumor, hemorrhage, infarction, congenital malformation, abscess, meningitis, demyelinating disorders, hydrocephalus, pseudotumor cerebri, seizure, Meniere disease, labyrinthitis, motion sickness, anxiety, depression, psychogenic vomiting, anorexia nervosa, bulimia nervosa, postconcussive syndrome
Drugs (only most common offenders listed)	Chemotherapy, nonsteroidal anti-inflammatory drugs (NSAIDs), opioids, antiarrhythmics, antihypertensives, diuretics, antibiotics, hormonal preparations, anticonvulsants, oral hypoglycemics, vitamins, ethanol
Metabolic and endocrinologic	Pregnancy, diabetic ketoacidosis, uremia, hyperparathyroidism, hypoparathyroidism, Addison disease, porphyria, uremia, alcoholic ketoacidosis
Cardiac	Cardiac ischemia, myocardial infarction, hypotension, hypertension, congestive heart failure
Other	Pain, gonadal torsion, renal colic, postoperative, overdose and toxins, emotional response, sepsis

Despite the heterogeneity in potential etiology, a thorough history and physical examination can often focus the approach and narrow the differential diagnosis. The American Gastroenterological Association (AGA) recommends a pragmatic 3-step approach to the management of the patient with nausea and vomiting.[6] After a complete history and physical examination, the clinician should first correct any complications of vomiting such as hypokalemia, metabolic alkalosis, hypovolemia, ketosis, or vitamin deficiencies. Second, the underlying cause should be sought with the intention of initiating targeted therapy. The third step is the initiation of treatment strategies to suppress the symptoms. Although there are no clinical guidelines in the initial workup of the patient with vomiting, pregnancy testing should be considered in women of reproductive age. Serum electrolytes, complete blood count, liver function tests, lipase, urinalysis, and electrocardiogram may also be considered depending on the clinical situation.

Antiemetics

Dopamine receptor antagonists
When a specific etiology of vomiting is diagnosed, targeted intervention toward the underlying process is important. For the empiric treatment of undifferentiated vomiting, the pharmaceutical armamentarium consists of many different drug classes primarily directed at 5 neurotransmitter receptor sites (**Table 2**). Before the recent increase in use of the serotonin 5-hydroxytryptamine-3 (5-HT$_3$) antagonists, the mainstay of therapy had been dopamine receptor antagonists. The literature on this class of

Table 2
Antiemetics

Drugs	Mechanism of Action	Special Considerations
Prochlorperazine, promethazine, chlorpromazine	Phenothiazines: predominantly D2-dopamine antagonism, also M1-muscarinic and H1-histamine antagonism	High incidence of extrapyramidal reactions, may cause hypotension, promethazine black box warning for children <2 y
Metoclopramide, domperidone	Benzamides: D2-dopamine antagonism, weak 5-HT$_3$ antagonism at higher doses, enhances acetylcholine at neuromuscular junction	Prokinetic properties, domperidone does not cross blood-brain barrier, metoclopramide pregnancy category B
Droperidol, haloperidol	Butyrophenones: D2-dopamine and α antagonism	Second-line agents, droperidol black box warning due to QT prolongation and torsades
Diphenhydramine, dimenhydrinate, cyclizine	H1-histamine antagonism	Primarily used for motion sickness, sedating
Ondansetron, granisetron, dolasetron, palonosetron	Selective 5-HT$_3$ antagonism	Favorable toxicity profile, high cost
Aprepitant, fosaprepitant	Selective NK1-substance P antagonism	Used for chemotherapy, synergistic effect with serotonin receptor antagonists and corticosteroids
Dexamethasone, methylprednisolone	Corticosteroid: inhibits inflammatory cytokines, produces glucocorticoid and mineralocorticoid effects	Prophylaxis for chemotherapy-induced vomiting
Lorazepam, alprazolam	Binds to benzodiazepine receptors, enhances GABA effects	Sedating, often used as adjunctive agent
Dronabinol, nabilone	Cannabinoids: exact mechanism unknown, possible interaction with vomiting control center	Multiple other effects, most studied in cancer patients

Abbreviations: 5-HT$_3$, 5-hydroxytryptamine-3; GABA, γ-aminobutyric acid.

medications is vast and at times contradictory. One of the most extensively studied drugs is metoclopramide (Reglan). Metoclopramide has been compared with prochlorperazine (Compazine), with some investigators finding similar efficacy[7,8] and others finding a modest benefit of one over the other.[9-11] Metoclopramide is often recommended for pregnant patients, as it is the only medication in this class with a pregnancy category B rating.

Similar inconclusive findings have been found when comparing promethazine (Phenergan) and prochlorperazine. Recently, however, one randomized, double-blind study of 84 ED patients found subjects who received promethazine had a treatment failure rate of 31% versus just 9.5% in the prochlorperazine group.[12] Of interest, both groups had a similar rate of akathisia although the promethazine group experienced increased drowsiness. Other studies have shown a higher rate of akathisia and dystonia with prochlorperazine compared with other antiemetics.[13,14] In an ED-based study of 229 patients receiving prochlorperazine, 16% developed akathisia and 4% developed acute dystonia.[15] Diphenhydramine (Benadryl) is the first-line choice to treat these reactions. A study of 82 patients with akathisia found diphenhydramine was effective in reducing akathisia from 9.8 to 1.2 on a scale of 0 to 17.[16] These findings have led some clinicians to administer diphenhydramine concurrently with prochlorperazine in an effort to prevent akathisia; however, this practice has not been validated with a randomized, placebo-controlled study.

As the literature does not consistently support one dopamine receptor antagonist over another, it is not surprising that practice patterns vary. A 2000 ED-based analysis found antiemetics to be used with the frequencies promethazine (55%), prochlorperazine (25.3%), metoclopramide (5.2%), and ondansetron (Zofran) (1.3%), reflecting the choice of antiemetic remains one of clinician preference.[17]

Serotonin 5-HT$_3$ antagonists

Over the past decade, there has been an increase in the use of 5-HT$_3$ antagonists due to a lower incidence of side effects. Although controversial, the 2001 black box warning by the Food and Drug Administration (FDA) of droperidol (Inapsine)[18] may also have contributed to shifting practice patterns. Of the currently approved drugs in the United States, ondansetron (Zofran), granisetron (Granisol, Kytril), and dolasetron (Anzemet) have all been shown to be equally effective and tolerated.[19–21] Palonosetron (Aloxi) differs from the others in this class by its longer half-life, and has been shown to reduce delayed chemotherapy-induced vomiting when compared with dolasetron.[22] Although the bulk of the research on this class of drugs comes from the oncology literature for chemotherapy-induced vomiting,[23,24] studies examining undifferentiated ED patients have recently been published. A randomized, placebo-controlled, double-blind trial found ondansetron was not superior to metoclopramide and promethazine in 163 patients presenting to the ED with undifferentiated nausea.[25] Furthermore, a 2008 study of 120 ED patients found no difference in the reduction of nausea between ondansetron and promethazine, however, the group that received ondansetron experienced less sedation.[26] A recent review article examined the evidence supporting the use of droperidol, promethazine, prochlorperazine, metoclopramide, and ondansetron for the treatment of nausea or vomiting in the ED. The investigators concluded that "based on the safety and efficacy of ondansetron, it may be used as a first-line agent for relief of nausea or vomiting for most patient populations in the ED."[27]

Pediatric Patients

Vomiting in the pediatric patient is an extremely common complaint in children presenting to the ED.[28] While most patients have a self-limiting disease process, vomiting may also be the presenting symptom for severe life-threatening conditions, and a thorough history and physical examination are therefore required to guide management. Clinicians have historically been cautious to prescribe antiemetics for children, a practice reinforced by the American Academy of Pediatrics' (AAP) recommendation to use oral rehydration as first-line therapy for both mildly and moderately dehydrated children with gastroenteritis.[29] In a recent study, 73 children ranging in age from 8 weeks to 3 years with moderate dehydration from viral gastroenteritis were randomized to either oral rehydration therapy (ORT) or intravenous fluids. While nearly 50% of both groups were successfully rehydrated at 4 hours, subjects receiving ORT had shorter ED stays and were hospitalized less often. Based on their findings, the investigators opined that ORT was the preferred treatment option.[30]

Despite these recommendations, a survey found 36% of pediatricians believed vomiting was a contraindication to ORT.[31] The FDA's 2006 black box warning on promethazine for pediatric patients younger than 2 years may have contributed to the hesitancy to use antiemetics and subsequently avoid ORT in children. Nonetheless, the past decade has also seen an increase in $5\text{-}HT_3$ antagonists in the pediatric population. A double-blind, placebo-controlled study from 2002 on intravenous ondansetron for gastroenteritis found a reduction in admission rates for pediatric patients presenting with vomiting and an initial serum carbon dioxide level of 15 mEq/L or more.[32]

Pharmacologic data demonstrating that orally administered ondansetron tablets are equivalent to its intravenous formulation have led to further investigations exploring whether intravenous access could be avoided. In 2006, investigators enrolled 215 children aged 6 months to 10 years treated in the ED for gastroenteritis-related dehydration. Compared with placebo, subjects who received ondansetron orally were less likely to vomit (14% vs 35%), had greater oral intake (239 mL vs 196 mL), and were less likely to require intravenous fluids (14% vs 31%).[33] Another pediatric study replicated these results, finding subjects who received oral ondansetron had a decreased need for intravenous fluids than those who received a placebo (21.6% vs 54.5%).[34] These results reinforce the practice of using oral ondansetron and ORT to treat pediatric patients with mild to moderate dehydration.

DIARRHEA

Diarrhea is classically thought of as a physical sign of a disease rather than a disease in itself; therefore, much of the pertinent literature focuses on its etiology and the supportive, empiric treatment of diarrhea. Nevertheless, while the majority of cases of diarrhea in the United States are self-limited, diarrhea continues to pose an enormous health challenge worldwide. The World Health Organization (WHO)[35] estimates approximately 4 billion cases of diarrhea worldwide per year, with such episodes responsible for a staggering 2.2 million deaths annually. Overall, in the United States, there are an estimated 211 million to 375 million cases of acute diarrhea, resulting in 900,000 hospitalizations.[36] Furthermore, diarrhea remains the most common and incapacitating symptom of patients with ulcerative colitis.[37] Diarrhea is an ailment that can be particularly severe in children, with the majority of the deaths worldwide caused by diarrheal illness occurring in children younger than 5 years old. A recent study found ED visits for pediatric patients with diarrhea nearly doubled from 1995 to 2004, with 25% of those presentations being due to rotavirus.[38,39] Diarrhea is also common in the military. More than three-quarters of troops deployed to Iraq and Afghanistan reported at least one diarrhea episode during their deployments, with 45% noting a decreased work performance for a median of 3 days.[40]

Although definitions vary, diarrhea is typically characterized as a change in normal bowel movements with the passage of 3 or more stools per day or at least 200 g of stool per day.[41] Acute diarrhea is defined as episodes lasting 14 days or less; persistent diarrhea lasts more than 14 days; and chronic diarrhea lasts for more than 30 days. Furthermore, diarrhea is broadly categorized as either secretory or osmotic. Osmotic diarrhea occurs when a nonabsorbable solute exerts an osmotic pressure effect across the intestinal mucosa, a process that produces excessive water output.

Secretory diarrhea, commonly caused by bacterial toxins or neoplasms that disrupt epithelial crypt cells in the gastrointestinal tract, is extremely difficult to control.

Differential Diagnosis

The differential diagnosis for diarrhea is broad, with several causes displaying overlapping signs and symptoms. A focused history including the onset, frequency, and character of the diarrhea (eg, presence of blood or mucus) as well as associated symptoms (eg, fever, vomiting), medical history (eg, human immunodeficiency virus [HIV], inflammatory bowel disease), medications, and travel history may aid in narrowing the differential. Nevertheless, there are several clinically noteworthy causes of diarrhea that have exceptional treatment regimens as well as important clinical ramifications to consider.

Clostridium difficile, which affects approximately 3 million patients yearly in the United States with a mortality rate of 1% to 2.5%,[42] is caused by a disruption of normal intestinal flora,[43] and is responsible for 15% to 20% of antibiotic-related cases of diarrhea.[44] Severe *C difficile* infection may result in life-threatening complications such as toxic megacolon, intestinal perforation, sepsis, or death. Furthermore, diarrhea caused by *C difficile* may present with severe abdominal pain, high fever, and more than 10 watery stools per day; however, as it is common among elderly patients many or all of these signs and symptoms may be absent. One study found 15% of patients with diarrhea hospitalized at an academic center tested positive for *C difficile*,[45] while during times of outbreak more than 50% of patients in an affected ward may become colonized.[46] Of interest, although *C difficile* historically has not been thought of as a pediatric illness, recent evidence suggests the contrary. A pediatric ED-based study found that of specimens that underwent complete testing, 12.4% tested positive for *C difficile* toxin,[47] and nearly 3% of children tested positive for *C difficile* toxin in another similar study from France.[48] Recently a new disease pattern, community-onset *C difficile*–associated diarrhea, has emerged, and may occur without exposure to the typical risk factors including antibiotic usage.[49]

Several agents have been implicated in the increased incidence of *C difficile*, including usage of antibiotics and proton pump inhibitors (PPIs). In one recent study, *C difficile* diarrhea among hospital inpatients was associated with the use of PPIs (9.3% of patients receiving PPIs vs 4.4% who did not receive PPIs) and receipt of 3 or more antibiotics.[50] Removing the inciting antibiotic treats up to 25% of cases of *C difficile* diarrhea.[51] Antibiotic treatment regimens have traditionally used oral metronidazole (Flagyl) or vancomycin (Vancocin) for 14 days; however, for recurrent *C difficile* infection some experts recommend oral tapered-pulsed vancomycin (125 mg once a day for 1 week, 125 mg 3 times a day for 1 week, 125 mg every day for 1 week, 125 mg every other day for 2 weeks, 125 mg every third day for 2 weeks).[52]

Traveler's diarrhea, which affects 20% to 50% of individuals traveling from developed to developing countries and 4% to 9% of individuals traveling from developing to developed countries, is typically caused by enterotoxigenic *Escherichia coli* (ETEC) and enteroaggregative *E coli*, which bind to the intestinal mucosa to cause diarrhea typically without fever.[53] Incubation periods for ETEC last between 10 hours and 3 days followed by 3 to 5 days of illness.[54] ETEC produces a noninvasive toxin that causes severe watery diarrhea, abdominal cramps, nausea, and (infrequently) fever.[55] *Shigella* species and *Salmonella* species are other important bacterial pathogens. *Campylobacter jejuni*, a bacteria that poses additional hazards because it has been implicated with acute cases of myocarditis, has emerged as another important cause of traveler's diarrhea.[56] Electrolyte disturbances for patients with traveler's diarrhea are rare, and therefore laboratory work is usually unnecessary.[57] Treatment of traveler's diarrhea is centered on antibiotic therapy, such as ciprofloxacin (Cipro), trimethoprim-sulfamethoxazole (Bactrim; resistance common), azithromycin (Zithromax), and rifaximin (Xifaxan).[58] If the patient with suspected traveler's diarrhea has more than 2 unformed stools per day, bloody stools, or fever (>37.8°C), treatment with antibiotics is advised.[59] A short, single-day course of ciprofloxacin, 500 mg twice a day, is usually successful at stopping the illness within 24 hours,[60] although other sources recommend a 3-day course of ciprofloxacin or rifaximin.[61] Prophylactic administration of antibiotics for those traveling to developing countries is not typically recommended. However, in one placebo-controlled trial performed on United States travelers in Mexico, subjects who took rifaximin prophylactically had significantly reduced rates of diarrhea (53.70% for those taking placebo vs 14.74% for those taking rifaximin).[62] Nonetheless, C difficile and Helicobacter pylori must also be on the differential among the traveler afflicted with diarrhea. Noninfectious origins need to be considered if there is no response to antimicrobials or antiparasitics and there is a protracted course. Nonbacterial causes include enteric viruses, viral hepatitis, influenza, giardia, Cryptosporidium, Cyclospora, Entamoeba, Strongyloides, and other less common parasites.

Cryptosporidiosis, which typically affects immunocompromised individuals (particularly HIV-infected persons) and may also affect immunocompetent persons (usually children younger than 5 years), causes diarrhea lasting 1 to 2 weeks, and may develop into life-threatening illnesses. Although it appears that nitazoxanide (Alinia) reduces the load of parasites and may be useful in immunocompetent persons, a recent review found there is no evidence for effective agents in the management of cryptosporidiosis.[63]

Pediatric Patients

The differential diagnosis for the pediatric patient with diarrhea is broad and includes pathogens such as E coli, Campylobacter, Shigella, Salmonella, and viruses. However, in recent years a newer strain of E coli has emerged in the pediatric population: enteroaggregative E coli. In a study of 1327 children younger than 1 year with acute gastroenteritis, enteroaggregative E coli was isolated significantly more often in inpatients (4.7%) and ED patients (10.0%) than from well children (1.4%).[64] Viral gastroenteritis caused by rotaviruses is another concern in the pediatric population. Among middle- and low-income countries, it is estimated rotaviruses are responsible for 600,000 to 870,000 pediatric deaths per year, resulting in up to 6% of all mortality in children younger than 5 years.[65] The majority of these deaths were due to dehydration, underscoring the importance of rehydration therapies for children. Implementation of the rotavirus vaccine shows promise. A 2004 review of 64 trials conducted on 21,070 children found the vaccine's effectiveness at preventing diarrhea caused by rotavirus ranged from 22% to 89%.[66]

Evaluation of hydration status often dictates the treatment of pediatric patients with diarrhea. While acute appendicitis must always remain on the differential diagnosis of the child with diarrhea, digital rectal examinations and nasogastric tubes rarely provide additional actionable information for pediatric patients.[66] Treatment of the pediatric patient with diarrhea centers on supportive care, with encouragement of fluids for mild to moderate cases, and in severe cases intravenous or nasogastric fluid replacement. Educating parents in the appropriate treatment of their child's diarrhea is crucial. Whereas 52% of parents treated their child's diarrhea with appropriate rehydration fluids and solutions, 13% of parents used treatments not recommended in the current Centers for Disease Control (CDC) guidelines, typically using antidiarrheal agents and fluids high in simple sugars.[67]

Developed in 1975, the WHO standard oral rehydration solution consists of a high content of sodium (90 mmol/L) and has been found to be effective in the treatment of dehydration from acute gastroenteritis regardless of the etiology of the diarrhea.[68] Several newer products with lower sodium levels, including the WHO revised formula (75 mmol/L) and Pedialyte (45 mmol/L), may be better tolerated among pediatric patients. However, these products may not be appropriate for patients suffering from diarrhea caused by cholera, one of the most serious types of diarrheal disease that can cause rapid electrolyte loss. In an analysis of 7 trials of patients with cholera, the investigators found an increased number of patients with hyponatremia treated with hypoosmolar solutions compared with standard oral rehydration solutions, although the outcomes were similar.[69]

Elderly Patients

Elderly patients afflicted with diarrhea tend to have longer hospital stays (7.4 days in patients older than 75 years versus 4.1 days in those patients 20 to 49 years old) and a higher mortality.[70] Age greater than 65 years is also considered an independent *C difficile* risk factor.[71] In one ED-based study of 174 patients with diarrhea, it was found that age greater than 40 years with constant abdominal pain and diarrhea was predictive of a surgical etiology for their symptoms.[72] Taken together, these factors should prompt the clinician to at times take a more aggressive and perhaps more comprehensive approach in attempting to search for the origin of diarrhea in the elderly patient.

Treatment

Rehydration and electrolyte replacement remain cornerstones of treatment for patients with diarrhea. To accomplish this, the "BRAT" diet (bananas, rice, apple sauce, and toast) is often recommended, although evidence supporting its practice is limited. Loperamide (Imodium) has been shown to be efficacious in reducing the symptoms of diarrhea in undifferentiated patients with mild symptoms[73]; however, there is scant evidence regarding its safety profile in patients with moderate or severe diarrhea.[74] A recent review did not find conclusive evidence supporting or refuting the usage of antimotility agents and adsorbents in controlling diarrhea in people with HIV/AIDS,[75] thus reinforcing the need for adjunct treatments such as fluid replacement. Nevertheless, one meta-analysis found that when combined with antibiotic therapy, loperamide was more efficacious than antibiotics alone in decreasing illness duration for adult patients with traveler's diarrhea.[76] Antidiarrheal agents are not recommended in the treatment of pediatric patients with diarrhea, as they have potentially serious side effects in this population.[77]

Antibiotics are the mainstay of treatment for patients with a suspected bacterial cause for their diarrheal symptoms. A study of 139 patients presenting with severe diarrhea characterized by one of either profuse watery diarrhea with dehydration, passage of stools containing mucus and blood, temperature greater than 38.4°C, passage of more than 6 soft stools in 24 hours, duration of illness of more than 48 hours, severe abdominal pain in a patient older than 50, or diarrhea in the elderly, found single-dose quinolone therapy shortened the duration of symptoms and was equally efficacious when compared with a 5-day antibiotic regimen.[78]

Probiotics, which are found in yogurts, fermented milks, and dietary supplements, may help treat diarrheal diseases. In one randomized, double-blind, placebo-controlled study, consumption of a 100-g drink containing *Lactobacillus casei*, *Lactobacillus bulgaricus*, and *Streptococcus thermophilus* twice daily during a course of antibiotics and 1 week after the antibiotic was finished resulted in an absolute risk reduction of 21.6% for the occurrence of antibiotic-associated diarrhea.[79] Another study noted probiotic organisms may be beneficial for 3 problems common in the elderly: undernutrition, constipation, and the capacity to resist infection.[80] A systematic review of the literature on probiotics, which examined 23 studies with 1917 participants, found probiotics reduced the risk of diarrhea at 3 days and the mean duration of diarrhea by 30 hours.[81]

Prevention

Most preventive measures aimed at limiting the spread of diarrheal diseases focus on improving the quality of available water sources. Two studies found the addition of household-based water filters reduced the prevalence of diarrhea by 60% in Columbia[82] and by 70% in rural Bolivia.[83] Further, one study found treating turbid water in rural Kenya with a disinfectant resulted in a 19% absolute reduction in the prevalence of diarrhea.[84] Communicable and diarrheal diseases are also major concerns for disaster-affected populations in camp settings. In treated households in Liberia, disinfectants reduced diarrheal prevalence by 83% compared with control households.[85] Other developing countries have instituted hand-washing campaigns. One, in urban squatter settlements in Pakistan, found campaigns promoting hand-washing reduced the incidence of diarrhea by 53% among children younger than 15 years.[86] A recent review, which examined 33 trials with more than 53,000 participants, found that interventions focused on improving the quality of drinking water were effective in preventing diarrhea, with interventions aimed at the household level more effective than those aimed at the source.[87]

CONSTIPATION

Constipation is the most common digestive complaint in the United States, affecting up to 27% of the North American population. Although constipation tends to be associated with increasing age,[88] children also may experience this problem. One review of 4157 children younger than 2 years found the prevalence of constipation was 2.9% in the first year of life and 10.1% in the second year of life. While the majority of these cases were diagnosed as functional constipation, in 1.6% of cases underlying disease was responsible.[89] Constipation is also the most common cause of acute abdominal pain in children. A study of 962 children seen in a pediatric office found 9% had a complaint of abdominal pain; chronic constipation was diagnosed in 35% of those patients and acute constipation was diagnosed in 13%. A surgical condition was found in only 2% of the children with abdominal pain.[90] Furthermore, pregnant women are also disproportionately afflicted with constipation, with 25% of healthy women experiencing symptoms during their pregnancy and up to 3 months postpartum.[91]

Etiology

The cause of constipation is often multifactorial. While a 2007 review revealed a small number of publications addressing the etiologic factors of this very common problem,[92] it was suggested that insufficient dietary fiber intake, inadequate fluid intake, decreased physical activity, side effects of drugs, hypothyroidism, sex hormones, and colorectal cancer obstruction may be responsible for constipation.[92] Furthermore, the cause of constipation may also be related to abnormal bowel motility, anatomical rectal disorders, neurological disorders, or psychosocial issues (Table 3). A thorough review of the patient's medications is advisable, as there are many different medications that secondarily contribute to constipation, such as calcium and iron supplements, opioids, anticonvulsants, antipsychotics, and

Table 3
Etiology of constipation

Category	Cause
Abnormal motility	Slow-transit constipation, irritable bowel syndrome
Anatomic disorders	Anal fissure, hemorrhoids, rectal polyps, rectocele, rectal stenosis, fistulas, colonic or rectal neoplasm
Drugs	Calcium, iron, opioids, anticonvulsants, antipsychotics, antihistamines
Neurologic	Hirschsprung disease, spinal cord injury, multiple sclerosis, diabetes mellitus, Parkinson disease
Endocrine	Hypothyroidism, pregnancy, hypercalcemia, diabetes mellitus
Psychosocial	Depression, anxiety
Systemic	Scleroderma, amyloidosis, lupus

antihistamines.[88] Constipation resistant to simple measures may be caused by painful anorectal conditions, irritable bowel syndrome (IBS), slow transit constipation, or obstructive defecation. Obstructed defecation is a broad term used to describe the inability to empty stool from the rectum, which may result from functional, metabolic, mechanical, or anatomical problems.[93] Mechanical and anatomical disorders causing obstructive defecation include Hirschsprung disease, rectocele, rectoanal intussusception, enterocele, sigmoidocele, and rectal prolapse.[94] Studies have found that obstructive defecation is a significant problem for middle-aged women. Obstructive defecation was self-reported and defined by difficulty in passing stool, hard stool, straining for more than 15 minutes, or incomplete evacuation, occurring at least weekly. In this study of 2109 subjects, 12.3% of women reported obstructive defecation at least once weekly. Risk factors correlated with patients developing obstructive defecation included a history of IBS, vaginal or laparoscopic hysterectomy, unemployment, use of 3 or more medications, symptomatic pelvic organ prolapse, history of urinary incontinence surgery, or other pelvic surgeries.[95]

IBS, characterized by chronic abdominal pain and altered bowel habits without a clearly defined organic cause,[96] affects 10% to 15% of North Americans.[97,98] Attempts to standardize the diagnosis of IBS have been made, and the American Gastroenterology Association recommends clinicians use the Rome III criteria, last revised in 2005, to diagnose IBS.[99] These criteria require the presence of recurrent abdominal pain or discomfort at least 3 days per month as well as 2 or more of the following: improvement with defecation, onset associated with a change in form of stool, or onset associated with a change in frequency of stool. The Rome III diagnostic criteria for IBS must be fulfilled for 3 consecutive months with symptom onset at least 6 months before diagnosis.[100] Other symptoms that are not part of the Rome criteria but support the diagnosis of IBS include defecation straining, urgency, a feeling of incomplete bowel movement, passing mucus, and bloating. Four subtypes of IBS are recognized: IBS with constipation (hard stools ≥25% and loose stools <25% of bowel movements), IBS with diarrhea (loose stools ≥25% and hard stools <25% of bowel movements), mixed IBS (hard stools ≥25% and loose stools ≥25% of bowel movements), and unsubtyped IBS (insufficient abnormality of stool consistency to meet the other subtypes).

Pharmacologic intervention must be tailored to the specific subtype of IBS. While antidepressant therapy has been explored as treatment for IBS, a trial of 51 patients randomized to placebo, imipramine, or citalopram found none of these agents significantly improved global IBS end points.[101] Antibiotics, specifically rifaximin, have also been tried in the treatment of IBS. A recent study of 80 patients randomized to rifaximin or placebo for 10 days found the group that received rifaximin had a greater improvement of IBS symptoms and a lower bloating score.[102]

Presenting Signs and Symptoms

Studies show a discrepancy among how physicians and patients define constipation, although they have a similar understanding of the symptoms.[88] Patients typically describe constipation as straining to have bowel movements, lumpy or hard stools, incomplete evacuation, anorectal obstruction, and a decreased frequency of bowel movements. To establish a standard for defining constipation, the Rome III criteria were created by a consortium of representatives from 18 countries.[88,100] These criteria include the aforementioned signs and symptoms frequently described by patients, while requiring at least 2 of the following over 3 months' duration: fewer than 3 bowel movements per week, at least 25% of bowel movements involving manual maneuvers to disimpact, straining, passing hard stools, or a sensation of anorectal obstruction. The Rome criteria excludes patients with loose stools as well as those meeting diagnostic criteria for IBS, given that there are separate Rome criteria for the diagnosis of IBS as mentioned previously.

Diagnostic Evaluation

The physical examination may include a digital rectal examination to determine presence of stool impaction or blood in the stool. The clinician should be aware of what the American College of Gastroenterology (ACG) refers to as "alarm" signs or symptoms, which include fever, nausea, vomiting, weight loss of more than 10 pounds, anorexia, blood in stool, anemia, family history of colon cancer, onset of constipation after the age of 50 years, or acute onset of constipation in the elderly.[88,103] If any of these symptoms are present a workup is advised, including a complete blood count, basic metabolic panel, thyroid tests, and possibly colonoscopy. If these signs are absent, the ACG recommends empiric treatment of the constipation.[88,103]

Radiographic studies are sometimes used to help determine the etiology of constipation. However, in a 2005 review article of the pediatric literature, the investigators found conflicting evidence for an association between a clinical and a radiographic diagnosis of constipation. The investigators therefore do not recommend performing routine abdominal films on pediatric patients presenting with constipation.[104]

Management and Treatment

The management of constipation depends on the degree to which the symptoms affect the patient's daily life, patient preference for type of treatment, efficacy of treatments tried in the past, and the provider's clinical judgment. If, for example, the patient is impacted then an enema or manual disimpaction is indicated. The ACG Chronic Constipation Task Force guidelines state exercise may help patients with constipation by reducing gastrointestinal transit time. Further, increasing water and fiber in the diet can increase frequency of bowel movements.[92,103,105] However, patient satisfaction surveys show dissatisfaction with initial treatment regimens of lifestyle and dietary changes for chronic constipation,[105] which highlights the importance of a multi-pronged approach in treating constipation.

When lifestyle changes fail, the options for medical treatment include bulking agents, osmotic agents, stimulant laxatives, and enemas (**Table 4**). Stool softeners are surface-acting agents that function as detergents, allowing water to interact more effectively with stool. Docusate sodium (Colace) is a stool softener that is frequently prescribed for the treatment of chronic constipation; however, there are insufficient data to support its use.[106] One placebo-controlled crossover trial of docusate calcium (Surfak) versus placebo demonstrated no differences in stool consistency or frequency between the 2 groups.[107] Another trial, which was a multicenter, randomized, double-blind study of 170 patients with chronic constipation, found psyllium was superior to docusate sodium for increasing the stool water content and frequency of bowel movements.[108]

Nevertheless, the ACG recommends osmotic laxatives to treat constipation if an increase in water and dietary fiber fails.[103,109] One double-blind, multicenter study randomized 100 patients who presented with chronic medication-induced constipation to receive either polyethylene glycol (PEG) 3350 (Miralax) or placebo for 28 days. The standard dosing of PEG, 17 g mixed with 8 ounces of water daily, was given to patients in the treatment group. PEG 3350 was found to be superior to placebo (78.3% vs 39.1%) in relieving constipation. Diarrhea and flatulence occurred more frequently with PEG treatment, although not to a statistically significant extent from placebo.[110] Based on this study and others supporting PEG's efficacy at improving stool frequency and consistency, the ACG Task Force gave PEG as well as lactulose (Cholac) grade A recommendations.[103,105]

Nevertheless, when osmotic laxatives fail to provide relief of symptoms of constipation, stimulant laxatives may be prescribed. Stimulant laxatives include compounds containing senna or bisacodyl, and are thought to act by stimulating the sensory nerve endings of the colonic mucosa. The FDA has approved these agents for treatment of occasional constipation; however, they should be used only as needed and for a brief time (<1 week), due to concerns regarding side effects with chronic use such as

Table 4
Medications used to treat constipation

Type	Agent	Mechanism
Bulking	Psyllium (Metamucil)	Increases stool bulk and intestinal motility, shortens transit time
	Methylcellulose (Citrucel)	Same as above
	Polycarbophil (FiberCon)	Same as above
	Docusate sodium (Colace)	Facilitates mixture of stool fat and water, softens stool
Osmotic	Lactulose	Osmotically active nonabsorbable sugars pull fluid into the gut
	Sorbitol	Same as above
	Polyethylene glycol (Golytely, Miralax)	Same as above
Stimulants	Bisacodyl (Dulcolax)	Stimulates the myenteric plexus, increasing intestinal motility
	Anthraquinones (Peri-Colace)	Same as above
	Senna (Senokot, Ex-lax)	Same as above
	Magnesium (milk of magnesia, magnesium citrate)	Shortens colonic transit time
	Glycerin suppository	Local rectal stimulation
Enemas	Tap water	Colonic distention prompts defecation
	Soap suds	Same as above, bowel wall irritant
	Monophosphate (Fleets)	Same as above, osmotic effect in small intestine, stimulates peristalsis

abdominal cramping, fecal incontinence, electrolyte imbalances, and reduced colonic motility.[88,105] One study, which evaluated sennosides (Sennakot) alone versus sennosides plus docusate sodium in the treatment of hospitalized oncologic patients, found that the sennosides group required fewer alternative laxative therapies (40% in the sennosides group versus 57% in the sennosides plus docusate sodium group) to treat constipation.[111] As there are no placebo-controlled trials of stimulant laxatives, insufficient data exist to make a recommendation about the effectiveness of stimulant laxatives in patients with chronic constipation.[106] A drug that has recently emerged for the treatment of chronic constipation is lubiprostone (Amitiza), which works by activating chloride channels that in turn increase secretion of intestinal fluid.[105,109] Patients treated with lubiprostone in phase 3 clinical trials experienced a median increase of 3 or 4 spontaneous bowel movements per week after 1 month of treatment.[112]

Treating constipation in pediatric patients is also challenging, although studies have demonstrated superior efficacy of PEG in this population as well.[113–117] In one study of 100 children aged 6 months to 15 years with constipation who received PEG or lactulose for 8 weeks, the investigators found a significant increase in the mean number of defecations per week in both groups. In terms of complete relief of symptoms after 18 weeks, however, 56% of patients who received PEG 3350 were successfully treated compared with 29% of patients who received lactulose.[114] Other studies have been performed to establish the most effective dose of PEG.[108,109] The results showed that 95% of patients receiving a higher dose (1–1.5 g/kg/d) achieved disimpaction versus 55% of patients receiving a lower dose (0.25–0.50 g/kg/d). However, diarrhea and bloating were more common in the higher-dose group.[117] A second study on PEG for children with constipation found low-dose PEG (0.2 g/kg/d) was successful in 77% of patients, mid-dose PEG (0.4 g/kg/d) was successful in 74% of patients, and high-dose PEG (0.8 g/kg/d) was successful in 73% of patients. All were more successful than placebo (42% success rate).[118] Nevertheless, a recent review stated that even though PEG achieved more treatment success compared with other laxatives, the studies were not of high enough quality to suggest laxative treatment is better than placebo in children with constipation.[119]

GASTROENTERITIS

Gastroenteritis is defined as a syndrome of vomiting, diarrhea, or the combination of both, that begins abruptly in otherwise healthy individuals.[120] Although the symptoms of vomiting and diarrhea convey a broad differential, it is clinically important to consider the diagnosis of gastroenteritis in patients with these symptoms for public health reasons. Worldwide, infectious gastroenteritis is a leading cause of morbidity and mortality.[120] In the United States, the highest incidence of infectious gastroenteritis is in patients younger than 5 years, whereas severe disease leading to hospitalization and resulting in mortality is most frequently observed in patients older than 60 years.[121] Even so, approximately 10% of hospitalizations in children younger than 5 years are caused by gastroenteritis and dehydration, accounting for nearly 220,000 hospitalizations yearly.[122] Gastroenteritis has many causes, including viral, bacterial, parasitic, and noninfectious (**Table 5**).

Norwalk Virus

The most prominent cause of acute gastroenteritis is viruses. Noroviruses account for more than 90% of the outbreaks in the United States, and affect both children and adults.[123,124] Outbreaks occur more commonly in cold-weather climates and in places where people are closely confined, such as schools, nursing homes, hospitals, and

Table 5
Gastroenteritis etiology

Viral (50%–70%)	Bacterial (15%–20%)	Parasitic (10%–15%)	Others	Drug-Associated
Norovirus	Shigella	Giardia	Ciguatera	Antibiotics
Calicivirus	Salmonella	Amebiasis	Scombroid	Laxatives
Rotavirus	Campylobacter	Cryptosporidium	—	Colchicine
Adenovirus	Yersinia	Cyclospora	—	Quinidine
Parvovirus	Escherichia coli	—	—	Sorbitol
Astrovirus	Vibrio cholera	—	—	—
Coronavirus	Aeromonas	—	—	—
Pestivirus	Bacillus cereus	—	—	—
Torovirus	Clostridium difficile	—	—	—
—	Clostridium perfringens	—	—	—
—	Listeria	—	—	—
—	Mycobacterium avium-intracellulare (MAI)	—	—	—
—	Providencia	—	—	—
—	Vibrio parahaemolyticus	—	—	—
—	Vibrio vulnificus	—	—	—

cruise ships.[125] The primary mode of transmission is through fecal-oral spread, but the virus can also be transmitted by respiratory droplet contact or ingestion of contaminated food or water. Up to 30% of exposed individuals shed the virus before developing the illness, and patients with underlying illnesses or immunocompromised states may continue to do so long after the illness resolves.[126] Noroviruses survive in a variety of temperatures, remaining live on environmental surfaces, in recreational and drinking water, and on raw fruits and vegetables. Although patients may develop illness year-round, outbreaks tend to peak during periods of cold weather.[124] Norovirus illness usually presents with both vomiting and diarrhea, as well as abdominal cramps, malaise, myalgias, and chills. Symptom onset is sudden, with vomiting being more common in children and diarrhea more common in adults.[124]

Fever, which is typically low grade, is present in 50% of patients. Symptoms usually last 24 to 60 hours and are typically mild and self-limited, while severe disease may develop in debilitated, elderly, or immunocompromised individuals.[123] Of particular concern, noroviruses may be associated with necrotizing enterocolitis (NEC). In one study of an outbreak of 8 infants with NEC in a neonatal intensive care unit, investigators found 4 (50%) of the infants had stool samples that tested positive for norovirus.[127]

Rotavirus

Although norovirus infection is the most common cause of gastroenteritis outbreaks in people of all ages worldwide, group A rotavirus is the leading cause of diarrheal illness in children younger than 5 years.[128] A cohort study from Europe of 2928 children younger than 5 years with more than 3 loose stools per day for more than 2 weeks found 43.4% of stool samples were positive for rotavirus.[129] A similar incidence was found in the United States. In a study of 516 children younger than 3 years with acute gastroenteritis, the investigators found 44% had rotavirus-positive stool samples.[130] Although rotavirus is more common in children, it can also affect adults. In a 4-year prospective study of 683 adults with acute diarrhea, 14% of subjects tested positive for rotavirus.[131] There is a wide spectrum of disease severity for adults presenting with rotavirus, from mild vomiting, diarrhea, or both, to dehydration and severe systemic disease. Vomiting is present in 90% of cases and 30% of patients have a fever (>39.0°C). Finally, while the illness is usually worst in the first 24 hours it is typically mild and self-limited in immunocompetent adults.[132]

Salmonella

Salmonella infection is the most common cause of bacterial gastroenteritis in the United States, with more than 95% of subjects infected by contaminated food. Usually the source is raw or undercooked eggs, but the bacteria may also be found in meats, unpasteurized dairy products, fruits, vegetables, and peanuts.[133–137] Transmission may also occur via contact with infected animals, such as turtles.[138] *Salmonella* infection has a short incubation period of approximately 6 to 48 hours. Symptoms typically persist for 24 hours to 1 week and may include vomiting, diarrhea, crampy abdominal pain, and fever. In patients infected with *Salmonella*, resistance can be a problem and susceptibility testing is recommended. While antibiotics are thought to increase carrier states in patients with *Salmonella* infection, in selected patients, or in patients with severe illness, recommended antibiotics include third-generation cephalosporins or fluoroquinolones.[139]

Campylobacter jejuni

C jejuni is the most common cause of bacterial gastroenteritis worldwide and the second most common in the United States after *Salmonella* infection. The CDC reported an incidence of *C jejuni* infection of 13.02 per 100,000 persons in 2009.[140] The highest incidence of disease is among children younger than 5 years. Although *C jejuni* infection may be acquired from contaminated drinking water or exposure to infected farm or domestic animals, 50% of cases are associated with the handling and consumption of undercooked poultry.[141] *Campylobacter* infection develops 1 to 10 days postexposure. The illness may start with a prodrome of fever, malaise, chills, and headache before the onset of abdominal symptoms, which include watery but sometimes bloody diarrhea, abdominal pain, nausea, and vomiting. Symptoms typically resolve within 5 days, but in some cases may persist for several weeks.[141] For patients infected with *C jejuni*, treatment with erythromycin (Erythrocin) or azithromycin (Zithromax) is recommended. Fluoroquinolones are no longer advised as there have been increasing resistance patterns, possibly resulting from the usage of fluoroquinolones for farm animals.[141,142]

Campylobacter infection has also been associated with the development of postinfectious Guillain-Barré Syndrome (GBS), with an incidence of 1 per 1000 individuals. Serological surveys have found anti–*C jejuni* antibodies in patients with GBS, a finding consistent with recent infection. Further, a high proportion of patients have *C jejuni* in their stools when they develop GBS. Finally, GBS has been shown to be more severe and more likely to be irreversible when it is preceded by *C jejuni* infection.[143]

Vibrio parahaemolyticus

Whereas gastroenteritis caused by the organism *Vibrio parahaemolyticus* is common in Japan, the CDC reports a total of just 4500 cases per year in the United States.[140] The organism lives in oysters, clams, and crabs, and is transmitted by the ingestion of contaminated saltwater seafood or direct exposure of an open wound to seawater. Cases in the United States have predominantly been linked to the consumption of raw oysters.[144] *V parahaemolyticus* has a 6-hour to 4-day incubation period and presents with the sudden onset of severe watery diarrhea, vomiting, abdominal cramping, and fever. Based on susceptibility testing of an outbreak of 10,000 patients infected with *V parahaemolyticus* in Chile in 2005, it is best treated with tetracycline (Sumycin), ciprofloxacin, or chloramphenicol. Of note, investigators found the organism was universally resistant to ampicillin.[145]

Shigella

Shigella infection primarily affects people in developing countries, and the majority of cases are in children younger than 5 years.[146] The incidence of *Shigella* in the United States in 2009 was 3.99 per 100,000.[140] The bacteria are transmitted mainly through person-to-person contact but may also be acquired from food, water, flies, and feces. *Shigella* invades the cells of the colonic epithelium, and the shiga toxin induces local inflammation, which in turn produces hemorrhagic colitis. Following an incubation period from 1 to 6 days, patients develop fever, crampy abdominal pain, and diarrhea, which often contains blood and mucus. Infants, on the other hand, present more often with nonbloody stool and lack of fever.[147] Although symptoms caused by *Shigella* infection are typically self-limiting and resolve within 2 to 3 days, most clinicians treat *Shigella* with antibiotic therapy. Fluoroquinolones are the mainstays of therapy, while azithromycin, trimethoprim-sulfamethoxazole (Bactrim), ampicillin, and ceftriaxone (Rocephin) are other options.

Yersinia

Yersinia is a prominent infection worldwide, but caused only 0.32 cases per 100,000 persons in the United States in 2009.[140] A primary risk factor for acquiring *Yersinia* is the consumption of contaminated foods, in particular raw pork.[148] *Yersinia* infection presents with a gradual onset of symptoms from several days to 1 week, which include bloody diarrhea, fever, vomiting, and severe right lower quadrant abdominal pain that may mimic appendicitis. Approximately 20% of patients also present with pharyngitis.[149] Treatment regimens for *Yersinia* include trimethoprim-sulfamethoxazole, fluoroquinolones, gentamycin, tobramycin, amikacin (Amikin), or cefotaxime (Claforan). *Yersinia*-infected individuals have a risk of developing bacteremia, liver or spleen abscesses, suppurative appendicitis, peritonitis, intussusception, and toxic megacolon.

Escherichia coli

E coli infections are categorized as enterohemorrhagic (O157:H7), enterotoxigenic (traveler's diarrhea), enteropathogenic (nontoxin mediated, uses an adhesin to attach and efface intestinal cells), or enteroinvasive. *E coli* O157:H7 primarily affects children younger than 10 years and elderly patients, with an incidence of 0.99 per 100,000 persons in the United States in 2009.[140] Transmission has been linked to the consumption of undercooked beef, contaminated drinking water, unpasteurized milk,[150,151] and from fecal contamination of raw vegetables and unpasteurized apple juice.[152,153] *E coli* O157:H7 bacteria cause a hemorrhagic colitis due to a shiga-like cytotoxin that destroys the colonic microvilli. Patients infected with *E coli* may develop an acute onset of watery diarrhea, which may progress to bloody diarrhea, abdominal cramps, and vomiting. Fever is typically absent or low grade. Approximately 6% of patients with *E coli* O157:H7 infection, particularly those younger than 5 years and elderly patients, develop hemolytic uremic syndrome.[154] This risk is increased with bloody diarrhea, leukocytosis, fever, and possibly the use of antimotility agents.[155,156]

Outbreaks

Gastroenteritis outbreaks have been studied to determine their causes. One study examined patients hospitalized with community-acquired gastroenteritis in Berlin, Germany. The investigators found *Campylobacter* in 35% of specimens, norovirus in 23%, *Salmonella* in 20%, rotavirus in 15%, and a noninfectious cause in 8% of patients, supporting the need to remain diligent in looking for other causes of diarrhea even in an outbreak. In this study, length of hospital stay (median: 5.5 days) was independent of the pathogen, but was associated with patients who had underlying medical conditions.[157] Another study evaluated 29 acute gastroenteritis outbreaks in childcare centers. Stool specimens from symptomatic children and environmental surface swabs found offending pathogens included rotavirus (17% of outbreaks), norovirus (10%), astrovirus (10%), and sapovirus (7%). In 3 of the outbreaks, 10% of patients were found to have multiple viruses responsible for their infection, highlighting the importance of surveillance monitoring during these occurrences.[128]

Assessment and Diagnostic Evaluation

The duration and severity of the patient's diarrhea and vomiting should be assessed, along with their fluid intake, urine output, and overall mental status. Malnourished and immunocompromised patients are more likely to have serious outcomes. Stool cultures in the ED are typically reserved for patients with severe illness or for patients presenting with diarrhea in times of community-wide outbreaks. While fecal leukocytes are 70% sensitive and 50% specific for detecting inflammation in studies examining the infectious etiology of diarrhea, white blood cells in the stool may also be present in other conditions such as ulcerative colitis and Crohn disease.[158] Sensitivities can be increased to 83% by testing for fecal calprotectin.[159] Nonetheless, clinicians may consider sending a stool sample if there is blood or mucus in the stool, persistent diarrhea of more than 2 weeks' duration, or to help exclude an intestinal infection.

Laboratory testing for patients with vomiting and diarrhea caused by viral illnesses is typically not helpful, as these patients may not demonstrate markers of infection in their blood work or stool cultures. However, in one study of patients with known norovirus illness, investigators found leukocytosis with a neutrophil predominance was common. Furthermore, 64% of subjects tested positive for fecal leukocytes. This finding was surprising, as it had been thought that leukocytosis and stool leukocytes were rare in patients with norovirus-induced gastroenteritis.[160]

Management

The mainstay of therapy for acute gastroenteritis is supportive care. No specific antiviral therapy exists for viral gastroenteritis. Rehydration and electrolyte replacement are the most important aspects of treatment. Severely ill, immunocompromised, or very young children with suspected bacterial infections should receive empiric treatment with antibiotics.[161] To help estimate the degree of fluid loss in children, investigators in Canada have created the Clinical Dehydration Scale (CDS) to identify pediatric patients with severe dehydration. The scale assesses 4 characteristics: general appearance, eyes, mucous membranes, and tears. If all of these are normal, the score is zero, and the child is determined to have no dehydration. A score of 1 is given in each category if the child appears thirsty or restless, has slightly sunken eyes, sticky mucous membranes, or decreased tears. A score of 2 is given in each category if the child has a drowsy, limp, cold, or sweaty appearance, has very sunken eyes, dry mucous membranes, or absent tears. A CDS score of 1 to 4 indicates some dehydration, whereas a score of 5 to 8 indicates moderate to severe dehydration.[162]

According to the CDC, children weighing less than 10 kg should receive 60 to 120 mL of oral rehydration solution per episode of vomiting or diarrheal stool, and those weighing more than 10 kg should receive 120 to 240 mL oral rehydration solution in addition to their daily requirements.[28,132] The original standard WHO oral rehydration solution had an osmolality of 311 mOsm/kg; however, in 2002 the formulation was changed to a lower osmolality solution (245 mOsm/kg) with lower concentrations of glucose (75 mmol/L) and sodium (75 mEq/L) based on several studies demonstrating a reduced osmolality solution, diminished stool volume, and the duration of diarrhea.[163] Most commercial oral rehydration solutions contain 2% to 3% carbohydrate. Common household fluids such as tea, fruit juice, sports drinks, and soft drinks have too little sodium along with a higher carbohydrate and osmolality content than suggested, and should therefore be avoided when attempting to hydrate a child with diarrhea.[28,29] In children with severe dehydration (more than 10% body weight loss), intravenous fluids are recommended. A 20 mL/kg bolus of intravenous fluid is suggested except in the case of a malnourished infant, where 10 mL/kg as a starting resuscitative amount is recommended to avoid overhydration or heart failure. After the initial intravenous therapy, 100 mL/kg oral rehydration solution over 4 hours or D5½NS (dextrose 5% in 0.45% normal saline) intravenously at a rate of twice maintenance may be administered.

Suggested indications for hospital admission for children with gastroenteritis include severe dehydration, neurological involvement, toxic state or shock, inability to tolerate oral rehydration, potential for surgery, failure of treatment despite oral rehydration therapy, or uncertain diagnosis. Providers should also consider admission for children younger than 2 months, febrile infants younger than 6 months with bloody stool, children with immunodeficiency or malnutrition, or if there is an inability to take care of the child at home.[132]

SUMMARY

Patients commonly present to the ED with symptoms of vomiting, diarrhea, constipation, and gastroenteritis. While management focuses largely on supportive care, the clinician needs to be aware that some patients, particularly infants, the elderly, and immunocompromised individuals, may need more aggressive care. New medications and treatment modalities continue to be developed for these conditions, with the latest pharmaceuticals offering promise in terms of their efficacy and side effect profiles.

ACKNOWLEDGMENTS

The authors would like to gratefully acknowledge Cynthia Clendenin, Medical Editor, for her assistance in preparing this article.

REFERENCES

1. Carpenter DO. Neural mechanisms of emesis. Can J Physiol Pharmacol 1990; 68:230.
2. Pitts SR, Niska RW, Xu J, et al. National Hospital Ambulatory Medical Care Survey: 2006 emergency department summary. Natl Health Stat Report 2008; 7:1–38.
3. Klebanoff MA, Koslowe PA, Kaslow R, et al. Epidemiology of vomiting in early pregnancy. Obstet Gynecol 1985;66(5):612–6.

4. Sandler RS, Everhart JE, Donowitz M, et al. The burden of selected digestive diseases in the United States. Gastroenterology 2002;122:1500–11.
5. Heilenbach T. Nausea and vomiting. In: Marx JA, editor. Rosens's emergency medicine concepts and clinical practice. 5th edition. St. Louis (MO): Mosby; 2002. p. 180.
6. Quigley EM, Hasler WL, Parkman HP. AGA technical review on nausea and vomiting. Gastroenterology 2001;120:263–86.
7. Braude D, Soliz T, Crandall C, et al. Antiemetics in the ED: a randomized controlled trial comparing 3 common agents. Am J Emerg Med 2006;24:177–82.
8. Gilbert CJ, Ohly KV, Rosner G, et al. Randomized double-blind comparison of a prochlorperazine-based versus a metoclopramide-based antiemetic regimen in patients undergoing autologous bone marrow transplantation. Cancer 1995; 76:2330–7.
9. Oliver IN, Wolf M, Laidlaw C, et al. A randomised double-blind study of high-dose intravenous prochlorperazine versus high-dose metoclopramide as antiemetics for cancer chemotherapy. Eur J Cancer 1992;28:1798–802.
10. Jamil M, Gilani SM, Khan SA. Comparison of metoclopramide, prochlorperazine and placebo in prevention of postoperative nausea and vomiting (PONV) following tonsillectomy in young adults. J Ayub Med Coll Abbottabad 2005; 17(4):40–4.
11. Gralla RJ, Itri LM, Pisko SE, et al. Antiemetic efficacy of high-dose metoclopramide: randomized trials with placebo and prochlorperazine in patients with chemotherapy-induced nausea and vomiting. N Engl J Med 1981;305:905–9.
12. Ernst AA, Weiss SJ, Park S, et al. Prochlorperazine versus promethazine for uncomplicated nausea and vomiting in the emergency department: a randomized, double-blind clinical trial. Ann Emerg Med 2000;36:89–94. Grade A.
13. Friedmann BW, Esses D, Solorzano C, et al. A randomized controlled trial of prochlorperazine versus metoclopramide for treatment of acute migraine. Ann Emerg Med 2008;52(4):399–406.
14. Gattera JA, Charles BG, Williams GM, et al. A retrospective study of risk factors of akathisia in terminally ill patients. J Pain Symptom Manage 1994;9:454–61.
15. Olsen JC, Keng JA, Clark JA. Frequency of adverse reactions to prochlorperazine in the ED. Am J Emerg Med 2000;18:609–11.
16. Vinson DR. Diphenhydramine in the treatment of akathisia induced by prochlorperazine. J Emerg Med 2004;26:265–70. Grade B.
17. Patel MM, Pitts SR. Pharmacotherapeutic approach to nausea and vomiting in the emergency department [abstract 113]. In: 2003 SAEM annual meeting abstracts. Acad Emerg Med 2003;10:460.
18. Koa LW, Kirk MA, Evers SJ, et al. Droperidol, QT prolongation, and sudden death: what is the evidence. Ann Emerg Med 2003;41:546–58.
19. Marty M, Kleisbauer JP, Fournel P, et al. Is Navoban (tropisetron) as effective as Zofran (ondansetron) in cisplatin-induced emesis? The French Navoban Study Group. Anticancer Drugs 1995;6(Suppl 1):15.
20. Hesketh P, Navari R, Grote T, et al. Double-blind, randomized comparison of the antiemetic efficacy of intravenous dolasetron mesylate and intravenous ondansetron in the prevention of acute cisplatin-induced emesis in patients with cancer. Dolasetron Comparative Chemotherapy-induced Emesis Prevention Group. J Clin Oncol 1996;14:2242.
21. Navari R, Candara D, Hesketh P, et al. Comparative clinical trial of granisetron and ondansetron in the prophylaxis of cisplatin-induced emesis. The Granisetron Study Group. J Clin Oncol 1995;13:1242.

22. Saito M, Aogi K, Sekine I, et al. Palonosetron plus dexamethasone versus granisetron plus dexamethasone for prevention of nausea and vomiting during chemotherapy: a double blind, double dummy, randomized, comparative phase III trial. Lancet Oncol 2009;10:115.

23. Aapro M. 5-HT(3)-receptor antagonists in the management of nausea and vomiting in cancer and cancer treatment. Oncology 2005;69(2):97–109.

24. Olver IN. Update on anti-emetics for chemotherapy induced emesis. Intern Med J 2005;35:478–81.

25. Barrett TW, DiPersio DM, Jenkins CA, et al. A randomized, placebo-controlled trial of ondansetron, metoclopramide, and promethazine in adults. Am J Emerg Med 2010. [Epub ahead of print]. DOI:10.1016/j.ajem.2009.09.028.

26. Braude D, Crandall C. Ondansetron versus promethazine to treat acute undifferentiated nausea in the emergency department: a randomized, double-blind, non-inferiority trial. Acad Emerg Med 2008;15:209–15. Grade A.

27. Patanwala AE, Amini R, Rosen P. Antiemetic therapy for nausea and vomiting in the emergency department. J Emerg Med 2010;39(3):330–6.

28. King CK, Glass R, Bresee JS, et al. Managing acute gastroenteritis among children: oral re-hydration, maintenance, and nutritional therapy. MMWR Recomm Rep 2003;52(RR–16):1–16. Grade A.

29. American Academy of Pediatrics, Provisional Committee on Quality Improvement and Subcommittee on Acute Gastroenteritis. Practice parameter: the management of acute gastroenteritis in young children. Pediatrics 1996;97:424–35.

30. Spandorfer PR, Alessandrini EA, Joffe MD, et al. Oral versus intravenous re-hydration of moderately dehydrated children: A randomized, controlled trial. Pediatrics 2005;115:295–301. Grade A.

31. Reis EC, Goepp JG, Katz S, et al. Barriers to use of oral re-hydration therapy. Pediatrics 1994;93:708–11.

32. Reeves JJ, Shannon MW, Fleisher GR. Ondansetron decreases vomiting associated with acute gastroenteritis: a randomized, controlled trial. Pediatrics 2002;109:e62. Grade A.

33. Freedman SB, Adler M, Seshadri R, et al. Oral ondansetron for gastroenteritis in a pediatric emergency department. N Engl J Med 2006;354:1698–705. Grade A.

34. Rossland G, Hepps TS, McQuillan KK. The role of oral ondansetron in children with vomiting as a result of acute gastritis/gastroenteritis who have failed oral re-hydration therapy: a randomized controlled trial. Ann Emerg Med 2008;52:22–9. e6. Grade A.

35. WHO Global water supply and sanitation assessment 2000 report. World Health Organization. Geneva (Switzerland). Available at: http://www.who.int/docstore/water_sanitation_health/Globassessment/Global1.htm#1.1, Accessed December 4, 2009.

36. Theilman NM, Guerrant RI. Acute infectious diarrhea. N Engl J Med 2004;350(1):38–47.

37. Payne CM, Fass R, Bernstein H, et al. Pathogenesis of diarrhea in the adult: diagnostic challenges and life-threatening conditions. Eur J Gastroenterol Hepatol 2006;18:1047–51.

38. Pont SJ, Carpenter LF, Griffin MR, et al. Trends in healthcare usage attributable to diarrhea, 1995-2004. J Pediatr 2008;153(6):777–82.

39. Pont SJ, Grijalva CG, Griffin MR, et al. National rates of diarrhea-associated ambulatory visits in children. J Pediatr 2009;155(1):56–61.

40. Sanders JW, Putnam SD, Riddle MS, et al. Military importance of diarrhea: lessons from the middle east. Curr Opin Gastroenterol 2004;21:9–14.

41. Sabol VK, Carlson KK. Diarrhea: applying research to bedside practice. AACN Adv Crit Care 2007;18(1):32–44.
42. Schroeder MS. *Clostridium difficile*-associated diarrhea. Am Fam Physician 2005;71(5):921–8.
43. Kyne L, Hammel MB, Polayaram R, et al. Health care costs and mortality associated with nosocomial diarrhea due to *Clostridium difficile*. Clin Infect Dis 2002; 34(3):346–53.
44. Hurley BW, Nguyen CC. The spectrum of pseudomembranous enterocolitis and antibiotic-associated diarrhea. Arch Intern Med 2002;162:2177–84.
45. Martirosian G, Szczesny A, Cohen S, et al. Analysis of *Clostridium difficile*-associated diarrhea among patients hospitalized in tertiary care academic hospital. Diagn Microbiol Infect Dis 2005;52:153–5.
46. Naaber P, Mikelsaar M. Interactions between lactobacilli and antibiotic-associated diarrhea. Adv Appl Microbiol 2004;54:231–60.
47. Klein EJ, Boster DR, Stapp JR, et al. Diarrhea etiology in a children's hospital emergency department: a prospective cohort study. Clin Infect Dis 2006;43: 807–13. Grade B.
48. Prere MF, Bacrie SC, Baron O, et al. Bacterial etiology of diarrhoea in young children: high prevalence of enteropathogenic *Escherichia coli* (EPEC) not belonging to the classical EPEC serogroups. Pathol Biol 2006;54:600–2.
49. Bauer MP, Goorhuis A, Koster T. Community-onset *Clostridium difficile*-associated diarrhoea not associated with antibiotic usage. Neth J Med 2008;66(5):207–11.
50. Dial S, Alrasadi K, Monoukian C. Risk of *Clostridium difficile* diarrhea among hospital inpatients prescribed proton pump inhibitors: cohort and case-control studies. CMAJ 2004;171(1):33–6.
51. Bouza E, Burillo A, Munoz P. Antimicrobial therapy of *Clostridium difficile*-associated diarrhea. Med Clin North Am 2006;90:1141–63.
52. Maroo S, Lamont JT. Recurrent *Clostridium difficile*. Gastroenterology 2006;130: 1311–6.
53. Adachi JA, Jiang ZG, Mathewson JJ, et al. Enteroaggregative *Escherichia coli* as a major etiologic agent in traveler's diarrhea in 3 regions of the world. Clin Infect Dis 2001;32:1706–9.
54. Gupta SK, Keck J, Ram PK, et al. Analysis of data gaps pertaining to enterotoxigenic *Escherichia coli* infections in low and medium human development index countries, 1984–2005. Epidemiol Infect 2008;136:721–38.
55. Richardson M, Elliman D, Maguire H, et al. Evidence base of incubation periods, periods of infectiousness and exclusion policies for the control of communicable diseases in schools and preschools. Pediatr Infect Dis J 2001; 20(4):380–91.
56. Mera V, Lopez T, Serralta J. Take traveller's diarrhoea to heart. Travel Med Infect Dis 2007;5:202–3.
57. Juarez J, Abramo TJ. Diarrhea in the recent traveler. Pediatr Emerg Care 2006; 22(8):602–9.
58. Taylor DN, Bourgeois AL, Ericsson CD, et al. A randomized, double-blind, multicenter study of rifaximin compared with placebo and with ciprofloxacin in the treatment of traveler's diarrhea. Am J Trop Med Hyg 2006;74(6):1060–6. Grade A.
59. Huang DB, Okhuysen PC, Jiang Z, et al. Enteroaggressive *Escherichia coli*: an emerging enteric pathogen. Am J Gastroenterol 2004;99:383–9.
60. Qadri F, Svennerholm A, Faruque AS, et al. Enterotoxigenic *Escherichia coli* in developing countries: epidemiology, microbiology, clinical features, treatment, and prevention. Clin Microbiol Rev 2005;18(3):465–83.

61. Huang DB, Mohanty A, DuPont HL, et al. A review of an emerging enteric pathogen: enteroaggregative *Escherichia coli*. J Med Microbiol 2006;55:1303–11.
62. DuPont HL, Jiang Z, Okhuysen PC, et al. A randomized, double-blind, placebo-controlled trial of rifaximin to prevent traveler's diarrhea. Ann Intern Med 2005; 142(10):805–12. Grade A.
63. Abubakar II, Aliyu SH, Arumugam C, et al. Prevention and treatment of cryptosporidiosis in immunocompromised patients [review]. Cochrane Database Syst Rev 2007;1:CD004932. DOI:10.1002/14651858.CD004932.pub2. Grade A.
64. Cohen MB, Natario JP, Bernstein DI, et al. Prevalence of diarrheagenic *Escherichia coli* in acute childhood enteritis: a prospective controlled study. J Pediatr 2005;146:54–61. Grade B.
65. Soares-Weiser K, Goldberg E, Tamimi G, et al. Rotavirus vaccine for preventing diarrhoea. Cochrane Database Syst Rev 2004;1:CD002848. DOI:10.1002/14651858.CD002848.pub2. Grade A.
66. Holtz LR, Neill MA, Tarr PI. Acute bloody diarrhea: a medical emergency for patients of all ages. Gastroenterology 2009;136:1887–98.
67. Li ST, Klein EJ, Tarr PI. Parental management of childhood diarrhea. Clin Pediatr 2009;48(3):295–303.
68. Sentongo TA. The use of oral re-hydration solutions in children and adults. Curr Gastroenterol Rep 2004;6:307–13.
69. Murphy CK, Hahn S, Volmink J. Reduced osmolarity oral re-hydration solution for treating cholera. Cochrane Database Syst Rev 2004;4:CD003754. DOI: 10.1002/14651858.CD003754.pub2.
70. Mounts AW, Holman RC, Clarke MJ, et al. Trends in hospitalizations associated with gastroenteritis among adults in the United States, 1979–1995. Epidemiol Infect 1999;123(1):1–8.
71. Trinh C, Prabhakar K. Diarrheal disease in the elderly. Clin Geriatr Med 2007;23: 833–56.
72. Chen EH, Shofer FS, Dean AJ, et al. Derivation of a clinical prediction rule for evaluating patients with abdominal pain and diarrhea. Am J Emerg Med 2008;26:450–3. Grade B.
73. Bruyn G. Diarrhoea in adults. BMJ 2008;03:1–38.
74. Bourne S, Petrie C. The management of acute diarrhoea in a healthy adult population deploying on military operations. J R Army Med Corps 2008;154(3):163–7.
75. Nwachukwu CE, Okebe JU. Antimotility agents for chronic diarrhoea in people with HIV/AIDS. Cochrane Database Syst Rev 2008;4:CD005644. DOI: 10:1002/14651858.CD00005644.pub2. Grade A.
76. Riddle MS, Arnold S, Tribble DR. Effect of adjunctive loperamide in combination with antibiotics on treatment outcomes in traveler's diarrhea: a systematic review and meta analysis. Clin Infect Dis 2008;47:1007–14. Grade A.
77. Harris C, Wilkinson F, Mazza D, et al. Evidence based guideline for the management of diarrhoea with or without vomiting in children. Aust Fam Physician 2008; 37(6):22–9.
78. Zamir D, Weiler Z, Kogan E, et al. Single-dose quinolone treatment in acute gastroenteritis. J Clin Gastroenterol 2006;40:186–90. Grade B.
79. Hickson M, D'Souza AL, Muthu N, et al. Use of probiotic *Lactobacillus* preparation to prevent diarrhoea associated with antibiotics: randomized double blind placebo controlled trial. BMJ 2007;335:80. Grade A.
80. Hamlton-Miller JM. Probiotics and prebiotics in the elderly. Postgrad Med J 2004;80:447–51.

81. Allen SJ, Okoko B, Martinez EG, et al. Probiotics for treating infectious diarrhea. Cochrane Database Syst Rev 2003;4:CD003048. DOI:10.1002/14651858. CD003048.pub2. Grade A.

82. Clasen T, Parra GG, Boisson S, et al. Household-based ceramic water filters for the prevention of diarrhea: a randomized, controlled trial of a pilot program in Columbia. Am J Trop Med Hyg 2005;73(4):790–5. Grade A.

83. Clasen TF, Brown J, Collin S, et al. Reducing diarrhea through the use of household-based ceramic water filers: a randomized, controlled trial in rural Bolivia. Am J Trop Med Hyg 2004;70(6):651–7. Grade A.

84. Crump JA, Otieno PO, Slutsker L, et al. Household based treatment of drinking water with flocculant-disinfectant for preventing diarrhoea in areas with turbid source water in rural western Kenya: cluster randomized controlled trial. BMJ 2005;331:478. Grade B.

85. Doocy S, Burnham G. Point-of-use water treatment and diarrhoea reduction in the emergency context: an effectiveness trial in Liberia. Trop Med Int Health 2006;11(10):1542–52.

86. Luby SP, Agboatwalla M, Painter J, et al. Effect of intensive handwashing promotion on childhood diarrhea in high-risk communities in Pakistan: a randomized controlled trial. JAMA 2004;291(21):2547–54. Grade A.

87. Clasen TF, Roberts IG, Rabie T, et al. Interventions to improve water quality for preventing diarrhoea. Cochrane Database Syst Rev 2006;3:CD004794. DOI: 10.1002/14651858.CD004794.pub2. Grade A.

88. Cash BD, Chang L, Sabesin S. Update on the management of adults with idiopathic chronic constipation. J Fam Pract 2007;56(Suppl 6):S1–8. Grade B.

89. Loening-Baucke V. Prevalence, symptoms and outcome of constipation in infants and toddlers. J Pediatr 2005;146(3):359–63.

90. Loening-Baucke V, Swidsinski A. Constipation as cause of acute abdominal pain in children. J Pediatr 2007;151(6):666–9.

91. Bradley C, Kennedy C, Turcea A. Constipation in pregnancy. Obstet Gynecol 2007;110(6):1351–7.

92. Leung FW. Etiologic factors of chronic constipation-review of the scientific evidence. Dig Dis Sci 2007;52(2):313–6.

93. Khaikin M, Wexner SD. Treatment strategies in obstructed defecation and fecal incontinence. World J Gastroenterol 2006;12(20):3168–73.

94. McCallum I, Ong S, Mercer-Jones M. Chronic constipation in adults. BMJ 2009; 338:b831.

95. Varma MG, Hart SL, Brown JS, et al. Obstructive defecation in middle-aged women. Dig Dis Sci 2008;53(10):2702–9.

96. Ringel Y, Sperber AD, Drossman DA. Irritable bowel syndrome. Annu Rev Med 2001;52:319–38.

97. Drossman DA, Zhiming L, Adruzzi E, et al. US householders survey of functional gastrointestinal disorders: prevalence, sociodemography, and health impact. Dig Dis Sci 1993;38:1569.

98. Brandt LJ, Chey WD, Foxx-Orenstein AE, et al, American College of Gastroenterology Task Force of Irritable Bowel Syndrome. An evidence-based position statement on the management of irritable bowel syndrome. Am J Gastroenterol 2009;104(Suppl):S1. Grade A.

99. American Gastroenterology Association. American Gastroenterology Association medical position statement: irritable bowel syndrome. Gastroenterology 2002;123:2105.

100. Longstreth GF, Thompson GW, Chey WD, et al. Functional bowel disorders. Gastroenterology 2006;130(5):1480–91.
101. Talley NJ, Kellow JE, Boyce P, et al. Antidepressant therapy (imipramine and citalopram) for irritable bowel syndrome: a double-blind, randomized, placebo-controlled trial. Dig Dis Sci 2008;53(1):108–15. Grade A.
102. Pimentel M, Park S, Mirocha J, et al. The effect of a nonabsorbed oral antibiotic (Rifaximin) on the symptoms of the irritable bowel syndrome. Ann Intern Med 2006;145:557–63.
103. American College of Gastroenterology Chronic Constipation Task Force. An evidence-based approach to the management of chronic constipation in North America. Am J Gastroenterol 2005;100(Suppl 1):S1–4. Grade A.
104. Reuchlin-Vroklage LM, Bierma-Zeinstra S, Benninga MA, et al. Diagnostic value of abdominal radiography in constipated children. Arch Pediatr Adolesc Med 2005;159(7):671–8. Grade B.
105. Bleser SD. Chronic constipation: let symptom type and severity direct treatment. J Fam Pract 2006;55(7):587–93. Grade B.
106. Brandt LJ, Prather CM, Quigley EM, et al. Systematic review on the management of chronic constipation in North America. Am J Gastroenterol 2005; 100(Suppl 1):S5–21.
107. Xing JH, Soffer E. Adverse effects of laxatives. Dis Colon Rectum 2001;44: 1201–9.
108. McRorie JW, Daggy BP, Morel JG. Psyllium is superior to docusate sodium for treatment of chronic constipation. Aliment Pharmacol Ther 1998;12:491–7. Grade B.
109. Wald A. Constipation in the primary care setting: current concepts and misconceptions. Am J Med 2006;119(9):736–9.
110. DiPalma JA, Cleveland MB, McGowan J, et al. A comparison of polyethylene glycol laxative and placebo for relief of constipation from constipating medications. South Med J 2007;100(11):1085–90. Grade A.
111. Hawley PH. A comparison of sennosides-based bowel protocols with and without docusate in hospitalized patients with cancer. J Palliat Med 2008; 11(4):575–81. Grade B.
112. Johanson JF, Gargano MA, Holland PC, et al. Phase III patient assessments of the effects of lubiprostone, a chloride channel-2 (ClC-2) activator, for the treatment of constipation. Presented at: American College of Gastroenterology 70th Annual Scientific Meeting; October 31-November 2, 2005; Honolulu, Hawaii. Abstract 899. Am J Gastroenterol 2005;100(Suppl 9):S329–30.
113. Phillips B. Towards evidence based medicine for paediatricians. Arch Dis Child 2005;90(11):1194–5.
114. Voskuijl W, De Lorijn F, Verwijs W, et al. PEG 3350 (Transipeg) versus lactulose in the treatment of childhood functional constipation: a double blind, randomized, controlled, multicentre trial. Gut 2004;53(11):1590–4. Grade A.
115. Thomson M. A placebo controlled crossover study of movicol in the treatment of childhood constipation. J Pediatr Gastroenterol Nutr 2004;39(Suppl 1):S16. Grade B.
116. Gremse DA, Hixon J, Crutchfield A. Comparison of polyethylene glycol 3350 and lactulose for treatment of chronic constipation in children. Clin Pediatr 2002;41(4):225–9. Grade B.
117. Youssef NN, Peters JM, Henderson W, et al. Dose response of PEG 3350 for the treatment of childhood fecal impaction. J Pediatr 2002;141(3):410–4. Grade B.

118. Nurko S, Youssef Nader N, Sabri M, et al. PEG3350 in the treatment of childhood constipation: a multicenter, double-blinded, placebo-controlled trial. J Pediatr 2008;153(2):254–61. Grade A.
119. Pijpers MAM, Tabbers MM, Benninga MA, et al. Currently recommended treatments of childhood constipation are not evidence based: a systematic literature review on the effect of laxative treatment and dietary measures. Arch Dis Child 2009;94(2):117–31. Grade B.
120. Musher DM, Musher BL. Contagious acute gastrointestinal infections. N Engl J Med 2004;351(23):2417–27.
121. Gangarosa RE, Glass RI, Lew JF, et al. Hospitalizations involving gastroenteritis in the United States, 1985: the special burden of the disease among the elderly. Am J Epidemiol 1992;135:281–90.
122. McConnochie KM, Conners GP, Lu E, et al. How commonly are children hospitalized for dehydration eligible for care in alternative settings? Arch Pediatr Adolesc Med 1999;153(12):1233–41.
123. Dolin R. Noroviruses-challenges to control. N Engl J Med 2007;357(11): 1072–3.
124. Glass RI, Parashar UD, Estes MK. Norovirus gastroenteritis. N Engl J Med 2009; 361(18):1776–85.
125. Atmar RL, Estes MK. The epidemiologic and clinical importance of norovirus infection. Gastroenterol Clin North Am 2006;35(2):275–90, viii.
126. Siebenga JJ, Beersma MFC, Vennema H, et al. High prevalence of prolonged norovirus shedding and illness among hospitalized patients: a model for in vivo molecular evolution. J Infect Dis 2008;198(7):994–1001.
127. Turcios-Ruiz RM, Axelrod P, St John K, et al. Outbreak of necrotizing enterocolitis caused by norovirus in a neonatal intensive care unit. J Pediatr 2008;153(3): 339–44.
128. Lyman W, Walsh J, Kotch J. Prospective study of etiologic agents of acute gastroenteritis outbreaks in child care centers. J Pediatr 2009;154(2):253–7.
129. Forster J, Guarino A, Parez N, et al. Hospital-based surveillance to estimate the burden of rotavirus gastroenteritis among European children younger than 5 years of age. Pediatrics 2009;123(3):e393–e400.
130. Payne DC, Staat MA, Edwards KM, et al. Active, population-based surveillance for severe rotavirus gastroenteritis in children in the United States. Pediatrics 2008;122(6):1235.
131. Nakajima H, Nakegomi T, Kamisawa T, et al. Winter seasonality and rotavirus diarrhoea in adults. Lancet 2001;357(9272):1950.
132. D'Agostino J. Considerations in assessing the clinical course and severity of rotavirus gastroenteritis. Clin Pediatr 2006;45(3):203–12. Grade B.
133. Trepka MJ, Archer JR, Altekrus SF, et al. An increase in sporadic and outbreak-associated *Salmonella enteritidis* infections in Wisconsin: the role of eggs. J Infect Dis 1999;180(4):1214–9.
134. CDC. Multistate outbreak of *Salmonella typhimurium* infections associated with eating ground beef—United States, 2004. MMWR Morb Mortal Wkly Rep 2006; 55(7):180–2.
135. Cody SH, Abbott SL, Marfin AA, et al. Two outbreaks of multidrug-resistant *Salmonella* serotype *typhimurium* DT104 infections linked to raw-milk cheese in Northern California. JAMA 1999;281(19):1805–10.
136. Van Beneden CA, Keene WE, Strang RA, et al. Multinational outbreak of *Salmonella enterica* serotype Newport infections due to contaminated alfalfa sprouts. JAMA 1999;281(2):158–62.

137. Kirk MD, Little CL, Lem M, et al. An outbreak due to peanuts in their shell caused by *Salmonella enterica* serotypes Stanley and Newport—sharing molecular information to solve international outbreaks. Epidemiol Infect 2004;132(4): 571–7.

138. Harris JR, Bergmire-Sweat D, Schlegel JH, et al. Multistate outbreak of salmonella infections associated with small turtle exposure, 2007–2008. Pediatrics 2009;124(5):1388–94.

139. Choice of antibacterial drugs. Treat Guidel Med Lett 2007;5(57):33–50 Grade B.

140. CDC. Preliminary FoodNet data on the incidence of infection with pathogens transmitted commonly through food—10 states, 2009. MMWR Morb Mortal Wkly Rep 2010;59(14):418–22.

141. Galanis E. *Campylobacter* and bacterial gastroenteritis. CMAJ 2007;177(6): 570–1. Grade B.

142. Smith KE, Besser JM, Hedberg CW. Quinolone-resistant campylobacter jejuni infections in Minnesota, 1992-1998. Investigation Team. N Engl J Med 1999; 340(20):1525–32. Grade B.

143. Allos BM. Association between *Campylobacter* infection and Guillian-Barre syndrome. J Infect Dis 1997;176(Suppl 2):S125–8.

144. McLaughlin JB, DePaola A, Bopp CA, et al. Outbreak of *Vibrio parahaemolyticus* gastroenteritis associated with Alaskan oysters. N Engl J Med 2005; 353(14):1463–70.

145. Heitmann I, Jofre L, Hormazabal JC. Review and guidelines for treatment of diarrhea caused by *Vibrio parahaemolyticus*. Rev Chilena Infectol 2005;22(2): 131–40 [in Spanish]. Grade B.

146. Ashkenazi S. *Shigella* infections in children: new insights. Semin Pediatr Infect Dis 2004;15(4):246–52.

147. Huskins WC, Griffiths JK, Faruque AS. Shigellosis in neonates and young infants. J Pediatr 1994;125(1):14–22.

148. Tauxe RV, Vandepitte J, Wauters G, et al. *Yersinia enterocolitica* infections and pork: the missing link. Lancet 1987;1(8542):1129–32.

149. Ostroff SM, Kapperud G, Lassen J. Clinical features of sporadic *Yersinia enterocolitica* infections in Norway. J Infect Dis 1992;166(4):812–7.

150. Mead PS, Finelli L, Lambert-Fair MA. Risk factors for sporadic infection with *Escherichia coli* O157:H7. Arch Intern Med 1997;157(2):204–8.

151. CDC. *Escherichia coli* O157:H7 infections in children associated with raw milk and raw colostrum from cows—California, 2006. MMWR Morb Mortal Wkly Rep 2008;57(23):625–8.

152. Mohle-Boetani JC, Farrar JA, Werner SB, et al. *Escherichia coli* O157 and *Salmonella* infections associated with sprouts in California, 1996-1998. Ann Intern Med 2001;135(4):239–47.

153. Cody SH, Glynn MK, Farrar JA. An outbreak of *Escherichia coli* O157:H7 infection from unpasteurized commercial apple juice. Ann Intern Med 1999;130(3): 202–9.

154. Boyce TG, Swerdlow DL, Griffin PM, et al. *Escherichia coli* O157:H7 and the hemolytic-uremic syndrome. N Engl J Med 1995;333(6):364–8.

155. Bell BP, Griffin PM, Lozano P. Predictors of hemolytic uremic syndrome in children during a large outbreak of *Escherichia coli* O157:H7 infections. Pediatrics 1997;100(1):E12.

156. Dundas S, Todd WT, Stewart AI, et al. The central Scotland *Escherichia coli* O157:H7 outbreak: risk factors for the hemolytic uremic syndrome and death among hospitalized patients. Clin Infect Dis 2001;33(7):923–31.

157. Jansen A, Stark K, Kunkel J, et al. Aetiology of community-acquired, acute gastroenteritis in hospitalised adults: a prospective cohort study. BMC Infect Dis 2008;8:143–50. Grade B.
158. Headstrom PD, Surawicz CM. Chronic diarrhea. Clin Gastroenterol Hepatol 2005;3(8):734–7.
159. Shastri YM, Bergis D, Povse N, et al. Prospective multicenter study evaluating fecal calprotectin in adult acute bacterial diarrhea. Am J Med 2008;121(12): 1099–106.
160. Yu C, Baker S, Morse LJ, et al. Clinical and laboratory findings in individuals with acute norovirus disease. Arch Intern Med 2007;167(17):1903–5.
161. Amieva M. Important bacterial gastrointestinal pathogens in children: a pathogenesis perspective. Pediatr Clin North Am 2005;52(3):749–77, vi. Grade B.
162. Goldman RD, Friedman JN, Parkin PC. Validation of the clinical dehydration scale for children with acute gastroenteritis. Pediatrics 2008;122(3):545–9. Grade B.
163. Hahn S, Kim Y, Garner P. Reduced osmolarity oral re-hydration solution for treating dehydration due to diarrhoea in children: systematic review. BMJ 2001; 323(7304):81–5. Grade A.

Gastrointestinal Bleeding

Ritu Kumar, MD, Angela M. Mills, MD*

KEYWORDS

- Gastrointestinal bleeding • Emergency department
- Gastrointestinal hemorrhage • Peptic ulcer disease

Gastrointestinal bleeding (GIB) is a common problem encountered in the emergency department (ED) and a significant cause of morbidity and mortality. The overall mortality rate is approximately 10% and has not changed significantly in the past several decades.[1,2] The significant morbidity and mortality associated with GIB requires clinicians to be equipped with the skills to promptly diagnose, aggressively resuscitate, risk stratify, and request timely consultations. For hemodynamically or clinically unstable patients, early resuscitative measures focus on infusion of intravenous fluids or transfusion of blood products to reverse the direct consequences of bleeding; prevent end-organ damage, such as hypoxia or prerenal azotemia; and promote hemostasis.[3] Although controversy exists regarding the management of gastrointestinal hemorrhage, the use of a treatment algorithm enables emergency medicine physicians to effectively care for these patients. This article reviews the initial assessment, management, differential diagnosis, and treatment modalities available for patients presenting to an ED with GIB.

EPIDEMIOLOGY

Gastrointestinal hemorrhage may be divided into upper GIB (UGIB) and lower GIB (LGIB) as defined by bleeding originating proximal or distal to the ligament of Treitz. Both UGIB and LGIB are more common in men and older adults.[2,4,5] In general, UGIB is more common, accounting for a greater proportion of admissions in adults. The annual incidence for UGIB is estimated at 50 to 150 per 100,000 population,[2,6] whereas that for LGIB is lower, at approximately 20 to 27 per 100,000 population.[5,6] The mortality associated with UGIB is estimated to be anywhere from 6% to 13%, and even with the advent of endoscopic intervention, this mortality rate has not substantially decreased within the past 30 years.[7] This is believed secondary to the increased number of older adults presenting with GIB, who are often on antiplatelet and anticoagulation agents and often have other comorbidities associated with their disease.[3]

Department of Emergency Medicine, University of Pennsylvania School of Medicine, 3400 Spruce Street, Ground Ravdin, Philadelphia, PA 19104, USA
* Corresponding author.
E-mail address: millsa@uphs.upenn.edu

Emerg Med Clin N Am 29 (2011) 239–252
doi:10.1016/j.emc.2011.01.003
0733-8627/11/$ – see front matter © 2011 Elsevier Inc. All rights reserved.

emed.theclinics.com

Other independent markers of increased morbidity and mortality associated with GIB include the requirement of more than 5 units of packed red blood cells, hemodynamic instability, recurrent bleeding, endoscopic stigmata of recent hemorrhage, melena or hematochezia, esophageal varices, and bloody nasogastric aspirate.[1,8,9] In general, most cases of GIB are self-limited, with the majority of patients having only one episode of bleeding.[6] Compared with UGIB, LGIB has a decreased mortality rate of approximately 4%.[5] Bleeds originating from the colon require fewer blood transfusions than those originating from the small intestine (36% vs 64%).[10] In general, patients with LGIB are more likely to have higher hemoglobin levels (84% vs 61%) and less likely to go into shock (19% vs 35%).[10,11]

ETIOLOGY OF UGIB

There are several causes of UGIB, with age playing a role in determining potential etiologies. The elderly are more likely to present with bleeds secondary to peptic ulcer disease, esophagitis, and gastritis. Together these account for 70% to 90% of hospital admissions for UGIB in this age group.[12] Younger patients account for a larger percentage of cases secondary to causes such as Mallory-Weiss tears, gastrointestinal varices, and gastropathy, which are all less likely in older adults. Common causes of UGIB with prevalence are summarized in **Table 1**.

Peptic ulcer disease (PUD) is the most common cause of UGIB, accounting for approximately half of all cases.[3] PUD occurs secondary to erosion of the gastric or duodenal tissue with symptoms of a gnawing epigastric discomfort and pain that worsens after eating and with lying down. Nausea and vomiting, along with anorexia and concomitant weight loss, are symptoms that are consistent with a diagnosis of PUD. Symptoms are often treated with the use of a proton pump inhibitor or H_2 receptor antagonist. Infection with helicobacter pylori is the most common cause of PUD, with nonsteroidal anti-inflammatory drug (NSAID) use coming in second. Aspirin use, history of PUD, smoking, and alcohol use are all risk factors for PUD.[13]

Table 1
Major causes of upper gastrointestinal bleeding

Causes	Prevalence
Peptic ulcer disease	55%
Gastric ulcer	21.3%–23.1%
Duodenal ulcer	13.9%–24.3%
Esophageal varices	10.3%–23.1%
Esophagitis	3.7%–6.3%
Duodenitis	3.7%–5.8%
Gastritis	4.7%–23.4%
Mallory-Weiss tears	5%–10.2%
Angiodysplasia	6%
Neoplasm	2%–4.9%
Stomal ulcer	1.8%
Esophageal ulcer	1.7%
Dieulafoy lesion	1%

Data from Cappell M, Friedel D. Initial management of acute upper gastrointestinal bleeding: from initial evaluation up to gastrointestinal endoscopy. Med Clin North Am 2008;92:491–509.

Zollinger-Ellison syndrome, a disorder resulting in excess production of the hormone gastrin, is an uncommon cause of PUD. Although the overall prevalence of PUD as a cause of UGIB has decreased, an increase in PUD incidence secondary to NSAID use is noted in the elderly.[14]

Varices are responsible for approximately 10% to 25% of UGIB overall and 60% of UGIB in patients with cirrhosis.[15] Cirrhotic patients develop portal hypertension secondary to blockage of the portal venous system, which lends itself to portosystemic collaterals, such as varices, and variceal bleeding. In patients with liver disease, the incidence of new esophageal varices is linear over time with a rate of approximately 9% per year.[16] In addition, 30% of patients with portal hypertension and cirrhosis have bleeding secondary to these varices. Patients with portal hypertension–related bleeding, which includes esophageal and gastric varices and portal hypertensive gastropathy, have mortality rates of greater than 50% as compared with a 4% rate with bleeding from PUD.[2] Other common causes of UGI bleeds are inflammatory pathologies, such as gastritis and duodenitis, and Mallory-Weiss tears. Less common causes include angiodysplasia and Dieulafoy lesions, which are large tortuous arterioles in the gastric wall that can erode and bleed.[3]

ETIOLOGY OF LGIB

LGIB has decreased morbidity in comparison to UGIB and is often self-limited. Similar to UGIB, there are several factors that may be responsible for the bleed. The most common cause of LGIB is colonic diverticulosis, which presents with painless hematochezia. It is estimated that more than two-thirds of the population over the age of 80 are affected by diverticular disease. Approximately 60% of diverticular bleeds are found in the left aspect of the colon on colonoscopy.[17] The recurrence rate of diverticular bleeds is 25% after 4 years.[5]

After colonic diverticulosis, angiodysplasia, colitis, and postpolypectomy bleeding follow in frequency of LGIB causes. Angiodysplasia is responsible for both acute and chronic LGIB but those are often asymptomatic because they do not frequently bleed. Patients taking NSAIDs, aspirin, and anticoagulants as well as coagulopathic patients or patients with platelet dysfunction are more likely to present with LGIB from angiodysplasia.[17]

Although there are poor data on the incidence of ischemic colitis, it is proposed that the disease is becoming more prevalent secondary to an increase in elderly patients with cardiovascular disease.[17] Ischemic colitis is caused by a decrease in mesenteric blood flow as a result of hypotension or vasospasm, and patients often present with sudden onset of abdominal pain followed by diarrhea mixed with blood or hematochezia. LGIB is also a common manifestation of colitis secondary to inflammatory bowel disease but uncommonly leads to acute major gastrointestinal hemorrhage, with ulcerative colitis and Crohn's disease responsible for 0.1% and 1.2% of massive bleeds, respectively.[18] **Table 2** lists common causes of LGIB with prevalence.

Determining the source of LGIB can be a challenging task for clinicians. Although most lesions responsible for LGIB are due to colonic or anorectal disease, diagnosis may be difficult because LGIB may be intermittent and may originate from the small intestine or an upper tract source of brisk bleeding. Lower tract sources of GIB have a rebleeding rate of approximately 10% to 20%, require operative intervention in 10% to 15% of cases, and have a mortality rate of 4%.[2,5,6] Chronic LGIB is responsible for 18% to 30% of patients with iron deficiency anemia presenting to the ED.[17]

Table 2 Major causes of lower gastrointestinal bleeding	
Causes	Prevalence
Diverticular disease	17%–40%
Angiodysplasia	9%–21%
Colitis	2%–30%
Inflammatory bowel disease	—
Ischemia	—
Infectious	—
Radiation	—
Postpolypectomy bleeding	11%–14%
Anorectal disease	4%–10%
Hemorrhoids	—
Rectal varices	—
Fissures	—
Small bowel bleeding	2%–9%
Upper gastrointestinal bleeding	0–11%

Data from Barnert J, Messmann H. Diagnosis and management of lower gastrointestinal bleeding. Nat Rev Gastroenterol Hepatol 2009;6:637–46.

INITIAL EVALUATION

The initial evaluation of patients presenting with GIB should focus on assessment of vital signs, the obtainment of a thorough yet focused medical history, a physical examination with particular attention paid to evidence of GIB and hemodynamic compromise, and laboratory diagnostic testing. Prompt and accurate assessment of these factors guides medical decision making, allowing for early diagnosis, aggressive resuscitation, and timely consultations. Vital signs, in particular heart rate and blood pressure, provide clinicians with diagnostic clues regarding the stability of patients. The loss of approximately less than 250 mL of blood does not usually affect heart rate or blood pressure. Greater than 800 mL of blood loss, however, may cause a drop in blood pressure of 10 mg Hg and a rise in heart rate of 10 beats per minute.[17] Significant tachycardia, tachypnea, hypotension, decreased mental status, and shock may result from blood loss totaling more than 1500 mL.[17] Although abnormal vital signs are concerning, normal vital signs do not preclude the presence of a significant bleed.

NATURE OF THE BLEED

The medical history can provide important diagnostic information with regards to the severity of disease and help focus triage and treatment of patients. Pertinent historical questions are detailed in **Box 1**. Historical questions include defining the nature of the bleed as hematemesis, hematochezia, or melena. Hematemesis usually signifies a UGIB and can be defined as bright red blood or darker coffee ground emesis. Approximately 50% of patients with UGIB present with hematemesis.[6] The return of bright red blood or coffee grounds through the passage of a nasogastric tube and subsequent nasogastric lavage has high predictive value for a bleed proximal to the ligament of Treitz; however, a negative lavage does not exclude UGIB.[3] Hematochezia is characterized by bright red or maroon-colored blood per rectum and suggests

Box 1
Pertinent historical questions

Bleeding location (distinguish upper from lower)

Bleeding severity

Nature, duration, and frequency of bleed

Risk factors (history of coagulopathy, prior GIB, alcohol intake, and liver disease)

a source distal to the ligament of Treitz. Approximately 14% of bleeds presenting with hematochezia are caused by a brisk upper source with rapid transit.[19] Hematochezia due to an upper tract source of bleeding has been shown associated with a higher transfusion requirement, need for surgery, and mortality rate.[6,19] Dark tarry or melanotic stools, which may also signify either an upper or lower source for the bleed, are associated with a lower mortality rate compared with hematochezia.[6] It is estimated that 90% of melanotic stools arise proximal to the ligament of Treitz and take on a dark tarry appearance secondary to prolonged transit and degradation of blood.[3] Approximately 70% of patients with UGIB present with melena in contrast to only 20% to 30% of patients with LGIB.[6,11] In addition to characterizing the nature of the bleed, it is important to define the duration, quantity, and frequency of bleeding episodes.

CLINICAL FEATURES

Although many patients may present with a chief complaint of hematemesis or blood in the stool, clinical suspicion for GIB must remain high in patients with signs or symptoms of hypovolemia or more subtle presentations, which may include hypotension, tachycardia, dizziness, angina, confusion, or syncope. Additional clinical features that should be ascertained as part of the medical history include questions pertaining to hypovolemia, including lightheadedness and dizziness, and symptoms suggestive of anemia, such as chest pain, dyspnea, and fatigue. Gastrointestinal historical features themselves may help delineate the possible etiology of the bleed. For example, epigastric pain is often associated with duodenal ulcers, whereas pain relieved with food intake is suggestive of a gastric ulcer. Mesenteric ischemia may present with significant abdominal pain out of proportion to physical examination findings. If a patient complains of streaks of blood present after vomiting, retching, or coughing, a Mallory-Weiss tear should be considered.

Medications and past medical, family, and social histories are also useful tools to help diagnose patients presenting with signs and symptoms suggestive of GIB. Medication history includes patient use of NSAIDs, aspirin, glucocorticoids, anticoagulants, and antiplatelet agents. Both aspirin and NSAID use have been shown to contribute to UGIB and LGIB, which are dependent on dose and duration of use.[11,20,21] Additionally, the use of aspirin (<100 mg/d), anticoagulation agents in the therapeutic range, and antiplatelet agents, such as clopidogrel, all increase the risk of UGIB threefold.[22,23] Important past medical history includes episodes of prior gastrointestinal hemorrhage, because up to 60% of UGI bleeds arise from prior gastrointestinal lesions that have bled.[24] Other relevant medical history includes presence of hemorrhoids, hepatic disease, coagulopathies, vascular disease, HIV infection, prior radiation therapy for prostate or pelvic cancer, inflammatory bowel disease, and recent colonoscopy with polypectomy. Family history of colon cancer and social history, specifically pertaining to alcohol and tobacco intake, also help to risk stratify patients. Both alcohol and cigarette smoking are associated with gastrointestinal malignancies.[25] Alcohol abuse is independently associated with an increased incidence of PUD and may also result in cirrhosis and varices.[25]

PHYSICAL EXAMINATION

Physical examination should include assessment of general appearance, mental status, examination of the conjunctiva (with pallor suggesting anemia), and skin characteristics, including color and temperature. Presence of petechiae or ecchymoses on skin examination may indicate a coagulopathy. Extremities should be evaluated for character of pulses and adequacy of capillary refill. Cool, clammy, pale extremities often indicate hypovolemic shock. Patients with cirrhosis may present with stigmata of liver disease, which include jaundice, caput medusa, palmar erythema, ascites, and hepatomegaly. Examination of the nasopharynx and oropharynx may reveal a source of blood that is being swallowed. A thorough abdominal examination is important and includes auscultation for bowel sounds and assessment of tenderness, masses, and signs of peritonitis. Blood from a proximal source can be irritating to the gastrointestinal tract and thereby stimulate peristalsis, leading to hyperactive bowel sounds. On the converse, LGIB presents with normoactive bowel sounds. Significant abdominal tenderness, involuntary guarding, or rebound tenderness should raise concern for a perforation, which needs to be excluded before endoscopy or colonoscopy is performed. Rectal examination should include inspection for anal fissures or hemorrhoids, assessment for rectal masses, and evaluation of stool for color and occult blood.

INITIAL DIAGNOSTIC TESTING

Laboratory studies to obtain in patients with GIB include a type and crossmatch, hemoglobin and hematocrit levels, blood urea nitrogen (BUN) and creatinine, coagulation profile, platelet count, and liver function tests. The initial hemoglobin level may not adequately reflect the true amount of blood loss in an acute bleed, because it often takes more than 24 hours to manifest a change in hemoglobin level. Infusion of intravenous fluids and movement of extracellular fluid into intravascular spaces can also confuse the initial and subsequent serial analyses of hemoglobin levels. If available, prior hemoglobin levels for comparison are helpful in determining the severity of the bleed. A hemoglobin level of less than 10 g/dL has been associated with increased rebleeding and mortality rates.[8] Because an elevation of the BUN concentration is associated with UGIB, the BUN-to-creatinine ratio has been used to distinguish UGIB from LGIB. In patients without renal failure, a BUN-to-creatinine ratio greater than 36 has a sensitivity of 90% to 95% in predicting UGIB.[26,27] Coagulation profile and platelet count may be beneficial in patients with liver disease or on anticoagulation therapy.

Because significant GIB may lead to decreased oxygen delivery and resultant myocardial ischemia and infarction, an electrocardiogram and cardiac markers should be obtained in patients at risk for acute coronary syndrome.[28,29] Patients with GIB who are diagnosed with concurrent myocardial infarction often do not complain of chest pain but rather dyspnea, dizziness, or abdominal pain.[30,31] In patients with GIB, routine abdominal radiographs have been shown of limited value.[32] In addition, routine chest radiographs have not been found to alter clinical outcomes or management decisions in the absence of pulmonary examination findings or known pulmonary disease.[33]

NASOGASTRIC ASPIRATION

Nasogastric aspiration detects active bleeding and may be helpful in the management of some patients with GIB. Once considered important in the initial management of GIB, there is now controversy surrounding its clinical utility, especially in light of the significant patient discomfort with its use. In patients with hematemesis and a clear upper source of GIB, nasogastric aspiration with lavage may be used to quantify active bleeding. In patients presenting without hematemesis and an unclear source of bleeding, a bloody nasogastric aspirate indicates an upper source of bleeding and may help direct management. In these patients without hematemesis, nasogastric aspiration has a limited sensitivity (42%) and accuracy (66%) in detecting UGIB, although a positive aspirate has been demonstrated in 23% of cases with a likelihood ratio of 11.[34] Bright red blood from the nasogastric lavage suggests an active bleed, whereas darker coffee grounds suggest a recent bleed and slow rate of bleeding. A massive hemorrhage should be suspected in patients with continued bright red blood in the aspirate. A bloody aspirate has been shown associated with the presence of a high-risk lesion at endoscopy.[35]

In contrast, a negative nasogastric aspirate is not helpful because it may miss various sources of UGIB and has been shown to miss up to 50% of patients with recent duodenal bleeding.[34,36] A nonbloody nasogastric aspirate may indicate that the source of the bleed is distal to the ligament of Treitz or that the bleeding has ceased. Although nasogastric tube placement is one of the more painful commonly performed procedures in the ED, use of lubrication, proper positioning (sitting up with head tilted forward), and patient involvement (swallowing during placement) may facilitate insertion.[37] In addition, topical anesthesia can decrease pain by two-thirds.[38] Complications of nasogastric tube insertion include epistaxsis, aspiration, pneumothorax, perforation, and gastric lesions.[39,40]

OTHER CAUSES OF GASTROINTESTINAL BLEEDING

Some patients who complain of vomiting blood or passing blood in the stool may not have GIB. The source of suspected UGIB may actually be due to blood from the naso-pharynx or oropharynx, which is being swallowed. Vomitus may appear as hematemesis due to red colored food products. Iron or bismuth ingestion may lead to the appearance of melena, whereas ingestion of beets may result in the appearance of hematochezia. In these cases, fecal occult testing is heme negative.

EMERGENCY DEPARTMENT MANAGEMENT

ED care encompasses timely assessment with immediate resuscitation and management of patients with GIB. Because the loss of oxygen-carrying capacity from hemorrhaging can lead to hypoxia and tissue ischemia, supplemental oxygen and pulse oximetry are recommended. If indicated, definitive airway management may be required in patients unable to support their airway and to prevent aspiration. It is also recommended that patients be placed on cardiac monitoring secondary to the risk of demand ischemia from decreased oxygen delivery to cardiac tissue. Patients with significant GIB should be kept nothing by mouth to facilitate the need for emergent endoscopy or surgical intervention.

FLUID RESUSCITATION AND TRANSFUSION OF BLOOD PRODUCTS

Two peripheral large-bore (18-gauge or larger) intravenous catheters are recommended with aggressive resuscitation initiated with crystalloid infusion. Assessment of volume status and hemodynamic stability should dictate the amount of fluid transfused. In hemodynamically unstable patients or patients with large hemorrhage, boluses of 500 mL of normal saline or lactated Ringer solution with continuous reassessment are appropriate. Transducing a central venous pressure via a central line or the use of a Swan-Ganz catheter is a more accurate method of determining volume status; however, determining the need for invasive monitoring should be based on the clinical presentation and need for close assessment and management of volume status.

Transfusion of blood products is recommended in those patients with hemodynamic instability despite crystalloid resuscitation and in those with continuous bleeding. A patient's age, comorbid conditions, briskness of bleed, baseline hemoglobin and hematocrit levels, and evidence of cardiac, renal, or cerebral hypoperfusion should all be taken into consideration when determining the quantity of blood to transfuse. Although there are no hard-set transfusion parameters for GIB, it has been suggested that patients with variceal bleeding do not benefit from aggressive transfusion, because this increases portal pressure and may lead to more bleeding.[41] A small study comparing 25 cirrhotic patients transfused with 2 units or more of packed red blood cells with 25 cirrhotic patients transfused only for a hemoglobin level of less than 8 g/dL or hemodynamic compromise demonstrated a higher risk of rebleed in the patients who were aggressively transfused.[42] Achieving a goal hematocrit level of 27 is recommended for patients with variceal bleeding.[3] Although a hematocrit level of 25 to 27 may be adequate to maintain perfusion in younger GIB patients with no comorbid conditions, older patients, in particular those with cardiovascular disease, may require more aggressive resuscitation and a higher hematocrit level.[43] Attention should be paid to the precipitation of flash pulmonary edema or worsening congestive heart failure in patients with pre-existing congestive heart failure, and blood should be transfused slowly if possible. Patients requiring more than 5 units of packed red cells have a much higher mortality rate and often require surgery.[1]

Coagulopathic patients may require platelets or fresh frozen plasma as appropriate. To replace coagulation factors, it is recommended that for every 4 units of packed red blood cells transfused, a patient be given 1 unit of fresh frozen plasma.[44] Patients with platelet counts in the range of 50,000 to 90,000 platelets/μL do not require platelet transfusion, whereas those with counts less than 50,000 platelets/μL and active bleeding may require transfusion.[45] Clinical parameters, including age, comorbid conditions, and severity of bleed, should be used to determine whether or not platelets should be administered to thrombocytopenic patients.

MEDICAL THERAPIES

Various medications have been demonstrated to improve outcome in GIB. Somatostatin and octreotide, its longer-acting derivative that inhibits mesenteric vasodilation induced by glucagon, have been shown to decrease the risk for persistent bleeding and rebleeding in patients with an upper source of bleed in both variceal and nonvariceal bleeding.[46,47] A large systematic review of the use of somatostatin analogs for acute esophageal variceal bleeding revealed no significant decrease in mortality but did demonstrate a reduction in bleeding and transfusion requirement.[48] The recommended dose for octreotide is a 50-μg bolus intravenously followed by a continuous infusion of 50 μg per hour.

Proton pump inhibitors have been shown to reduce the risk of rebleeding and the need for surgical intervention and blood transfusions, with conflicting evidence for mortality reduction, in patients with UGIB due to PUD.[49,50] Proton pump inhibitors are recommended before endoscopy, because they reduce the likelihood of bleeding or need for intervention (cauterizing of vessels or injection of medications) during endoscopy.[51] Vasopressin has also been used for GIB, most often for variceal bleeding, but is associated with a significant rebleeding rate and a high rate of complications, which include hypertension, dysrhythmias, myocardial and peripheral ischemia, and decreased cardiac output.[52] The use of H_2-receptor antagonists in UGIB has not been shown to be of significant value, with a lack of benefit in bleeding duodenal ulcers and a possibly weak benefit in bleeding gastric ulcers.[53,54]

CONSULTATION AND DISPOSITION

Gastroenterology should be consulted promptly for significant GIB. The decision for emergent versus nonemergent endoscopic evaluation may be based on clinical parameters, including severity of the bleed and hemodynamic stability of the patient. Unstable patients, including those with hemodynamic instability, patients in shock, patients demonstrating a change in mental status, and those with signs of end-organ ischemia secondary to volume loss, may require intensive care unit admission and intensivists should be involved early in the care. Surgical consultation for continued hemorrhage may be necessary in those patients with UGIB or LGIB who fail to respond to standard therapies. Patients with signs of cardiac ischemia or infarction may require cardiology consultation. Hospital admission is needed for patients with significant GIB. Various studies have demonstrated a subset of low-risk patients who may be discharged safely with UGIB, although short observation and endoscopy were performed in all of these study patients before discharge home. These low-risk patients were under 60 years of age with follow-up care and had no significant comorbid conditions, no signs of shock, no history of liver disease or varices, no severe anemia, and no frequent hematemesis or melena.[55–57] Risk stratification for patients with lower sources of bleeding has not been well studied; therefore, most patients with significant LGIB are admitted for further management.

UPPER ENDOSCOPY

Although endoscopy is often performed once resuscitation is achieved, urgent endoscopy may be necessary if clinically warranted. After hemodynamic stabilization, upper endoscopy is the most accurate intervention in UGIB patients and allows for the diagnosis of the bleeding site with achievement of hemostasis in more than 90% of cases.[58] Endoscopic therapies, including sclerotherapy and band ligation, are useful in UGIB due to varices. Early esophagoduodenoscopy (EGD), performed within 12 to 24 hours of bleeding, reduces the risk of rebleeding and hospital length of stay for patients with UGIB.[59] Endoscopic findings are also useful in risk stratification and aid in the decision-making process regarding patient disposition.[59] Balloon tamponade with a Sengstaken-Blakemore tube is rarely used due to its high complication rate, but it may be helpful in exsanguinating patients due to active variceal bleeding when endoscopy is not available.

COLONOSCOPY

In patients with acute LGIB, the treatment goal is localization of the bleeding site for therapy, to ultimately avoid a subtotal colectomy. As a brisk UGIB may be the source of hematochezia, EGD may be performed before colonoscopy in unstable patients with bright red blood per rectum.[17] Otherwise, colonoscopy is indicated to attempt to identify the source of the LGIB. Colonoscopy is often performed in stabilized patients with self-limited bleeding or in those with a higher likelihood of a localized lesion. Although urgent colonoscopy requires both rapid bowel preparation and availability of the endoscopist, it may be both diagnostic and therapeutic in cases of LGIB.[5,60] Severe hemorrhage may necessitate an urgent colonoscopy without bowel preparation, but it is recommended that the bowel be purged before evaluation to facilitate visualization and decrease the incidence of bowel perforation from poor visualization. Bowel preparation consists of administering 3 to 6 L of polyethylene glycol solution, which may be difficult for patients to tolerate. Administration of the solution through a nasogastric tube or adding an antiemetic with promotility properties, such as metoclopramide (10 mg intravenously), may be helpful. Urgent colonoscopy without bowel preparation is diagnostic approximately 89% to 97% of the time.[61,62] Colonoscopy is usually performed 24 to 48 hours after initial presentation.[61] The risk of serious complications for patients undergoing colonoscopy is 1:1000.[17] If neither EGD nor colonoscopy allows for visualization of the source of bleeding, other endoscopic techniques may be used. These include push enteroscopy, where approximately 100 cm of the proximal jejunum may be visualized, and wireless video capsule endoscopy, where 80% of the small bowel may be seen.[63] Patients with clinical signs of severe hemorrhage may be more likely to undergo radiographic interventions than urgent colonoscopy.[64]

NUCLEAR SCINTIGRAPHY

Nuclear scans, in particular those involving technetium Tc 99m–labeled red blood cells, are a noninvasive technique that may be used in localizing an obscure source of LGIB. Nuclear scintigraphy is less specific but more sensitive than angiography for detecting bleeds and requires active hemorrhage at a rate of at least 0.1 mL per minute.[6,65–67] On average, approximately 45% of technetium Tc 99m–labeled red blood cell scans performed for LGIB are positive.[10] The source of the bleed is identified correctly approximately 95% to 100% of the time with a positive scan within 2 hours of erythrocyte injection, with the accuracy dropping to 57% to 67% with a positive scan 2 hours after the injection.[10] Nuclear scintigraphy is useful for bleeds that are difficult to visualize using EGD or colonoscopy and in recurrent bleeds. Technetium scans are then used to direct therapy through the use of angiography or surgery.

ANGIOGRAPHY

Angiography may also be used to localize obscure lower bleeding but requires a brisker rate of hemorrhage of at least 0.5 to 1 mL per minute. The sensitivity of angiography has been demonstrated to be 46% for acute bleeds and 30% for recurrent bleeds, whereas the specificity approaches 100%.[68] Although angiography has the advantage of allowing for therapeutic intervention, it also has the disadvantage of complications, which include acute renal failure, contrast reactions, arterial thrombosis or dissection, and bowel infarction. The complication rate for visceral angiography is approximately 9.3%.[68] Angiography is often reserved for massive, continuous LGIB, particularly when endoscopy is unfeasible or difficult secondary to the briskness of the bleed.[6,15] The management of LGIB is controversial as to which diagnostic test should be performed initially, and management may be influenced by institutional availability and expertise, and the preference of the consulting physician.

OTHER STUDIES

Barium studies do not play a role in the evaluation of LGIB. CT or plain film radiography might be indicated when an acute abdomen is suspected, such as with bowel perforation, or for further evaluation of bowel pathology, such as inflammatory bowel disease. Chronic bleeds may benefit from CT colonography, but lesions such as angiodysplasia are not visualized using this method.

SUMMARY

GIB is a common complaint encountered in an ED and frequent cause of hospitalization. Important diagnostic factors that increase morbidity and mortality include advanced age, serious comorbid conditions, hemodynamic instability, esophageal varices, significant hematemesis or melena, and marked anemia. Because GIB carries a 10% overall mortality rate, emergency physicians must perform timely diagnosis, aggressive resuscitation, risk stratification, and early consultation for these patients.

REFERENCES

1. Hussain H, Lapin S, Cappell MS. Clinical scoring systems for determining the prognosis of gastrointestinal bleeding. Gastroenterol Clin North Am 2000;29(2): 445–64.
2. Wilcox CM, Clark WS. Causes and outcome of upper and lower gastrointestinal bleeding: the Grady Hospital experience. South Med J 1999;92:44.
3. Cappell M, Friedel D. Initial management of acute upper gastrointestinal bleeding: from initial evaluation up to gastrointestinal endoscopy. Med Clin North Am 2008;92:491–509.
4. Longstreth GF. Epidemiology of hospitalization for acute upper gastrointestinal hemorrhage: a population-based study. Am J Gastroenterol 1995;90:206.
5. Longstreth GF. Epidemiology and outcome of patients hospitalized with acute lower gastrointestinal hemorrhage: a population-based study. Am J Gastroenterol 1997;92:419–24.
6. Peter DJ, Dougherty JM. Evaluation of the patient with gastrointestinal bleeding: an evidence based approach. Emerg Med Clin North Am 1999;17:239.
7. van Leerdam ME, Vreeburg EM, Rauws EA, et al. Acute upper GI bleeding. Did anything change? Am J Gastroenterol 2003;98:1494–9.
8. Rockall TA, Logan RF, Devlin HB, et al. Risk assessment after acute upper gastrointestinal haemorrhage. Gut 1996;38:316.
9. Kollef MH, O'Brien JD, Zuckerman GR, et al. BLEED: a classification tool to predict outcomes in patients with acute upper and lower gastrointestinal hemorrhage. Crit Care Med 1997;25:1125.
10. Zuckerman GR, Prakash C. Acute lower intestinal bleeding: part I: clinical presentation and diagnosis. Gastrointest Endosc 1998;48:606–17.
11. Peura DA, Lanza FL, Gostout CJ, et al. The American College of Gastroenterology Bleeding registry: preliminary findings. Am J Gastroenterol 1997;92:924–8.
12. Tariq S, Mekhjian G. Gastrointestinal bleeding in older adults. Clin Geriatr Med 2007;23:769–84.
13. Bayyurt N, Abasiyanik MF, Sander E, et al. Canonical analysis of factors involved in the occurrence of peptic ulcers. Dig Dis Sci 2007;52(1):140–6.
14. Boonpongmanee S, Fleischer DE, Pezzulo JC, et al. The frequency of peptic ulcer disease as a cause of upper-GI bleeding is exaggerated. Gastrointest Endosc 2004;59(7):788–94.
15. Fallah MA, Prakash C, Edmundowicz S. Acute gastrointestinal bleeding. Med Clin North Am 2000;84(5):1183–208.
16. Merli M, Nicolini G, Angeloni S, et al. Incidence and natural history of small esophageal varices in cirrhotic patients. J Hepatol 2003;38:266–72.

17. Barnert J, Messmann H. Diagnosis and management of lower gastrointestinal bleeding. Nat Rev Gastroenterol Hepatol 2009;6:637–46.
18. Pardi DS, Loftus EV Jr, Tremaine WJ, et al. Acute major gastrointestinal hemorrhage in inflammatory bowel disease. Gastrointest Endosc 1999;49:153–7.
19. Wilcox CM, Alexander LN, Cotsonis G. A prospective characterization of upper gastrointestinal hemorrhage presenting with hematochezia. Am J Gastroenterol 1997;92:231.
20. Hernandez-Diaz S, Rodriguez LA. Association between nonsteroidal anti-inflammatory drugs and upper gastrointestinal tract bleeding/perforation: an overview of epidemiologic studies published in the 1990s. Arch Intern Med 2000;160:2093.
21. Foutch PG. Diverticular bleeding: are nonsteroidal anti-inflammatory drugs risk factors for hemorrhage and can colonoscopy predict outcome for patients? Am J Gastroenterol 1995;90:1779.
22. Lana A, Garcia-Rodriguez LA, Arroyo MT, et al. Risk of upper gastrointestinal ulcer bleeding with selective cyclo-oxygenase-2 inhibitors, traditional non-aspirin non-steroidal anti-inflammatory drugs, aspirin and combinations. Gut 2006;55(12):1731–8.
23. Cryer B. The role of cyclooxygenase inhibitors in the gastrointestinal tract. Curr Gastroenterol Rep 2003;5(6):453–8.
24. McGuirk TD, Coyle WJ. Upper gastrointestinal tract bleeding. Emerg Med Clin North Am 1996;14(3):523–45.
25. Andersen IB, Jorgensen T, Bonnevie O, et al. Smoking and alcohol intake as risk factors for bleeding and perforated peptic ulcers: a population-based cohort study. Epidemiology 2000;11(4):434–49.
26. Ernst AA, Haynes ML, Nick TG, et al. Usefulness of the blood urea nitrogen/creatinine ratio in gastrointestinal bleeding. Am J Emerg Med 1999;17:70.
27. Chalasani N, Clark WS, Wilcox CM. Blood urea nitrogen to creatinine concentration in gastrointestinal bleeding: a reappraisal. Am J Gastroenterol 1997;92:1796.
28. Bellotto F, Fagiuoli S, Pavei A, et al. Anemia and ischemia: myocardial injury in patients with gastrointestinal bleeding. Am J Med 2005;118:548.
29. Prendergast HM, Sloan EP, Cumpston K, et al. Myocardial infarction and cardiac complications in emergency department patients admitted to the intensive care unit with gastrointestinal hemorrhage. J Emerg Med 2005; 28:19.
30. Bhatti N, Amoateng-Adjepong Y, Qamar A, et al. Myocardial infarction in critically ill patients presenting with gastrointestinal hemorrhage: retrospective analysis of risks and outcomes. Chest 1998;114(4):1137–42.
31. Cappell MS. A study of the syndrome of simultaneous acute upper gastrointestinal bleeding and myocardial infarction in 36 patients. Am J Gastroenterol 1995;90(9):1444–9.
32. Andrews AH, Lake JM, Shorr AF. Ineffectiveness of routine abdominal radiography in patients with gastrointestinal hemorrhage admitted to an intensive care unit. J Clin Gastroenterol 2005;39:228.
33. Tobin K, Klein J, Barbieri C, et al. Utility of routine admission chest radiographs in patients with acute gastrointestinal hemorrhage admitted to an intensive care unit. Am J Med 1996;101:349.
34. Witting MD, Magder L, Heins AE, et al. Usefulness and validity of diagnostic nasogastric aspiration in patients without hematemesis. Ann Emerg Med 2004; 43:525–32.

35. Aljebreen AM, Fallone CA, Barkun AN. Nasogastric aspirate predicts high-risk endoscopic lesions in patients with acute upper-GI bleeding [see comment]. Gastrointest Endosc 2004;59:172.
36. Leung FW. The venerable nasogastric tube. Gastrointest Endosc 2004;59:255.
37. Singer S, Richman P, LaVefre R, et al. Comparison of patient and practitioner assessments of pain from commonly performed emergency department procedures. Acad Emerg Med 1997;4:404–5.
38. Cullen L, Taylor D, Taylor S, et al. Nebulized lidocaine decreases the discomfort of nasogastric tube insertion: a randomized double-blind trial. Ann Emerg Med 2004;44:131–7.
39. Pancorbo-Hidalgo PL, Garaciaia-Fernandez FP, Ramiairez-Pea C. Complications associated with enteral nutrition by nasogastric tube in an internal medicine unit. J Clin Nurs 2001;10:482–90.
40. Pillai JB, Vegas A, Briste S. Thoracic complications of nasogastric tube: review of safe practice. Interact Cardiovasc Thorac Surg 2005;4:429–33.
41. Kravetz D, Bosch J, Arderiu M, et al. Hemodynamic effects of blood volume restitution following a hemorrhage in rats with portal hypertension due to cirrhosis of the liver: influence of the extent of portal-systemic shunting. Hepatology 1989;9(6):808–14.
42. Blair SD, Janvrin SB, McCollum CN, et al. Effect of early blood transfusion on gastrointestinal haemorrhage. Br J Surg 1986;73(10):783–5.
43. Klein HG, Spahn DR, Carson JL. Red blood cell transfusion in clinical practice. Lancet 2007;370(9585):415–26.
44. Maltz GS, Siegel JE, Carson JL. Hematologic management of gastrointestinal bleeding. Gastroenterol Clin North Am 2000;29(1):169–87.
45. Conteras M. Final statement from the consensus conference on platelet transfusion. Transfusion 1998;38:796–7.
46. Imperiale TF, Birgisson S. Somatostatin or octreotide compared with H2 antagonists and placebo in the management of acute nonvariceal upper gastrointestinal hemorrhage: a meta-analysis. Ann Intern Med 1997;127:1062.
47. Jenkins SA, Shields R, Davies M, et al. A multicentre randomised trial comparing octreotide and injection sclerotherapy in the management and outcome of acute variceal haemorrhage. Gut 1997;41:526.
48. Gotzsche PC. Somatostatin or octreotide for acute bleeding oesophageal varices [update in Cochrane Database Syst Rev 2002;1:CD000193; PMID: 11869569]. Cochrane Database Syst Rev 2000;2:CD000193.
49. Leontiadis GI, Sharma VK, Howden CW. Systematic review and meta-analysis: proton pump inhibitor treatment for ulcer bleeding reduces transfusion requirements and hospital stay-results from the Cochrane Collaboration. Aliment Pharmacol Ther 2005;22(3):169–74.
50. Bardou M, Toubouti Y, Benhaberou-Brun D, et al. Meta-analysis: proton-pump inhibition in high-risk patients with acute peptic ulcer bleeding. Aliment Pharmacol Ther 2005;21:677.
51. Andrews CN, Levy A, Fishman M, et al. Intravenous proton pump inhibitors in bleeding peptic ulcer disease with high-risk stigmata: a multicenter comparative study. Can J Gastroenterol 2005;19(11):667–71.
52. Grace ND, Bhattacharya K. Pharmacologic therapy of portal hypertension and variceal hemorrhage. Clin Liver Dis 1997;1:59.
53. Levine JE, Leontiadis GI, Sharma VK, et al. Meta-analysis: the efficacy of intravenous H2-receptor antagonists in bleeding peptic ulcer. Aliment Pharmacol Ther 2002;16:1137.

54. Walt RP, Cottrell J, Mann SG, et al. Continuous intravenous famotidine for haemorrhage from peptic ulcer. Lancet 1992;340:1058.

55. Rockall TA, Logan RF, Devlin HB, et al. Selection of patients for early discharge or outpatient care after acute upper gastrointestinal haemorrhage. National Audit of Acute Upper Gastrointestinal Haemorrhage. Lancet 1996;347:1138.

56. Longstreth GF, Feitelberg SP. Outpatient care of selected patients with acute non-variceal upper gastrointestinal haemorrhage. Lancet 1995;345:108.

57. Courtney AE, Mitchell RM, Rocke L, et al. Proposed risk stratification in upper gastrointestinal haemorrhage: is hospitalisation essential? Emerg Med J 2004; 21:39.

58. Van Dam J, Brugge WR. Endoscopy of the upper gastrointestinal tract. N Engl J Med 1999;341:1738.

59. Cooper GS, Chak A, Way LE, et al. Early endoscopy in upper gastrointestinal hemorrhage: associations with recurrent bleeding, surgery, and length of hospital stay. Gastrointest Endosc 1999;49:145.

60. Jensen DM, Machicado GA, Jutabha R, et al. Urgent colonoscopy for the diagnosis and treatment of severe diverticular hemorrhage. N Engl J Med 2000; 342:78.

61. Chaudhry V, Hyser MJ, Gracias VH, et al. Colonoscopy: the initial test for acute lower gastrointestinal bleeding. Am Surg 1998;64:723–8.

62. Ohyama T, Sakurai Y, Ito M, et al. Analysis of urgent colonoscopy for lower gastrointestinal tract bleeding. Digestion 2000;61:189–92.

63. Eliakim R. Video capsule endoscopy of the small bowel. Curr Opin Gastroenterol 2008;24:159–63.

64. Strate LL, Orav EJ, Syngal S. Early predictors of severity in acute lower intestinal tract bleeding. Arch Intern Med 2003;163:838.

65. Dusold R, Burke K, Carpentier W, et al. The accuracy of technetium-99m-labeled red cell scintigraphy in localizing gastrointestinal bleeding. Am J Gastroenterol 1994;89:345–8.

66. Levy R, Barto W, Gani J. Retrospective study of the utility of nuclear scintigraphic-labelled red cell scanning for lower gastrointestinal bleeding. ANZ J Surg 2003; 73:205.

67. Suzman MS, Talmor M, Jennis R, et al. Accurate localization and surgical management of active lower gastrointestinal hemorrhage with technetium-labeled erythrocyte scintigraphy. Ann Surg 1996;224:29.

68. Browder W, Cerise EJ, Litwin MS. Impact of emergency angiography in massive lower gastrointestinal bleeding. Ann Surg 1986;204:530–6.

Vascular Abdominal Emergencies

Resa E. Lewiss, MD*, Daniel J. Egan, MD, Ashley Shreves, MD

KEYWORDS

- Abdominal aorta • Mesenteric ischemia
- Abdominal aortic aneurysm • Embolus • Arterial thrombus
- Venous thrombus

Each shift, the emergency physician must consider the uncommon diagnoses grouped together as abdominal vascular emergencies in the differential diagnosis of the patient with nausea, vomiting, diarrhea, or with abdominal, back, or flank pain. Identification of vascular emergencies is made even more difficult by clinical findings often being nonspecific or equivocal.

Vascular abdominal emergencies are not common but, when present, are often catastrophic. Most of the conditions are time sensitive, putting perfusion of critical organs (eg, the bowel) at risk, leading to the potential for ischemia, infarction, and translocation of enteric microbes, bacteremia, and sepsis. Aneurysmal dilation of the aorta with rupture leads to rapid hypovolemic shock and death if not diagnosed.

A high index of suspicion is critical to the successful diagnosis of abdominal vascular emergencies. Because most emergencies ultimately require surgical intervention, diagnostic testing should be performed in parallel with resuscitation, consultation, and involvement of the vascular or general surgeon.

VASCULAR ABDOMINAL ANATOMY

The aorta gives rise to several paired and unpaired vessels within the abdomen. The adrenal, renal, and gonadal arteries are paired, and provide blood flow to their respective organs. The unpaired branches (celiac artery, superior mesenteric artery [SMA], and inferior mesenteric artery [IMA]) deliver blood to most of the digestive tract. The celiac trunk branches off the aorta at approximately 90 degrees, making it less susceptible to embolic phenomena compared with the SMA and IMA. The 3 branches of the celiac trunk (the splenic, left gastric, and common hepatic arteries) supply the foregut structures from the distal esophagus to the second part of the duodenum, the spleen, the liver, and parts of the pancreas (**Fig. 1**).[1]

No financial support was provided for this paper.
Department of Emergency Medicine, St Luke's Roosevelt Hospital Center, 1111 Amsterdam Avenue, New York, NY 10025, USA
* Corresponding author.
E-mail address: resaelewiss@yahoo.com

Emerg Med Clin N Am 29 (2011) 253–272
doi:10.1016/j.emc.2011.02.001
0733-8627/11/$ – see front matter

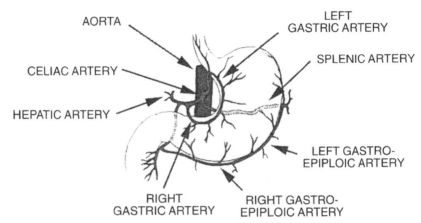

AORTA

LEFT
GASTRIC ARTERY

SPLENIC ARTERY

CELIAC ARTERY

HEPATIC ARTERY

LEFT GASTRO-
EPIPLOIC ARTERY

RIGHT
GASTRIC ARTERY

RIGHT GASTRO-
EPIPLOIC ARTERY

Fig. 1. The celiac artery and its 3 major branches: the splenic, left gastric, and hepatic arteries. (*From* Walker JS, Dire DJ. Vascular abdominal emergencies. Emerg Med Clin North Am 1996;14(3):573; with permission.)

The SMA typically arises about 1 cm below the celiac trunk, at the approximate level of the first lumbar vertebra.[2] The SMA gives rise to several branches that supply the midgut structures extending from the second part of the duodenum to the distal third of the transverse colon. The SMA leaves the aorta at an angle of less than 30 degrees, making it susceptible to thromboembolism (**Fig. 2**).[1]

Just before the bifurcation of the aorta at the level of the fourth lumbar vertebra, the IMA branches off the aorta and supplies all of the structures of the hindgut, which extend from the transverse colon to the rectum. It terminates in the superior rectal artery (see **Fig. 2**).[2] Although each branch is separate, there is extensive collateral blood flow

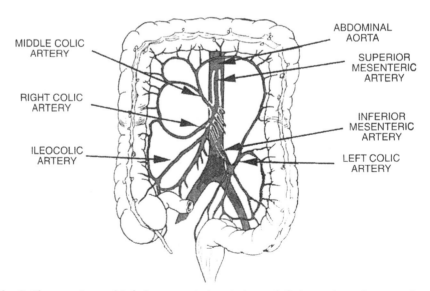

MIDDLE COLIC
ARTERY

ABDOMINAL
AORTA

SUPERIOR
MESENTERIC
ARTERY

RIGHT COLIC
ARTERY

INFERIOR
MESENTERIC
ARTERY

ILEOCOLIC
ARTERY

LEFT COLIC
ARTERY

Fig. 2. The superior and inferior mesenteric arteries and their anastomotic connections. (*From* Walker JS, Dire DJ. Vascular abdominal emergencies. Emerg Med Clin North Am 1996;14(3):574; with permission.)

between the celiac artery and SMA via the pancreaticoduodenal artery, and between the SMA and the IMA by way of the marginal artery of Drummond and arc of Riolan.[1]

The venous system of the gastrointestinal tract differs from the arterial system in that, rather than draining into the inferior vena cava (IVC), it passes via the portal vein into the liver. Blood passes through the hepatic lobules into the hepatic veins, which pass into the IVC. In normal health, portal blood is sequestered from the systemic venous circulation. Pathologic conditions (eg, cirrhosis, obstruction, thrombosis) that obstruct portal flow cause anastomoses to form between systemic and portal vessels in tissues that are at the watershed junction between the 2 systems. These locations are the lower esophagus, the umbilicus, and the rectum.[3] When anastomoses become very large they are referred to as varices.

ABDOMINAL VASCULAR THROMBOSES
Aortic Thrombosis

Acute occlusive aortic thrombosis is a rare condition that is lethal if not diagnosed. Nonocclusive aortic thrombosis is more common and occurs in the setting of aneurysmal disease, dissection, or severe atherosclerotic disease.[4–6] Other conditions associated with aortic thrombotic disease include diabetes, cardiomyopathy, blunt and penetrating abdominal trauma,[7–9] spinal surgery, polycythemia,[4] thrombocytosis,[4] nephrotic syndrome, exogenous estrogens, the classic hypercoagulable conditions (protein C and S deficiency, factor V Leiden deficiency, antithrombin III deficiency), malignancy,[5] use of certain chemotherapeutic agents,[10] antiphospholipid antibody syndrome,[5] and previous aortic grafting.[4] Because of the large diameter of the aorta, emboli (typically from the left ventricle) rarely lead to aortic occlusion. Patients with an acute thrombotic event typically present with symptoms of lower extremity ischemia: bilateral lower extremity pulselessness, pallor, pain, paresthesias, and possible paralysis.[4,11] Mesenteric ischemia may also be present. If the occlusion involves the artery of Adamkowicz, patients may also develop spinal cord infarction.[12] Signs of the anterior spinal artery syndrome include paralysis and loss of sensation to both light touch and pinprick, but preservation of vibratory sensation and proprioception.[12] In cases of chronic occlusion caused by atherosclerotic disease, there is time for the formation of collateral circulation to the distal structures.[6] Leriche syndrome results from chronic obstruction of the distal aorta leading to chronic ischemia of the pelvis and lower extremities. Classically described in men, the triad of symptoms includes claudication, abnormal or absent lower extremity pulses, and erectile dysfunction.[13,14] Acute ischemia from aortic occlusive disease warrants emergent consultation with a vascular surgeon. Patients will likely need emergent laparotomy for thrombectomy or embolectomy, often with aortic bypass.[4] The cause of the thrombus and other associated conditions (eg, aneurysm or dissection) determine the vascular surgery approach to treatment. In one series of 14 patients, mortality after surgery was 14%.[4] Overall mortality in a retrospective case series of 48 patients by Babu and colleagues[15] was 52%. Dossa and colleagues[11] reported a 40-year experience of 46 patients with an in-hospital mortality of 35%. The urgency of surgical consultation and intervention in patients with subacute or chronic occlusive disease is determined by the severity and progression of symptoms. Most patients will be admitted for observation, often with anticoagulant or antiplatelet agents.

Renal Artery Thrombosis

Renal artery thrombosis is also a rare condition, most commonly seen in individuals aged 30 to 50 years.[16] Similar to the other thromboses, the most common cause involves the development of a clot in situ on established atherosclerotic lesions. Thrombosis is also a known complication after renal transplantation because of both the surgical anastomoses, and immunosuppressive drugs being prothrombotic.[17] Intra-aortic catheter or balloon pump placement,[18] intravenous (IV) cocaine use,[16] and renal angiography are also risk factors. The transplanted renal artery graft may also develop thrombosis secondary to surgical technique including torsion of the artery, kinking of the anastomosis, or dissection into the wall.[19] Large case series have described rates of thrombosis after transplant between 0.5% and 3.5%.[19,20]

Patients with acute renal artery occlusion typically present with flank pain, which may be associated with hypertension.[16,21] Accompanying symptoms may include nausea, vomiting, and upper abdominal pain on the affected side. Hematuria only occurs in between 30% and 50% of patients.[16] An untreated occlusion of the renal artery leads to renal infarction. In the setting of renal infarct, the serum lactate dehydrogenase (LDH) is typically increased.[22] Symptoms may be difficult to distinguish from renal colic. When renal colic is suspected, unenhanced computed tomography (CT) is the initial study. However, with severe symptoms and a CT without renal stones, the study can be repeated with intravenous contrast if renal artery thrombosis is a consideration. In the renal transplant recipient, duplex ultrasound is the preferred initial test.

Renal artery occlusion can also occur in the setting of trauma. Blunt trauma to the abdomen can lead to compression of the artery, as well as dissection and thrombosis.[23] Patients typically require surgical revascularization, and the timeliness of this intervention is linked with improved outcomes.[21,24,25]

Nontraumatic thrombosis is treated with surgical revascularization or sometimes thrombolysis. Long-term sequelae of both traumatic and nontraumatic thromboses include renal artery stenosis, renal insufficiency or failure (more likely with bilateral disease), and hypertension.

Renal Vein Thrombosis

Renal vein thrombosis may be either an acute or chronic process. Diagnosis depends on a high level of clinical suspicion, because the clinical findings mimic those of renal colic, renal artery occlusion, and pyelonephritis.[26] With acute thrombosis, patients experience flank pain often associated with nausea and vomiting. Hematuria and proteinuria may also be noted. In the setting of chronic thrombosis, the diagnosis may not be made until the development of complications such as impaired renal function or pulmonary embolism.[27] The left renal vein is affected more often than the right, but up to two-thirds of patients have bilateral thrombosis.[27]

In contrast to occlusive arterial disease, renal vein thrombosis is also a disease of children and neonates. In the setting of severe volume depletion, dehydration, or sustained hypotension, blood flow is shunted from the renal vein, leading to sluggish flow that may eventually lead to the formation of a clot.[26–28] In children, a palpable mass in the flank may be present because of the enlargement of the kidney on the affected side.[28] The classic triad of symptoms in children includes a palpable mass, gross hematuria, and thrombocytopenia, although most patients do not have all three.[29]

Thrombosis of the renal vein may occur as a result of the hypercoagulable, post-transplant, and postoperative states mentioned in previously. In addition, blunt trauma[30] and infection play roles in its development. The most common disease associated with the development of renal vein thrombosis is nephrotic syndrome.[27,28] Patients have direct loss of protein S and antithrombin III in their urine.[26] With excessive proteinuria, the liver is stimulated to produce new proteins, many of which are prothrombotic.[27]

In patients receiving transplants, color Doppler sonography should be used to evaluate the flow in the graft. In all other patients, CT scan is the diagnostic study of choice. Intravenous contrast should be administered to visualize the vascular structures. In addition to visualizing the thrombus, the kidney on the affected side is typically engorged because of impaired venous drainage. Delayed images show a persistent enhancement from the contrast on CT scan because of the limited venous outflow.

Treatment of renal vein thrombosis is generally medical with systemic anticoagulation. Patients with, or at risk for, severe disease (eg, extensive clot progressing to the IVC, renal failure, bilateral disease, renal transplant) may be candidates for systemic or catheter-directed thrombolytic therapy.[27]

Portal Vein Thrombosis

The estimated lifetime risk of developing portal vein thrombosis in the general population is 1%.[31] Up to 15% of cirrhotics develop this condition. It is rarely seen in patients without known liver disease or other risk factors that include adjacent inflammatory conditions (eg, pancreatitis, cholecystitis, diverticulitis, inflammatory bowel disease, appendicitis), malignancies (local or systemic), or hypercoagulable conditions (especially sepsis).[32,33] Mortality caused by portal vein thrombosis itself is low; however, these patients frequently have other significant comorbidities that combine to give them poor outcomes with this condition.

The mechanism by which cirrhosis leads to portal vein thrombosis is not clear. It is believed that decreased portal blood flow, periportal inflammation and fibrosis, and impaired production of anticoagulation factors lead to thrombosis.[34] Fifty percent of portal vein thrombosis in children and neonates is associated with an intra-abdominal infection, including umbilical infections in the very young.[34]

With clot in the portal vein, the liver loses approximately two-thirds of its blood supply. In the acute phase, several compensatory mechanisms occur, including dilation of the hepatic artery to increase blood supply, the development of variceal collaterals between the portal and systemic venous systems, and collateral cavernoma formation. The cavernomas are a matted plexus of collateral vessels that form at the porta hepatis, often leading to secondary biliary effects including cholecystitis, biliary obstruction, and jaundice. Although collateral formation ultimately restores some degree of splanchnic circulation, hepatocytes often continue to be underperfused, leading to ongoing ischemia and cell death.[32,35]

Acute portal vein thrombosis may present with abdominal pain (which may be localized in the right upper quadrant, but is frequently diffuse), nausea, and fever. Signs of intestinal ischemia (discussed later), which is a secondary effect of acute portal vein thrombosis, may also be present.[32,34] With chronic thrombosis, patients may remain clinically silent until the secondary effects of the thrombosis occur. These effects include worsening hepatic function, worsening portal hypertension, and hematemesis from esophageal varices.[32,34,36]

Ultrasound with Doppler is the diagnostic modality of choice for portal vein thrombosis. The absence of flow within the lumen and, in some cases, the presence of a cavernoma identifies the disease. If suspicion exists for extension of the clot into the mesenteric venous system, CT with intravenous contrast is indicated to evaluate the vasculature and intestines.

Patients with portal vein thrombosis without complications of bleeding or intestinal ischemia are managed with systemic anticoagulation.[31,32,37] Empiric thrombolytic therapy in cases of acute thrombosis may be indicated in severely ill patients in consultation with a gastroenterologist, although there may be significant complication rates.[38] Thrombolytics are also considered when standard anticoagulation does not lead to recanalization.[32] A transjugular intrahepatic portosystemic shunt (TIPS) procedure may be considered in patients having liver transplants or as an alternative to thrombolytic therapy.

Mesenteric Artery and Venous Thrombosis

Mesenteric arterial and venous thromboses are discussed later.

ISCHEMIC BOWEL

Ischemic bowel can be caused by 1 of 4 mechanisms: arterial thrombosis, arterial embolism, venous thrombosis, or nonocclusive mesenteric ischemia (NOMI). Survival rates vary depending on the mechanism. Overall mortality is as high as 60% to 80%, especially with delays in diagnosis or presentation of greater than 24 hours.[39–42] Park and colleagues[43] reported worse survival rates in older patients, those not candidates for bowel resection, and those whose cause is NOMI. The overall survival rates for patients with mesenteric ischemia have improved according to a review that analyzed 45 studies and 3692 patients according to cause in almost 4 decades (1966–2002).[44,45] Mesenteric ischemia is categorized as occlusive or nonocclusive in origin. Occlusive mesenteric ischemia either involves the SMA or the superior mesenteric vein (SMV). Arterial occlusion may be embolic or thrombotic in origin.

Mesenteric ischemia and ischemic colitis are different clinical entities. The former refers to occlusion of the SMA and SMV, whereas the latter refers to ischemia in the distribution of the IMA. Patients with mesenteric ischemia primarily present with abdominal pain.[1,43,46] Patients with ischemic colitis present with lower gastrointestinal bleeding and are less likely to report abdominal pain as the primary complaint. Ischemic colitis has been reported in marathon runners with similar clinical presentations.[47] Patients with ischemic colitis tend to be older (77 vs 61 years in a retrospective review of 100 patients presenting to the emergency department [ED]) and show lower overall mortality.[48] Angiography is not indicated in cases of ischemic colitis.

Between 40% and 50% of patients with mesenteric ischemia have an arterial embolus as the cause. Emboli typically lodge in the SMA because of the narrow angle it subtends as it branches off the abdominal aorta. Less commonly, emboli lodge in the IMA and, rarely, in the celiac artery.[39,46,49] In most cases, a patient with underlying cardiac abnormalities presents with acute onset of pain. Predisposing cardiac conditions include arrhythmia (most commonly atrial fibrillation), myocardial infarction, cardiomyopathy, recent angiography, valvular disorder (eg, rheumatic valve disease), or ventricular aneurysm.[42,50,51] Following surgical embolectomy, the mortality from analyzed results from 4 decades is 54%.[44]

Thrombotic Occlusion of the Mesenteric Artery

Atherosclerosis is the major cause of arterial thrombosis leading to ischemia of the SMA and is the cause of mesenteric ischemia in 25% of patients.[39,42] The onset of pain is usually more insidious and may be initially intermittent and eventually becoming constant. Other causative factors are hypercoagulability, estrogen therapy, and prolonged hypotension.[50] Patients with chronic ischemia may present with intestinal angina (typically epigastric pain precipitated by eating) and describe food fear and ensuing weight loss.[42] Chronic mesenteric ischemia is usually caused by atherosclerosis and is more common in women and smokers. It is also associated with radiation arteritis, autoimmune arteritides, and fibromuscular dysplasia.[52] Mortality is high for this disorder and, following surgical treatment, is reportedly 77% (**Fig. 3**).[44]

Thrombotic Occlusion of the Mesenteric Vein

Mesenteric venous thrombosis accounts for 10% to 15% of mesenteric ischemia cases. Risk factors for mesenteric venous thrombosis include oral contraceptives or estrogen therapy, malignancy, hypercoagulability, portal hypertension, portal vein thrombosis or other deep vein thrombosis, sickle cell disease, clotting disorders, hepatosplenomegaly, hepatitis, pancreatitis, coagulopathic states, sepsis, cigarette smoking, prior abdominal surgery, and alcohol use.[42,50,52–56] Twenty percent of mesenteric venous thrombosis cases are found to be idiopathic. Patients may present in a subacute fashion with abdominal pain and diarrhea. Clinical findings are likely to be more severe, with frank peritonitis and bleeding in patients with extensive transmural ischemia. With chronic mesenteric vein thrombosis, the collateral circulation usually allows for adequate venous drainage, limiting symptoms and consequent secondary effects of portal hypertension and varix formation. Mesenteric venous thrombosis is usually diagnosed by CT with intravenous contrast. This modality has the advantage compared with color Doppler ultrasound of also allowing for assessment of the bowel and other intra-abdominal conditions. Most mesenteric venous ischemia is treated nonoperatively with anticoagulation. As with portal vein thrombosis, a consideration of the harm-to-benefit profile of thrombolytics can be undertaken in consultation with a gastroenterologist as clinical indications dictate. The pooled reported mortality following surgical treatment of venous thrombosis is 32%.[44]

NOMI

NOMI is defined as ischemia in the absence of identifiable occlusive lesions in the splanchnic arteries or veins. It tends to be precipitated by low-flow states such as hypotension, hypovolemia, heart failure, or sepsis, in which a vicious cycle develops with hypoperfusion leading to vasoconstriction, which leads to ischemia, followed

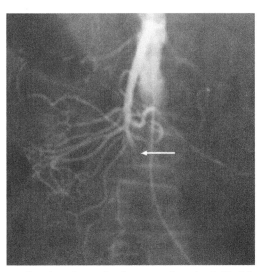

Fig. 3. Selective conventional angiography shows an abrupt cutoff of the SMA secondary to embolus (*arrow*). (*From* Martinez JP, Hogan GJ. Mesenteric ischemia. Emerg Med Clin North Am 2004;22(4):912; with permission.)

by elaboration of inflammatory mediators that further exacerbate hypotension and hypoperfusion. Mechanical processes, such as obstructive tissue bands, intussusception, volvulus, and incarcerated hernias, are nonocclusive causes of mesenteric infarction but are nonvascular in nature and therefore not considered in this article.[57] Twenty percent of cases of mesenteric ischemia have nonocclusive causes. Many patients with NOMI have underlying illness, which contributes to the high mortality. Medications associated with NOMI include cocaine, digitalis (splanchnic vasoconstriction), ergot alkaloids and vasopressors, α constricting agents, and β-blockers.[39,42,50,52]

Clinical Findings

Abdominal pain is the chief complaint in most patients with mesenteric ischemia, followed by associated nausea, vomiting, and diarrhea.[40,41,51] In one retrospective study of 83 patients, hypertension and diabetes mellitus were the most common risk factors. The features of the abdominal pain tend to vary depending on the mechanism of occlusion. Pain caused by embolic disease is often acute in onset and the patient may have associated nausea, vomiting, or diarrhea (both may be either bloody or nonbloody). Bleeding per rectum is reported in 14% to 16% of cases.[43,51] On examination, the patient may have remarkably mild abdominal tenderness compared with the severity of symptoms. With progression of ischemia, patients may be hypotensive with peritoneal signs on abdominal examination. Thrombotic ischemia is likely to have a more insidious onset that may progress to being constant in nature. Patients with NOMI have more varied presentation with underlying illness, abdominal distension, hypertension, and nausea.[41,57]

Laboratory Evaluation

There is no single specific test for the diagnosis of mesenteric ischemia.[39] Most commonly, an anion gap acidosis, leukocytosis, and hemoconcentration are found with mesenteric ischemia. Increased lactate is independently associated with higher mortality.[40] Studies evaluating the association between mesenteric ischemia and D-dimer note a high sensitivity but low specificity. There is no correlation between D-dimer value and severity of mesenteric ischemia.[58]

Diagnostic Imaging

Deciding on the most appropriate diagnostic imaging test once the possibility of mesenteric ischemia has been recognized is challenging. Plain abdominal radiographs, CT, ultrasound, magnetic resonance imaging (MRI), multislice CT angiography, and angiography are all radiographic modalities for consideration.

Plain radiographs may show pathognomonic findings of mesenteric ischemia (eg, thumb-printing or bowel loop thickening) in up to 40% of cases.[39] Often, these are useful as a first test to evaluate for obstruction or free air. Commonly, plain films show nonspecific findings. Abdominal radiographs have low sensitivity for the detection of air in the splanchnic vascular system and underestimate its extent if it is seen.[59] If portal gas is identified, mesenteric ischemia is the most likely diagnosis and emergent surgical intervention is indicated.

Doppler ultrasound has limited usefulness in the acute and emergent evaluation of mesenteric ischemia because of the time required and operator-dependent nature of this modality. Air-filled bowel makes ultrasound difficult to interpret, although more proximal occlusions in the celiac and SMA may be visualized. MRI is a time-consuming and costly measure whose accuracy has not been confirmed but may in the future prove to be sensitive.[39]

In the early phase of mesenteric ischemia, CT with IV contrast may show vascular opacification in the vessel lumen as with SMA thrombosis (**Fig. 4**). Dilated loops of bowel, air-fluid levels, and changes in bowel wall enhancement, or a combination of these, are nonspecific findings but may indicate more advanced stages of mesenteric ischemia. In later phases of ischemia, CT shows thickened bowel and air in the bowel wall or pneumotosis intestinalis (**Fig. 5**).[39] Mesenteric venous gas seen on CT alone is not pathognomonic and does not mark the extent of mesenteric ischemia. It can occur in more benign inflammatory or infectious abdominal processes such as ulcer disease, pancreatitis, diabetes mellitus, and caustic ingestions.[59–61] On CT, it is typically appreciated ventrally first, appearing in the left lobe peripherally and in the subcapsular region of the liver.[59,62] Therefore, mesenteric vascular gas, although sensitive, is not specific for mesenteric ischemia and occurs more commonly in mesenteric venous thrombosis (**Fig. 6**).[61,63]

Angiography is still the gold standard in the diagnosis of mesenteric ischemia, but multidetector CT angiography may emerge as a preferred imaging modality because of its ability to assess the bowel wall (**Fig. 7**). When angiography is performed, a catheter is left in the SMA for administration of vasodilators or papaverine, which is particularly useful in embolic mesenteric ischemia or NOMI.[39,42]

Treatment

Treatment is tailored to the cause of the mesenteric ischemia. All patients require hemodynamic monitoring, resuscitation, intravenous fluid, broad-spectrum antibiotic administration, and pain management.[39,46] Emergent surgical consultation is warranted in acute ischemia, and the patient should not be given anything to eat or drink by mouth. Without contraindications, heparin therapy should be initiated, and, if

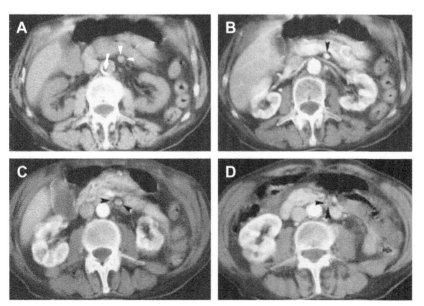

Fig. 4. Embolic occlusion of SMA. (*A*) Unenhanced CT scan; the SMA is normal (*arrowhead*). (*B*) Contrast-enhanced CT scan at the same level; the SMA has a regular enhancement. (*C, D*) Contrast-enhanced CT at a lower level; unenhanced aspect of the SMA caused by endoluminal embolus (*arrowhead*). (*From* Angelelli G, Scardapane A, Memeo M, et al. Acute bowel ischemia: CT findings. Eur J Radiol 2004;50(1):39; with permission.)

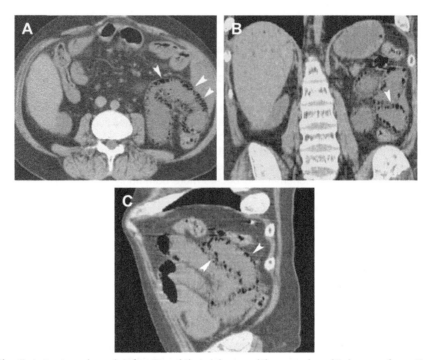

Fig. 5. Late-stage bowel infarction. (*A*) Axial scan, (*B*) coronal multiplanar reformation (MPR) image, and (*C*) sagittal MPR image. Pneumatosis; gas within bowel walls (*arrowheads*). (*From* Angelelli G, Scardapane A, Memeo M, et al. Acute bowel ischemia: CT findings. Eur J Radiol 2004;50(1):44; with permission.)

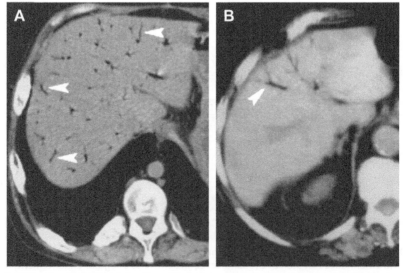

Fig. 6. Patients with bowel infarction. Gas in hepatic portal branches is peripherally located (*arrowheads*). (*From* Angelelli G, Scardapane A, Memeo M, et al. Acute bowel ischemia: CT findings. Eur J Radiol 2004;50(1):45; with permission.)

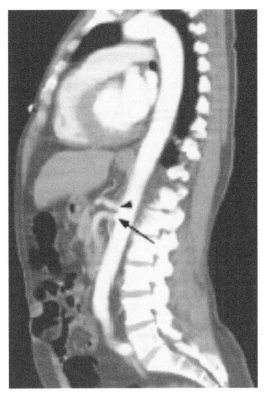

Fig. 7. Sagittal CT angiography of the aorta shows normal origins of the celiac axis (*arrowhead*) and SMA (*arrow*). (*From* Martinez JP, Hogan GJ. Mesenteric ischemia. Emerg Med Clin North Am 2004;22(4):919; with permission.)

vasopressors are indicated, pure α agonists should be avoided to minimize vasospasm and exacerbation of ischemia. Vasopressors and digitalis should be avoided when possible.[42]

A patient with peritoneal signs usually requires emergent laparotomy.[42,50] A patient with mesenteric ischemia caused by embolic phenomena would require surgical intervention for embolectomy, excision of infarcted bowel, and consideration of intra-arterial papaverine. The patient with an arterial thrombus is a candidate for similar interventions: thrombectomy and revascularization. Similarly, if the patient has mesenteric venous thrombosis, thrombectomy and excision of gangrenous bowel may be indicated, and heparin therapy should be initiated. Patients with NOMI should have the underlying cause treated as well as resection of the affected segment of bowel. With angiographic evidence of occlusion, intra-arterial papaverine may be injected directly via the catheter.[50]

Risk Management Strategy

Factors affecting mortality from mesenteric ischemia include older age, delay in presentation, signs of peritonitis, and delay in surgical intervention. One retrospective study of 60 patients who underwent surgery for mesenteric ischemia noted that age greater than 70 years conferred a 3.8-fold increased risk of mortality compared with those less than this age.[40] Another series reported an overall survival rate of 40% at 30 days after surgery, with an 81% survival rate for patients less than 71 years of age, compared with a 30% survival rate in those aged 71 to 84 years. Surgical inter-vention within 6 hours also resulted in significantly improved survival.[64]

ANEURYSM

A vascular aneurysm is defined by the focal dilatation of an artery to at least 1.5 times its normal diameter. A true aneurysm involves all 3 layers: the intima, media, and adventitia of the vessel wall; otherwise the dilated segment is referred to as a pseudoaneurysm.[65] There is a broad spectrum of disease severity associated with arterial aneurysms in the abdominal cavity. Some present as catastrophic abdominal emergencies, whereas others are asymptomatic and incidental for the life-time of the patient. With the increased use of abdominal imaging modalities, earlier diagnosis of these lesions is more common. Emergency physicians should understand their natural history as well as their management if they rupture.

Abdominal Aortic Aneurysm

The aorta is the most common location of an aneurysm in the abdominal cavity. Most abdominal aortic aneurysms (AAAs) occur in the infrarenal region. Most aneurysms are fusiform rather than saccular, meaning that the entire circumference of the vessel is involved.[65] The mean diameter of the infrarenal aorta is 1.66 to 2.16 cm in older women and 1.99 to 2.39 cm in older men. By convention, an anteroposterior diameter of greater than 3.0 cm is classified as an aneurysm.[65,66]

The prevalence of AAA in men between 65 and 79 years of age is 5% to 10% but less common in women at 2%.[67,68] The most important complication of AAA is rupture, which occurs almost exclusively in aneurysms larger than 4 cm.[69] According to one recent population-based study, the prevalence of aneurysms of this magnitude in men is 1.1% for age 55 to 64 years, 4.1% for age 65 to 74 years, and 8.6% for age 75 to 84 years. Larger aneurysms are present in only 0.4% of women older than 55 years.[68] AAA is very rare before the age of 50 years. Ruptured AAA is estimated to cause 15,000 deaths in the United States each year.[70]

A large prospective cohort of more than 120,000 veterans undergoing screening for AAA has elucidated the risk factors for this disease (**Table 1**). For clinically significant aneurysms (>3.9 cm), the most important risk factors are smoking, family history of AAA, increasing age, and history of atherosclerotic diseases. Factors that were not associated with the development of AAA included chronic obstructive pulmonary disease (COPD) and hypertension. This latter finding is surprising in view of the clear association between AAA and atherosclerosis. In addition, this study also showed that

Table 1 Associated positive and negative factors for AAA	
Factors	Odds Ratio (95% Confidence Interval)
Smoking	5.07 (4.13–6.21)
Family history of AAA	1.94 (1.63–2.32)
Age, per 7 y	1.71 (1.61–1.82)
History of atherosclerotic disease	1.66 (1.49–1.84)
Female sex	0.18 (0.07–0.48)
Diabetes	0.52 (0.45–0.61)
Black race	0.53 (0.40–0.69)

female sex, black race, and diabetes were traits associated with a decreased risk of AAA.[71]

The pathophysiology of AAA development and subsequent rupture is incompletely understood at this time. The aortic wall consists of 3 layers: the intima, media, and adventitia. Within the media and adventitia, elastin and collagen are the most important components for maintaining the mechanical integrity of the vessel wall. Elastin is highly concentrated in the medial layer, whereas collagen is concentrated in the adventitia. Damage to and loss of elastin fibers and an associated reduction in the density of smooth muscle cells seem to be integral to the early development of AAA, whereas collagen degradation in the adventitia might be the most important factor in rupture. There seems to be an inflammatory component to this process that ultimately results in the destruction of elastin and collagen. Matrix metalloproteinases have been implicated as one of the key enzymes responsible for the breakdown of these structural proteins.[65,66,72]

In most patients, the natural history of AAA is one of expansion. Size is the most important predictor of AAA rupture. Accordingly, determining the rate of growth and the size at which aneurysms are at significant risk for rupture are important for predicting who will benefit from elective repair. These principles are also valuable to the emergency physician managing patients with AAA. First, understanding the association between AAA size and rupture can aid in estimating the likelihood that a patient's symptoms are related to an aortic rupture or some other abdominal process. Second, it can guide the type and urgency of follow-up needed in asymptomatic patients in whom AAA is detected in the ED.

The average growth rate of AAAs is from 0.2 to 0.6 cm/y, with larger aneurysms growing at a faster rate than smaller ones. It is currently impossible to predict which aneurysms will undergo significant growth.[73] Although it seems that there is a substantial increase in rupture risk for aneurysms greater than 5.0 to 6.0 cm, estimating the precise risk associated with a specific aneurysm diameter is challenging. The Joint Council of the American Association for Vascular Surgery and Society for Vascular Surgery have pooled results from various studies and predicted annual rupture risks based on AAA diameter: size less than 4 cm, 0%; size 4 to 5 cm, 0.5% to 5%; size 5 to 6 cm, 3% to 15%; size 6 to 7 cm, 10% to 20%; size 7 to 8 cm, 20% to 40%; larger than 8 cm, 30% to 50%.[74] Because the mortality associated with surgical repair of AAA is considerable (2.1%–5.5%), elective repair is generally not recommended until aneurysms have reached 5.5 cm (or increase at a rate >1 cm/y), at which point the annual risk of rupture outweighs the risks associated with surgery.[75] Other factors, including female sex, current smoking, and hypertension, have been associated with an increased risk for rupture and should be factored on a case-by-case basis into decisions regarding elective operative repair versus ongoing ultrasound surveillance for AAA growth.[69] Two large trials have addressed the question of whether elective repair versus surveillance for small aneurysms (4.0–5.5 cm) decreases mortality, and it seems that early repair does not improve survival.[75]

As previously mentioned, the most widely accepted and feared complication of AAA is rupture. It is estimated that 50% of patients with a ruptured AAA die before reaching the hospital.[65] Of those who reach the hospital alive, the overall mortality is 80%.[76] This figure comes from one of the few studies reporting on all patients with ruptured AAA arriving to the hospital rather than just those undergoing operative repair. In this same cohort, 43% did not undergo operative repair, all of whom died. Fifty-seven percent received surgery, with a subsequent mortality of 64%.[76] A recent meta-analysis including more than 21,000 patients with ruptured AAA taken for operative repair suggests a lower mortality of close to 50%.[77]

Ruptured or leaking AAA should be suspected in any older patient presenting to the ED with the clinical findings, in isolation or combination, of abdominal pain, back pain, and shock. Based on the cohort examined, these symptoms and signs are variably present. One of the larger case series suggests that abdominal pain or back pain is present in 95% of patients with a ruptured AAA.[78] Based on another large series, most patients presenting with a ruptured AAA are hypotensive in the prehospital setting.[79] Of patients who arrive at the hospital alive with a ruptured AAA, about two-thirds have ruptured into the retroperitoneal space, a quarter intraperitoneal, with the remaining rupturing into the IVC or duodenum.[78] Before leaking or rupture, aortic aneurysms rarely produce prodromal symptoms; therefore, most patients presenting to the ED with this vascular emergency are unaware that they have this disease.[76]

The early management of patients with suspected unstable AAA, either leaking or ruptured, should focus on rapid diagnosis and early definitive treatment. The presence of known risk factors for the disease (such as male gender, advanced age, and a history of smoking) in conjunction with acute abdominal or back pain should heighten suspicion for an unstable AAA. Abdominal palpation for a pulsatile mass has a widely ranging sensitivity of 44% to 97%.[80]

At this time, bedside ultrasound is the most useful tool in the diagnostic evaluation of AAA. For emergency physicians, ultrasound is a highly accurate test, with a sensitivity and specificity approaching 100% in detecting AAA.[81] Ultrasound has the added advantage of being able to detect free fluid in the abdomen, associated with a free intraperitoneal rupture. However, sonography does not reliably distinguish between ruptured and asymptomatic aneurysms because hemorrhage (in patients who have not already exsanguinated into the peritoneum) most frequently occurs into the retroperitoneal tissues, where ultrasound assessment is limited. Regarding the mechanics of the test, the low-frequency abdominal probe should be used and measurements taken in a plane perpendicular to the axis of the vessel. CT might be a useful imaging modality for asymptomatic patients with a newly diagnosed AAA to fully define the anatomic details of the aneurysm; however, it is generally not considered as the initial test of choice for patients with suspected ruptured AAA if ultrasound is rapidly available. CT may be appropriate if the ultrasound is technically limited or cannot distinguish between a symptomatic or incidental AAA.

For those with a suspected ruptured AAA, resuscitation, diagnostic measures, and consultation with appropriate specialties, ideally vascular surgery, should occur simultaneously. With large-bore intravenous lines in place, judicious fluid and blood replacement should begin for patients in shock, while recognizing that the underlying disorder is an arterial rupture and hemorrhage that can only be corrected by prompt surgical repair. Although prognosis for a ruptured AAA is poor, there do not seem to be early prognostic factors that reliably predict who can and cannot survive a ruptured AAA; therefore, most patients should be aggressively resuscitated.[82]

When aneurysms are detected in asymptomatic ED patients and rupture has been excluded, referral for outpatient follow-up is adequate in most cases. For patients with an aneurysm greater than 5.4 cm, referral should be made to vascular surgery. For those between 4.0 and 5.4 cm, surveillance with ultrasound is recommended every 6 to 12 months, and, for those less than 4.0 cm, every 2 to 3 years is probably sufficient.[66]

Iliac Artery Aneurysm

Iliac artery aneurysms are defined by a focal dilatation in the vessel greater than 1.5 cm. In most case series, symptoms and rupture do not occur until aneurysm size is much larger, usually greater than 4 cm.[83] The risk factors and pathophysiology associated with aneurysms at this site are similar to those for AAA. About 10% to 20% of patients with AAA also have an iliac artery aneurysm.[84,85] Isolated iliac artery aneurysms are rare but, when present, the common iliac artery is the most commonly affected site.[85] There are a few key factors regarding this disease of which the emergency physician should be aware. Compared with AAA, they are more likely to present with urologic symptoms consistent with renal colic.[84,85] In addition, they are more difficult to visualize with sonography, with one cohort study suggesting that up to 50% of isolated iliac artery aneurysm are missed with this imaging modality.[84] When patients with a ruptured iliac artery aneurysm are taken for operative repair, the mortality is about 60%, higher than for AAA, potentially explained by the increased technical difficulties associated with an operation at this site.[84] Unlike AAA, there are no large-scale studies to inform the management of this disease in asymptomatic individuals; however, elective surgery is generally considered when aneurysm size is greater than 3.5 cm, and strongly recommended when greater than 5 cm.[85]

Visceral Artery Aneurysms

Visceral artery aneurysms, which include renal and splanchnic lesions, receive less attention than AAA because they are rare and usually asymptomatic.[66] The prevalence of these aneurysms is unknown. Based on one of the larger case series, 95% of the visceral artery aneurysms are detected during routine investigation into unrelated abdominal symptoms.[86] Of those detected, splenic and hepatic artery aneurysms are by far the most common, comprising 80% of visceral artery aneurysm.[87] The natural history is not well understood, and the clinical presentation poorly defined. In about one-third of patients, multiple aneurysms are present.[88] Most patients are diagnosed or present with symptoms in the sixth decade of life.[88] Aneurysms that rupture are typically greater than 2 cm, so this is often considered the threshold for repair in patients with asymptomatic disease.[86] Because of the low prevalence of these aneurysms, their investigation is most likely to be prompted by high-risk clinical findings in patients whose abdominal symptoms have not been otherwise explained.

Splenic Artery Aneurysm

Splenic artery aneurysm accounts for 60% of visceral artery aneurysms.[89] Most are true aneurysms. Common risk factors include arteriosclerosis, portal hypertension, pancreatitis, and trauma.[88] There is an increased prevalence of the disease in women, particularly those who are multiparous. With the increased use of high-resolution ultrasonography in pregnancy, more of these aneurysms are being detected in otherwise healthy pregnant women.[89]

Most patients are asymptomatic until the time of rupture, which is a rare occurrence. Pregnancy and aneurysm size greater than 2 cm increase the risk of rupture. Patients in whom the aneurysm has ruptured most commonly present with abdominal pain. Shock can be delayed if the initial aneurysm rupture is contained within the lesser peritoneal sac, leading to a double-rupture phenomenon. The treatment of rupture is both resuscitative and operative, historically including a splenectomy.[88] Endovascular techniques, specifically transarterial embolization, have also been successfully used.[90] There is no consensus on the management of asymptomatic aneurysms.

Hepatic Artery Aneurysm

Aneurysms of the hepatic artery are the second most common visceral artery aneurysm, comprising 20%. More than half (77%) occur in the common hepatic artery, and most of the rest in the extrahepatic segment of the proper hepatic artery. In contrast with splenic aneurysms, these aneurysms are more common in men.[87] About 50% of these lesions are pseudoaneurysms, most likely related to complications of interventional biliary procedures.[88] Vascular diseases, in particular fibromuscular dysplasia and polyarteritis nodosa, are associated with both aneurysm formation and rupture. Although abdominal pain and shock suggest rupture, even unruptured hepatic artery aneurysms can be symptomatic secondary to compression on the biliary tree. About 50% of aneurysms rupture into the biliary tract and can present with the classic triad of biliary colic, hematemesis (caused by hemobilia), and jaundice.[88] The mortality of 40% associated with rupture seems to be consistent across case series data.[91] As with splenic artery aneurysm rupture, the treatment has historically been surgical repair; however, transarterial embolization is an increasingly used technique.[91]

Renal Artery Aneurysm

Like other visceral artery aneurysms, renal artery aneurysms are most commonly incidental findings during abdominal imaging or investigations into renovascular hypertension. Similar to splenic aneurysms, there is an association with multiparous women. Arterial fibrodysplasia is the most common vascular disorder associated with these aneurysms.[92] Based on case series data, about 20% are bilateral. Rupture seems to be extremely rare.[92,93]

SUMMARY

The emergency physician should consider the possibility of vascular disorders in patients presenting with abdominal complaints. These clinical entities tend to be dangerous and time urgent. In maintaining an appropriate level of suspicion and assessing a patient's risk, the factors associated with the various diseases need to be considered. If a vascular emergency is deemed likely, the appropriate diagnostic studies need to be initiated promptly and consultants engaged early. Clinician-performed bedside ultrasonography is an invaluable tool, particularly if the concern is for ruptured or leaking AAA. CT angiography is becoming the initial imaging test of choice for abdominal vascular diseases caused by occlusive thrombosis. With rapid diagnosis and appropriate resuscitation, many of these vascular emergencies are correctable.

REFERENCES

1. Martinez JP, Hogan GJ. Mesenteric ischemia. Emerg Med Clin North Am 2004; 22(4):909–28.
2. Skandalakis J, Colborn G, Weidman T. Skandalakis' surgical anatomy. 2004 [internet]. Available at: www.accesssurgery.com/content/aspx?aID=70499. Accessed January 20, 2010.
3. Paula R. Hepatic Disease. In: Adams JG, Barton ED, Collings J, et al, editors. Emergency medicine. Philadelphia: Saunders Elsevier; 2008. p. 395–406.
4. Bradbury AW, Stonebridge PA, John TG, et al. Acute thrombosis of the non-aneurysmal abdominal aorta. Eur J Vasc Surg 1993;7(3):320–3.
5. Poirée S, Monnier-Cholley L, Tubiana J, et al. Acute abdominal aortic thrombosis in cancer patients. Abdom Imaging 2004;29(4):511–3.
6. Bhardwaj R. Total occlusion of the abdominal aorta and the severity of angiographically-proven coronary artery disease. Singapore Med J 2009; 50(10):967–70.

7. Jeddy TA, Buckenham TM, Taylor RS, et al. Abdominal aortic thrombosis following a fall. Br J Surg 1993;80(2):214.
8. Roehm EF, Twiest MW, Williams RC. Abdominal aortic thrombosis in association with an attempted Heimlich maneuver. JAMA 1983;249(9):1186–7.
9. Martin TJ, Bobba RK, Metzger R, et al. Acute abdominal aortic thrombosis as a complication of the Heimlich maneuver. J Am Geriatr Soc 2007;55(7):1146–7.
10. Dieckmann K, Gehrckens R. Thrombosis of abdominal aorta during cisplatin-based chemotherapy of testicular seminoma - a case report. BMC Cancer 2009; 9:459.
11. Dossa CD, Shepard AD, Reddy DJ, et al. Acute aortic occlusion. A 40-year experience. Arch Surg 1994;129(6):603–7 [discussion: 607–8].
12. Kelley CE. Nontraumatic abdominal aortic thrombosis presenting with anterior spinal artery syndrome and pulmonary edema. J Emerg Med 1991;9(4):233–7.
13. Lee W, Cheng Y, Lin H. Leriche syndrome. Int J Emerg Med 2008;1(3):223.
14. Krankenberg H, Schlüter M, Schwencke C, et al. Endovascular reconstruction of the aortic bifurcation in patients with Leriche syndrome. Clin Res Cardiol 2009; 98(10):657–64.
15. Babu SC, Shah PM, Nitahara J. Acute aortic occlusion–factors that influence outcome. J Vasc Surg 1995;21(4):567–72 [discussion: 573–5].
16. Campbell JP, Lane PW. Spontaneous renal artery thrombosis associated with altered mental status. Ann Emerg Med 1992;21(12):1505–7.
17. Samara EN, Voss BL, Pederson JA. Renal artery thrombosis associated with elevated cyclosporine levels: a case report and review of the literature. Transplant Proc 1988;20(1):119–23.
18. Baciewicz FA, Kaplan BM, Murphy TE, et al. Bilateral renal artery thrombotic occlusion: a unique complication following removal of a transthoracic intraaortic balloon. Ann Thorac Surg 1982;33(6):631–4.
19. Dimitroulis D, Bokos J, Zavos G, et al. Vascular complications in renal transplantation: a single-center experience in 1367 renal transplantations and review of the literature. Transplant Proc 2009;41(5):1609–14.
20. Salehipour M, Salahi H, Jalaeian H, et al. Vascular complications following 1500 consecutive living and cadaveric donor renal transplantations: a single center study. Saudi J Kidney Dis Transpl 2009;20(4):570–2.
21. Ouriel K, Andrus CH, Ricotta JJ, et al. Acute renal artery occlusion: when is revascularization justified? J Vasc Surg 1987;5(2):348–55.
22. Huang C, Lo H, Huang H, et al. ED presentations of acute renal infarction. Am J Emerg Med 2007;25(2):164–9.
23. Haas CA, Dinchman KH, Nasrallah PF, et al. Traumatic renal artery occlusion: a 15-year review. J Trauma 1998;45(3):557–61.
24. Spirnak JP, Resnick MI. Revascularization of traumatic thrombosis of the renal artery. Surg Gynecol Obstet 1987;164(1):22–6.
25. Knudson MM, Harrison PB, Hoyt DB, et al. Outcome after major renovascular injuries: a Western trauma association multicenter report. J Trauma 2000;49(6): 1116–22.
26. Seupaul RA, Stepsis TM, Doehring MC. Idiopathic renal vein thrombosis in a healthy young woman with flank pain and fever. Am J Emerg Med 2005; 23(3):417–9.
27. Asghar M, Ahmed K, Shah SS, et al. Renal vein thrombosis. Eur J Vasc Endovasc Surg 2007;34(2):217–23.
28. Witz M, Korzets Z. Renal vein occlusion: diagnosis and treatment. Isr Med Assoc J 2007;9(5):402–5.

29. Zigman A, Yazbeck S, Emil S, et al. Renal vein thrombosis: a 10-year review. J Pediatr Surg 2000;35(11):1540–2.
30. Kau E, Patel R, Fiske J, et al. Isolated renal vein thrombosis after blunt trauma. Urology 2004;64(4):807–8.
31. Sogaard KK, Astrup LB, Vilstrup H, et al. Portal vein thrombosis; risk factors, clinical presentation and treatment. BMC Gastroenterol 2007;7:34.
32. Ponziani FR, Zocco MA, Campanale C, et al. Portal vein thrombosis: insight into physiopathology, diagnosis, and treatment. World J Gastroenterol 2010;16(2): 143–55.
33. Plessier A, Darwish-Murad S, Hernandez-Guerra M, et al. Acute portal vein thrombosis unrelated to cirrhosis: a prospective multicenter follow-up study. Hepatology 2010;51(1):210–8.
34. Wang J, Zhao H, Liu Y. Portal vein thrombosis. Hepatobiliary Pancreat Dis Int 2005;4(4):515–8.
35. Webster GJ, Burroughs AK, Riordan SM. Review article: portal vein thrombosis-new insights into aetiology and management. Aliment Pharmacol Ther 2005; 21(1):1–9.
36. Fimognari FL, Violi F. Portal vein thrombosis in liver cirrhosis. Intern Emerg Med 2008;3(3):213–8.
37. Sobhonslidsuk A, Reddy KR. Portal vein thrombosis: a concise review. Am J Gastroenterol 2002;97(3):535–41.
38. Malkowski P, Pawlak J, Michalowicz B, et al. Thrombolytic treatment of portal thrombosis. Hepatogastroenterology 2003;50(54):2098–100.
39. Berland T, Oldenburg WA. Acute mesenteric ischemia. Curr Gastroenterol Rep 2008;10(3):341–6.
40. Kassahun WT, Schulz T, Richter O, et al. Unchanged high mortality rates from acute occlusive intestinal ischemia: six year review. Langenbecks Arch Surg 2008;393(2):163–71.
41. Dahlke MH, Asshoff L, Popp FC, et al. Mesenteric ischemia–outcome after surgical therapy in 83 patients. Dig Surg 2008;25(3):213–9.
42. Tekwani K, Sikka R. High-risk chief complaints III: abdomen and extremities. Emerg Med Clin North Am 2009;27(4):747–65, x.
43. Park WM, Gloviczki P, Cherry KJ, et al. Contemporary management of acute mesenteric ischemia: factors associated with survival. J Vasc Surg 2002;35(3):445–52.
44. Schoots IG, Koffeman GI, Legemate DA, et al. Systematic review of survival after acute mesenteric ischaemia according to disease aetiology. Br J Surg 2004;91: 17–27.
45. Mamode N, Pickford I, Leiberman P. Failure to improve outcome in acute mesenteric ischaemia: seven-year review. Eur J Surg 1999;165(3):203–8.
46. Walker JS, Dire DJ. Vascular abdominal emergencies. Emerg Med Clin North Am 1996;14(3):571–92.
47. Sanchez LD, Tracy JA, Berkoff D, et al. Ischemic colitis in marathon runners: a case-based review. J Emerg Med 2006;30(3):321–6.
48. Ullery BS, Boyko AT, Banet GA, et al. Colonic ischemia: an under-recognized cause of lower gastrointestinal bleeding. J Emerg Med 2004;27(1):1–5.
49. Demirpolat G, Oran I, Tamsel S, et al. Acute mesenteric ischemia: endovascular therapy. Abdom Imaging 2007;32(3):299–303.
50. Oldenburg WA, Lau LL, Rodenberg TJ, et al. Acute mesenteric ischemia: a clinical review. Arch Intern Med 2004;164(10):1054–62.
51. Sreedharan S, Tan YM, Tan SG, et al. Clinical spectrum and surgical management of acute mesenteric ischaemia in Singapore. Singapore Med J 2007;48(4):319–23.

52. Barkhordarian S. Mesenteric ischemia: identification and treatment. ACC Curr J Rev 2003;12(1):19–21.
53. Kumar S, Sarr MG, Kamath PS. Mesenteric venous thrombosis. N Engl J Med 2001;345(23):1683–8.
54. Cenedese A, Monneuse O, Gruner L, et al. Initial management of extensive mesenteric venous thrombosis: retrospective study of nine cases. World J Surg 2009;33(10):2203–8.
55. Brunaud L, Antunes L, Collinet-Adler S, et al. Acute mesenteric venous thrombosis: case for nonoperative management. J Vasc Surg 2001;34(4):673–9.
56. Hassan HA. Oral contraceptive-induced mesenteric venous thrombosis with resultant intestinal ischemia. J Clin Gastroenterol 1999;29(1):90–5.
57. Bartone G, Severino BU, Armellino MF, et al. Clinical symptoms of intestinal vascular disorders. Radiol Clin North Am 2008;46(5):887–9, v.
58. Chiu Y, Huang M, How C, et al. D-dimer in patients with suspected acute mesenteric ischemia. Am J Emerg Med 2009;27(8):975–9.
59. Hou S, Chern C, How C, et al. Hepatic portal venous gas: clinical significance of computed tomography findings. Am J Emerg Med 2004;22(3):214–8.
60. Nelson AL, Millington TM, Sahani D, et al. Hepatic portal venous gas: the ABCs of management. Arch Surg 2009;144(6):575–81 [discussion: 581].
61. Chiu H, Chen C, Lu Y, et al. Hepatic portal venous gas. Am J Surg 2005;189(4): 501–3.
62. Schindera ST, Triller J, Vock P, et al. Detection of hepatic portal venous gas: its clinical impact and outcome. Emerg Radiol 2006;12(4):164–70.
63. Angelelli G, Scardapane A, Memeo M, et al. Acute bowel ischemia: CT findings. Eur J Radiol 2004;50(1):37–47.
64. Wadman M, Syk I, Elmståhl S. Survival after operations for ischaemic bowel disease. Eur J Surg 2000;166(11):872–7.
65. Sakalihasan N, Limet R, Defawe OD. Abdominal aortic aneurysm. Lancet 2005; 365(9470):1577–89.
66. Hirsch AT, Haskal ZJ, Hertzer NR, et al. ACC/AHA guidelines for the management of patients with peripheral arterial disease (lower extremity, renal, mesenteric, and abdominal aortic): a collaborative report from the American Associations for Vascular Surgery/Society for Vascular Surgery, Society for Cardiovascular Angiography and Interventions, Society for Vascular Medicine and Biology, Society of Interventional Radiology, and the ACC/AHA Task Force on Practice Guidelines (writing committee to develop guidelines for the management of patients with peripheral arterial disease)–summary of recommendations. J Vasc Interv Radiol 2006;17(9):1383–97 [quiz: 1398].
67. Vardulaki KA, Prevost TC, Walker NM, et al. Incidence among men of asymptomatic abdominal aortic aneurysms: estimates from 500 screen detected cases. J Med Screen 1999;6(1):50–4.
68. Singh K, Bønaa KH, Jacobsen BK, et al. Prevalence of and risk factors for abdominal aortic aneurysms in a population-based study: the Tromsø study. Am J Epidemiol 2001;154(3):236–44.
69. Brown LC, Powell JT. Risk factors for aneurysm rupture in patients kept under ultrasound surveillance. UK Small Aneurysm Trial Participants. Ann Surg 1999; 230(3):289–96 [discussion: 296–7].
70. Gillum RF. Epidemiology of aortic aneurysm in the United States. J Clin Epidemiol 1995;48(11):1289–98.
71. Lederle FA, Johnson GR, Wilson SE, et al. The aneurysm detection and management study screening program: validation cohort and final results. Aneurysm

Detection and Management Veterans Affairs Cooperative Study Investigators. Arch Intern Med 2000;160(10):1425–30.

72. Weintraub NL. Understanding abdominal aortic aneurysm. N Engl J Med 2009; 361(11):1114–6.

73. Ernst CB. Abdominal aortic aneurysm. N Engl J Med 1993;328(16):1167–72.

74. Brewster DC, Cronenwett JL, Hallett JW, et al. Guidelines for the treatment of abdominal aortic aneurysms. Report of a subcommittee of the Joint Council of the American Association for Vascular Surgery and Society for Vascular Surgery. J Vasc Surg 2003;37(5):1106–17.

75. Ballard DJ, Filardo G, Fowkes G, et al. Surgery for small asymptomatic abdominal aortic aneurysms. Cochrane Database Syst Rev 2008;4:CD001835.

76. Basnyat PS, Biffin AH, Moseley LG, et al. Mortality from ruptured abdominal aortic aneurysm in Wales. Br J Surg 1999;86(6):765–70.

77. Bown MJ, Sutton AJ, Bell PRF, et al. A meta-analysis of 50 years of ruptured abdominal aortic aneurysm repair. Br J Surg 2002;89(6):714–30.

78. Davidović L, Marković M, Kostić D, et al. Ruptured abdominal aortic aneurysms: factors influencing early survival. Ann Vasc Surg 2005;19(1):29–34.

79. Johansen K, Kohler TR, Nicholls SC, et al. Ruptured abdominal aortic aneurysm: the Harborview experience. J Vasc Surg 1991;13(2):240–5 [discussion: 245–7].

80. Lederle FA, Simel DL. The rational clinical examination. Does this patient have abdominal aortic aneurysm? JAMA 1999;281(1):77–82.

81. Bentz S, Jones J. Towards evidence-based emergency medicine: best BETs from the Manchester Royal Infirmary. Accuracy of emergency department ultrasound scanning in detecting abdominal aortic aneurysm. Emerg Med J 2006;23(10): 803–4.

82. Johnston KW. Ruptured abdominal aortic aneurysm: six-year follow-up results of a multicenter prospective study. Canadian Society for Vascular Surgery Aneurysm Study Group. J Vasc Surg 1994;19(5):888–900.

83. Santilli SM, Wernsing SE, Lee ES. Expansion rates and outcomes for iliac artery aneurysms. J Vasc Surg 2000;31(1 Pt 1):114–21.

84. Vammen S, Lindholt J, Henneberg EW, et al. A comparative study of iliac and abdominal aortic aneurysms. Int Angiol 2000;19(2):152–7.

85. Sandhu RS, Pipinos II. Isolated iliac artery aneurysms. Semin Vasc Surg 2005; 18(4):209–15.

86. Pulli R, Dorigo W, Troisi N, et al. Surgical treatment of visceral artery aneurysms: a 25-year experience. J Vasc Surg 2008;48(2):334–42.

87. Berceli SA. Hepatic and splenic artery aneurysms. Semin Vasc Surg 2005;18(4): 196–201.

88. Pasha SF, Gloviczki P, Stanson AW, et al. Splanchnic artery aneurysms. Mayo Clin Proc 2007;82(4):472–9.

89. Sadat U, Dar O, Walsh S, et al. Splenic artery aneurysms in pregnancy–a systematic review. Int J Surg 2008;6(3):261–5.

90. Liu C, Kung C, Liu B, et al. Splenic artery aneurysms encountered in the ED: 10 years' experience. Am J Emerg Med 2007;25(4):430–6.

91. Abbas MA, Fowl RJ, Stone WM, et al. Hepatic artery aneurysm: factors that predict complications. J Vasc Surg 2003;38(1):41–5.

92. Henke PK, Cardneau JD, Welling TH, et al. Renal artery aneurysms: a 35-year clinical experience with 252 aneurysms in 168 patients. Ann Surg 2001;234(4): 454–62 [discussion: 462–3].

93. Tham G, Ekelund L, Herrlin K, et al. Renal artery aneurysms. natural history and prognosis. Ann Surg 1983;197(3):348–52.

Gastric and Esophageal Emergencies

Alessandro Mangili, MD

KEYWORDS

• Gastric • Esophageal • Emergency • Dysphagia • GERD

ESOPHAGEAL ANATOMY AND PHYSIOLOGY

The esophagus is a hollow muscular tube extending from the pharynx to the stomach. Its primary role is to carry solids and liquids from the mouth to the stomach. In the adult the esophagus measures 23 to 25 cm and runs in the mediastinum posterior and lateral to the trachea. Along its course 3 areas of luminal narrowing exist: (1) proximally at the level of the cricoid cartilage; (2) at the level of the aortic arch and left main stem bronchus; and (3) distally at the gastroesophageal junction, where the esophagus penetrates the diaphragm.

The walls of the esophagus are composed of different layers. From internal to external they include a mucosa, submucosa, muscularis propria, and adventitia. The mucosa is composed of nonkeratinizing, stratified squamous epithelial cells. Melanocytes, endocrine cells, and Langerhans cells are present in small numbers in the deeper epithelial layer. The proximal 5% of the esophagus contains striated muscle alone. The remaining 30% to 40% of the upper esophagus contains both smooth and striated muscle. The remaining distal portion of the esophagus is composed of smooth muscle only.

The esophagus has 2 high-pressure areas known as sphincters that help regulate flow. The upper esophageal sphincter (UES) consists of a 3-cm segment composed primarily of the cricopharyngeus muscle. It functions primarily to prevent aspiration and swallowing of large amounts of air. The lower esophageal sphincter (LES) is a 2-cm to 4-cm segment located just proximal to the gastroesophageal junction at the level of the diaphragm, and its primary function is to prevent retrograde flow of gastric contents into the esophagus (reflux).

Swallowing occurs in 3 stages: oral, pharyngeal, and esophageal. In the oral stage food is chewed, formed into a bolus, and moved to the posterior pharynx by the tongue. During the pharyngeal phase the bolus is moved across the UES from the pharynx into the proximal esophagus. In the final stage the food moves from the proximal esophagus into the stomach across the relaxed LES via peristalsis.

Department of Emergency Medicine, Oregon Health and Science University, 3181 SW Sam Jackson Park Road, CDW-EM, Portland, OR 97239-3098, USA
E-mail address: mangili@ohsu.edu

Emerg Med Clin N Am 29 (2011) 273–291
doi:10.1016/j.emc.2011.01.007
0733-8627/11/$ – see front matter © 2011 Elsevier Inc. All rights reserved.

DYSPHAGIA

Dysphagia is the sensation of impaired passage of food from the mouth to the stomach that occurs after swallowing. In contrast, globus refers to the constant sensation of a lump or fullness in the throat regardless of swallowing. In individuals older than 50 years the prevalence of dysphagia is estimated to be 16% to 22%.[1–3] Dysphagia occurs more commonly in older adults and in patients who have had cerebrovascular accidents, head injuries, esophageal cancers, and neuromuscular disorders. In addition, 60% to 87% of residents of nursing homes experience some form of feeding difficulty, and of those residents with oropharyngeal dysphagia and aspiration, 12-month mortality is estimated at 45%.[1,4–6]

Dysphagia is generally divided into 2 types based on the stage of swallowing during which it occurs: oropharyngeal, or transfer, dysphagia and esophageal dysphagia. Oropharyngeal dysphagia occurs during the oral and pharyngeal phases of swallowing when food is transferred from the mouth to the upper esophagus, hence symptoms generally occur within 1 second of swallowing. Esophageal dysphagia occurs during passage of a bolus from the esophagus to the stomach. Dysphagia is further characterized by the mechanism that causes it. Functional causes refer to disordered motor function, whereas mechanical causes include obstruction or narrowing of the esophageal lumen.

Oropharyngeal Dysphagia

Causes of oropharyngeal dysphagia include inflammatory, rheumatologic, neuromuscular, and infectious disorders (**Table 1**). Symptoms of oropharyngeal dysphagia may include drooling, difficulty in initiating swallowing, need to swallow repetitively to clear food from the mouth and pharynx, coughing, gagging, nasal or oral regurgitation, dysarthria, dysphonia, and aspiration.[1,6,7] Chronic oropharyngeal dysphagia may also lead to weight loss, failure to thrive, malnutrition, and recurrent pneumonia.

Esophageal Dysphagia

Esophageal dysphagia results from an obstructive process secondary to either a structural lesion, neuromuscular disorder, or inflammatory process (**Table 2**). In contrast to oropharyngeal dysphagia, symptoms typically occur 10 to 15 seconds after swallowing, and patients describe a sensation of fullness or pressure located in the substernal or epigastric region. Studies indicate that in approximately 75% of cases patients are able to localize the site of the obstruction based on the location of their symptoms.[8] Symptoms associated with esophageal dysphagia may include chest pain, late regurgitation, and odynophagia. Clinical history can be helpful in differentiating between neuromuscular and mechanical causes of esophageal dysphagia. In general, dysphagia that is present equally with solids and liquids suggests a neuromuscular disorder, whereas dysphagia that is present only with solids, or that has progressed from solids to liquids, is more consistent with a mechanical cause. Onset, progression, relief of symptoms, and sensitivity to food temperature also help to distinguish neuromuscular from mechanical causes (**Table 3**).

Neuromuscular Causes of Dysphagia

Achalasia

Achalasia is a primary motility disorder that affects men and women equally, most commonly between the ages of 25 and 60 years. The estimated prevalence in the United States is 10 cases per 100,000.[9] The disease results from the degeneration of neurons in the myenteric plexus enervating the esophagus secondary to an

Table 1
Common causes of oropharyngeal dysphagia

Structural Lesions	Examples
Pharyngeal diverticula	Zenker diverticulum Lateral pharyngeal pouch or diverticula
Intrinsic lesions	Oropharyngeal or laryngeal carcinoma Surgical resection Cricopharyngeal achalasia Cricopharyngeal bar and rings Proximal esophageal webs (Plummer-Vinson) Radiation injury
Extrinsic compression	Osteophytes, skeletal abnormalities Thyromegaly
Neuromuscular Diseases	Examples
Central nervous system	Cerebrovascular accidents, head injury, neoplasm, Parkinson disease, multiple sclerosis, amyotrophic lateral sclerosis, Huntington chorea
Peripheral nervous system	Poliomyelitis, amyotrophic lateral sclerosis Tabes dorsalis Glossitis, pharyngitis, thrush (sensory)
Neuromuscular transmission myopathies	Myasthenia gravis Polymyositis, dermatomyositis Muscular dystrophies Alcoholic myopathy Thyrotoxicosis, hypothyroidism Amyloidosis, Cushing syndrome

Data from Lind CD. Dysphagia: evaluation and treatment. Gastroenterol Clin North Am 2003;32:561.

inflammatory process. This loss of enervation leads to impaired LES relaxation, decreased esophageal peristalsis, and esophageal dilatation. In addition, there is decreased synthesis of important mediators affecting LES relaxation, nitric oxide, and vasoactive intestinal polypeptide.[10]

The most common presenting symptom of patients with achalasia is a progressive dysphagia to both solids and liquids. Sixty percent of patients also report regurgitation, which typically occurs after meals and can occur nocturnally and lead to cough and aspiration, resulting in significant bronchopulmonary complications in 10% of patients.[11] Chest pain is also reported in 20% to 60% of patients. Other symptoms include difficulty belching and heartburn. Weight loss is a rare finding and is generally associated with end-stage disease.

Diagnosis is typically delayed because symptoms are often attributed to gastro-esophageal reflux disease (GERD) or other disorders. Secondary causes of achalasia include Chagas disease secondary to infection with *Trypanosoma cruzi*, esophageal or gastric cancer, paraneoplastic syndrome from small-cell lung cancer, eosinophilic esophagitis (EE), and postfundoplication achalasia.

Numerous imaging modalities exist to aid in the evaluation of dysphagia. The barium esophagram is typically the initial study performed. Esophagram findings consistent with achalasia are a tapering of the distal esophagus with contrast in the distal esophageal lumen, classically described as a bird's beak, as well as dilation of the distal esophagus (**Fig. 1**). Esophageal manometry has the highest sensitivity for diagnosing

Table 2	
Common causes of esophageal dysphagia	
Structural Lesions	
Intrinsic lesions	Peptic stricture, Schatzki ring
	Esophageal carcinoma
	Leiomyoma, lymphoma
	Hiatal hernia
Extrinsic compression	Mediastinal tumors (lung cancer, lymphoma)
	Vascular structures (dysphagia lusoria)
	Surgical changes (fundoplication)
Motor Disorders	
Primary motor disorders	Achalasia
	DES
	Hypertensive LES
	Nutcracker esophagus
	Ineffective esophageal motility
Secondary motor disorders	Collagen vascular diseases or scleroderma, CREST
	Diabetes mellitus
	Alcoholism
Mucosal Diseases	
Esophagitis	GI reflux diseases
	Infectious esophagitis
	Pill induced
	Radiation injury
	Caustic ingestion

Data from Lind CD. Dysphagia: evaluation and treatment. Gastroenterol Clin North Am 2003;32:562.

achalasia; however, patients presenting with dysphagia typically first undergo upper endoscopy, which may reveal retained food and secretions. However, up to 44% of patients have a normal upper endoscopy.[11] Upper endoscopy is especially useful in evaluating for other mechanical causes of dysphagia. Diagnostic findings of esophageal manometry include aperistalsis of the distal esophagus and decreased or absent LES relaxation. Vigorous achalasia is a manometric variant of achalasia in which aperistalsis of the distal esophagus is replaced by normal or high-amplitude esophageal body contractions.[12] High-resolution esophageal manometry (HRM) combined with

Table 3		
Esophageal dysphagia: mechanical versus motor disorders		
History	**Mechanical Disorder**	**Motor Disorder**
Onset	Gradual or sudden	Usually gradual
Progression	Often	Usually not
Type of bolus	Solid (unless high-grade obstruction)	Solids or liquids
Response to bolus	Often must be regurgitated	Usually passes with repeated swallowing or drinking liquids
Temperature dependent	No	Worse with cold liquids; may improve with warm liquids

Data from Lind CD. Dysphagia: evaluation and treatment. Gastroenterol Clin North Am 2003;32:564.

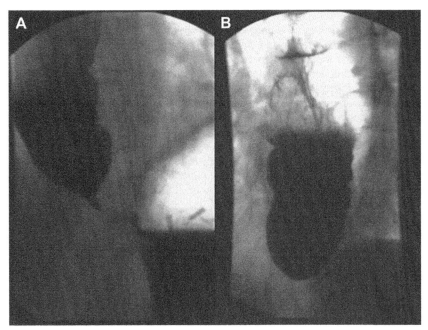

Fig. 1. (*A*) Barium esophagram showing the typical bird's beak appearance of the distal esophagus in a patient with achalasia. (*B*) Esophagram showing a significantly dilated esophagus with an air-fluid level. (*From* Woltman TA, Pellegrini CA, Oelschlager BK. Achalasia. Surg Clin North Am 2005;85:485; with permission.)

contour plot topographic analysis enhances the sensitivity of conventional manometry in the diagnosis of achalasia.[12]

Treatment of achalasia centers on decreasing basal LES pressure. Medical and surgical treatments exist and include medications, botulinum toxin injection, pneumatic dilatation, and myotomy. Treatment is oriented toward symptom relief and improvement in dysphagia as well as in objective measures of esophageal and LES function. As a result of inefficacy and many side effects, medical therapy with calcium channel blockers such as nifedipine is generally considered a temporizing measure while awaiting definitive management with more invasive therapy. Botulinum toxin injection into the LES decreases basal pressure by targeting acetylcholine-releasing neurons and carries a low side effect profile. Several studies have shown good efficacy and improved symptoms with this treatment, although benefits tend to be short lived and additional injections are required.[13,14] Balloon pneumatic dilatation has been used for many years with good success, and numerous long-term outcome studies have shown it to be an effective first-line treatment of achalasia.[10,12] The most serious complication from pneumatic dilation is esophageal rupture, which occurs at a mean rate of 2.6%. Laparoscopic myotomy has been shown to have a 90% success rate. However, it can lead to significant GERD and its associated complications. Consequently, myotomy is often performed in conjunction with a GERD-reducing procedure such as fundoplication.

Diffuse esophageal spasm

Like achalasia diffuse esophageal spasm (DES) is a primary motor disorder; however, the true pathophysiology is poorly understood. In general DES is characterized by simultaneous contractions of the distal esophageal smooth muscle, which result in dysphagia and chest pain. Decreased levels of nitric oxide in the myenteric plexus have also been implicated in the pathophysiology. The true prevalence of DES is not known because most of the epidemiologic data are derived from patients referred for a variety of complaints, including noncardiac chest pain and dysphagia. In these patients the prevalence was estimated at 4% to 4.5%.[15,16] Furthermore, studies do not reveal a clear relationship between the prevalence of the disease and factors such as age, gender, or race, although data suggest an association with mitral valve prolapse, obesity, and psychiatric illness.[17]

The diagnosis of DES is made by esophageal manometry criteria and specifically requires synchronous pressure waves (>8 cm/s propagation) with a minimum amplitude of 30 mm Hg.[18–20] However, a clear relationship between these manometric criteria and symptoms has not been established. The use of high-resolution manometry may help in diagnosing DES.

Treatment of DES involves medical and surgical options, with varying degrees of success. Trials of acid suppression with proton pump inhibitors (PPIs), anticholinergic medications, calcium channel blockers, and long-acting nitrates can result in improvement of symptoms, although not with any consistency. Treatment with antidepressants, most commonly trazodone, has been shown to decrease the pain associated with DES in some patients. Botulinum toxin injection in the distal esophageal body has been effective, although there are no large trials to evaluate long-term outcomes. Balloon dilation, bougienage, and esophagomyotomy are reserved for patients who have failed medical therapy.

Nutcracker esophagus

Nutcracker esophagus is a neuromuscular disorder characterized by high-amplitude peristaltic contractions of prolonged duration that may result in dysphagia and chest pain.[21] The diagnosis is frequently made in patients undergoing manometry for evaluation of noncardiac chest pain. Diagnosis is confirmed with manometry when distal esophageal body contractions reach an amplitude of more than 180 mm Hg. Some studies have suggested that changing the diagnostic criteria to require amplitudes as high as more than 260 mm Hg may increase the sensitivity for nutcracker esophagus.[22] Much like in DES and other spastic esophageal disorders, manometric findings often do not correlate with symptoms, and the cause of associated pain is unclear. Treatment is similar to that for DES and includes treatment of anxiety and depression.

Mechanical Causes of Dysphagia

Benign esophageal strictures

Benign esophageal strictures form in the setting of chronic inflammation and as a consequence of mucosal and epithelial injury, leading to collagen deposition and fibrous tissue formation.[23] Most benign strictures (70%–75%) result from chronic inflammation of the esophageal mucosa by gastric acid from peptic ulcer disease (PUD) and GERD.[24] Esophageal strictures may also be caused by Schatzki rings, pill esophagitis, corrosive ingestions, reaction to chronic foreign bodies (nasogastric tubes), sclerotherapy, radiation therapy, and surgery. Benign strictures are further characterized as simple and complex based on their length, angulation, luminal narrowing, and ability to pass an endoscope.[23]

Peptic esophageal strictures have a prevalence of 0.1%, and male gender, increased age, and white race are associated with higher rates.[25,26] Peptic strictures typically occur in the distal esophagus, where acid reflux is most frequent.

Midesophageal to upper esophageal strictures should heighten suspicion of Barrett esophagus and malignancy. Schatzki rings are membranous mucosal rings formed in the distal esophagus at the gastroesophageal junction and represent a variant of peptic stricture disease. Patients often present with dysphagia to solids greater than liquids. Diagnosis can often be made by history alone but is supplemented by barium esophagram and upper endoscopy findings.

Treatment of benign strictures aims both to relieve the obstruction as well as to prevent recurrence. Dilation of the stricture and esophageal lumen is the mainstay of therapy and can be accomplished with balloon dilators, mechanical dilators, and stents, depending on the nature and location of the stricture. Complications include esophageal perforation (0.1%–0.4%),[23] bleeding, and bacteremia. Patients often require repeat dilation for recurrence. Treatment of GERD and PUD with antihistamines and PPIs is essential to prevent formation of strictures.

Diverticula

Esophageal diverticula are a rare cause of mechanical dysphagia. The true prevalence of this disease is unknown, but an association with increased age and male gender has been noted.[27] Diverticula are characterized by location, wall structure, origin, and mechanism of formation. Most adult diverticula are acquired rather than congenital and have false walls lacking a full muscularis layer. Although midesophageal diverticula occur, most diverticula occur in the distal 10 cm of the esophagus in the epiphrenic region and are formed by pulsion.[28] Risk factors for diverticular formation include esophageal dysmotility, obstruction, and focal wall weakness.

Dysphagia associated with diverticula is generally felt to be secondary to the motility disorder and obstruction that led to the diverticula formation rather than to the diverticula itself. Most patients with diverticula are asymptomatic, and the size of the diverticulum does not correlate with the presence of symptoms. If present, symptoms are typically progressive and include dysphagia, regurgitation, vomiting, aspiration, halitosis, chest pain, dyspnea, and dysrhythmias.[27] Furthermore, diverticular rupture can lead to significant complications. Diverticula can be diagnosed on chest radiographs but are often discovered on esophagrams and upper endoscopy in patients being evaluated for dysphagia. Endoscopy should be performed to evaluate for associated malignancy.

Treatment is reserved for symptomatic patients and requires diverticulectomy with or without myotomy. Complications include recurrence of diverticula, esophageal leaks, and postoperative GERD.

Esophageal neoplasms

Two types of esophageal cancer exist: esophageal squamous cell carcinoma (ESCC) and esophageal adenocarcinoma (EAC). Over the last 30 years there has been a significant change in the epidemiology of esophageal cancer; EAC has become more prevalent than ESCC in the United States and among white individuals in most of the world.[29,30] ESCC remains the most prevalent esophageal cancer in nonwhites. The increased prevalence of EAC has been attributed to a concomitant increase in GERD related to higher rates of obesity and fat ingestion in white individuals.[31] Risk factors for EAC include male gender, smoking, excess alcohol consumption, obesity, GERD, Barrett esophagus, and excess fat consumption.

Barrett esophagus refers to a metaplastic change in the esophageal lining from squamous epithelium to intestinal columnar epithelium.[32] This change is preceded by destruction of the squamous epithelium, most commonly by chronic acid exposure. Barrett esophagus is considered a precancerous condition and predisposes individuals to developing EAC; however, the precise absolute risk is unclear. Management of Barrett esophagus is guided by the degree of cellular atypia noted on biopsy results and includes antacid medications, antireflux surgical procedures, endoscopic surveillance, and esophageal resection.[30,31] Much controversy still exists regarding the role of screening for EAC in patients with Barrett esophagus.

Patients with esophageal neoplasms generally present with dysphagia that starts with solids and rapidly progresses to liquids. Dysphagia is often associated with significant weight loss. Definitive diagnosis of esophageal cancer is made by pathologic analysis of endoscopic biopsy samples.

Treatment of esophageal neoplasms is determined by staging. Endoscopic ultrasound, computed tomography (CT), and fludeoxyglucose F 18 positron emission tomography (PET) can be used to assess local wall infiltration, lymph node involvement, and the presence of metastases.[33] Treatment of local minimally invasive cancer including high-grade interepithelial neoplasia, Barrett esophagus, and cancer limited to the mucosa can be treated with ablative techniques such as argon plasma coagulation as well as with endoscopic mucosal resection. In contrast, surgical resection is still considered the treatment of choice for advanced esophageal cancers. Other treatment options include neoadjuvant chemotherapy, chemotherapy alone, and radiation therapy. However, the benefits and efficacy of these therapies are still unclear because of limited data, and their use must be carefully weighed against the detriment they can cause to the patient's quality of life.[33]

EMERGENCY DEPARTMENT EVALUATION AND MANAGEMENT OF DYSPHAGIA

Evaluation and treatment of dysphagia in the emergency department (ED) are limited. A thorough history can often allow the emergency physician to differentiate between oropharyngeal and esophageal dysphagia and subsequently between mechanical and neuromuscular causes. All patients older than 40 years presenting with rapidly progressive dysphagia and weight loss should be suspected of having esophageal cancer.

Physical examination should focus on general appearance, head, nose, mouth, oropharynx, neck, chest, and abdomen. Neck examination should include auscultation for stridor and palpation for lymphadenopathy and thyromegaly. Cranial nerve examination is essential in the evaluation of oropharyngeal dysphagia. If available, nasopharyngoscopy may be helpful in the evaluation of patients presenting with symptoms concerning for proximal obstruction. If they can tolerate it, patients should be observed swallowing.

Plain radiographs of the chest and soft tissues of the neck may reveal obstructive masses typically in the setting of esophageal dysphagia. Laboratory testing is of little usefulness in the emergent evaluation of dysphagia but should be considered in patients with signs of dehydration and significant malnutrition.

Although a barium esophagram should be the initial radiographic test performed in the evaluation of dysphagia, it is seldom performed in the ED and should be arranged on an outpatient basis by a primary care physician. Further outpatient evaluation can include upper endoscopy and manometry.

ED treatment of dysphagia is also limited and should be aimed at addressing acute issues such as dehydration, electrolyte abnormalities, and acute obstruction. Gastroenterology consultation should be obtained on all patients with signs and symptoms of acute esophageal obstruction and inability to tolerate oral intake. These patients often require emergent endoscopy to relieve the obstruction. A trial of nitrates can be considered in patients in whom DES is suspected, whereas motility disorders can be treated initially with calcium channel blockers such as diltiazem or nifedipine if no contraindications exist.

All stable patients should be referred to a primary care physician for a complete workup.

GERD

GERD is the most common gastroesophageal disorder encountered in the ED. Nevertheless, clinicians have struggled to devise definite criteria for the diagnosis of GERD. Some degree of gastroesophageal reflux (GER) and heartburn is physiologic and alone is not felt to constitute a disease. GERD is now defined as the presence of GER in association with troublesome symptoms and/or complications.[26] Diagnosis can be made based on clinical symptoms alone or by showing reflux of gastric contents as well as its associated injuries.

Prevalence in the Western world is estimated at 15% to 25%, with a steadily increasing incidence.[34,35] In contrast, the prevalence in Asia is estimated at less than 5%. In the United States alone the annual cost of managing the disease is estimated at more than $14 billion.[36] The true prevalence of reflux esophagitis is unknown, and studies indicate that up to one-third of patients diagnosed with reflux esophagitis are asymptomatic.[37] The most recognized risk factor for GERD is obesity, although the precise causal mechanism is unclear. Although gender does not seem to be a risk factor for symptomatic GER, endoscopic studies indicate that males seem to have a higher incidence of esophagitis.[26] In addition, the escalating incidence of GERD has also been attributed to a decline in *Helicobacter pylor* infection.[38] It has been suggested that *H pylori*–associated gastritis reduces GERD by decreasing parietal cell mass and gastric acid secretion.

Heartburn and acid reflux are the typical symptoms reported by patients with GERD. Symptoms classically occur after large meals, and heartburn is exacerbated by intake of alcohol, fats, spicy food, and citrus. The supine position and bending over also tend to exacerbate both heartburn and acid regurgitation. Dysphagia, odynophagia, burping, water brash, and cough are additional symptoms associated with GERD. Complications of GERD include esophagitis, peptic strictures, and Barrett esophagus. It is also believed that GERD can exacerbate asthma, chronic cough, recurrent pneumonitis, and dental erosion.[39]

Abundant diagnostic tests for GERD exist, and consequently efficient testing is paramount. Testing for GERD may involve evaluation for reflux, esophageal mucosal injury, and esophageal and LES function with a combination of endoscopy, esophageal pH monitoring, and manometry. In patients with symptomatic GER, improvement after a trial of PPIs is also diagnostic.

Dietary and lifestyle modifications, medications, and surgical procedures are all used in the spectrum of GERD treatment. Although smoking, alcohol intake, fats, chocolate, and citrus are believed to exacerbate GERD, studies have not shown that avoiding these substances leads to significant symptom improvement.[40] Over-the-counter antacids and H2 receptor antagonists are effective in the treatment of mild disease, whereas PPIs have been shown to decrease gastric acid production for longer times and constitute the mainstay of therapy for moderate disease. PPIs have also been shown to reverse esophagitis and the changes associated with Barrett esophagus.[41] Chronic use of PPIs has been associated with gastric polyp formation, recurrent pneumonias, and enteric infections. There are some data to suggest that baclofen may also help reduce esophageal acid reflux by decreasing LES relaxation.[26] Various endoscopic techniques and surgery are typically reserved for severe and intractable disease, although it is unclear whether these procedures are more effective than medical therapy.

ED evaluation and management of patients presenting with symptoms suggestive of GERD can be difficult. Initial evaluation requires exclusion of life-threatening cardiac and abdominal conditions. Acute coronary syndrome and angina can masquerade as GERD especially in diabetic and elderly patients. Consequently, heartburn should warrant a thorough evaluation in such patients. Physicians should be wary of excluding cardiac disease because of symptomatic improvement with antacids, H2 blockers, and PPIs. Gastrointestinal (GI) disorders such as pancreatitis, peptic ulcer disease, and biliary colic may also present with similar symptoms. Clinicians should rely on a thorough history and physical examination to guide their management. Laboratory testing and imaging are nondiagnostic and of little usefulness in the ED management of GERD but may be helpful in excluding other conditions. ED treatment of GERD typically includes use of antacids, H2 blockers, and PPIs. In cases in which GERD is deemed the most likely diagnosis, patients should be started on a trial of H2 blockers or PPIs and advised to follow up with a primary care physician for further evaluation.

ESOPHAGITIS

Inflammation of the esophagus, referred to in general as esophagitis, has many causes, including infection, radiation exposure, GERD, sclerotherapy, and medications; it can also be immune mediated. Infectious esophagitis can be caused by a variety of pathogens, including viruses, fungi, and bacteria, and is most commonly encountered in immunocompromised hosts. Candida, herpes simplex, and cytomegalovirus are the most common causative organisms in such patients. In addition, diabetic patients, patients on chronic steroids, and those undergoing treatment with broad-spectrum antibiotics are all at increased risk for candidal esophagitis.

Patients suffering from infectious esophagitis typically present with complaints of dysphagia, odynophagia, and chest pain. Only in the most severe cases do patients present with dehydration from inability to tolerate liquids. Accurate diagnosis requires endoscopy and culture.

Treatment of candidal esophagitis depends on the host. Diabetic patients and patients on chronic corticosteroids who are deemed not to be severely immunocompromised can be treated as outpatients with oral nystatin solution. In contrast, severely immunocompromised patients require admission for treatment with systemic antifungal medications such as ketoconazole and amphoteracin B. Similarly, systemic antivirals such as acyclovir are indicated in the treatment of esophagitis secondary to herpes simplex.

Radiation-induced esophagitis is a common complication of patients undergoing localized radiation therapy for oral, neck, lung, esophageal, and mediastinal cancers. Severity is directly related to radiation exposure. Diagnosis is mostly clinical and should be suspected in patients undergoing radiation therapy who present with dysphagia and odynophagia, with the caveat that infectious causes should be ruled out. Early endoscopic findings include an erythematous and friable esophageal mucosa that can progress to more extensive fibrinous tissue deposition and frank strictures. Initial treatment is with topical anesthetics such as viscous lidocaine and xylocaine. Endoscopic dilation may be required in patients who develop significant strictures.

Medication-induced esophagitis occurs when an ingested substance remains in contact with the esophageal mucosa for a prolonged period. Such prolonged contact leads to localized mucosal irritation and inflammation. Antibiotics are most often implicated with tetracycline and its derivatives, accounting for more than half of cases.[42] Other medications known to cause esophagitis include iron and potassium preparations, quinidine, nonsteroidal antiinflammatory drugs (NSAIDs), and alendronate. Capsule size, fluid intake, swallowing position (taking the medication when lying down or lying down immediately after ingestion), and age are additional risk factors. Treatment is conservative, with removal of the offending medication and instruction on proper medication ingestion.

EE refers to a syndrome in which the esophageal mucosa is infiltrated by eosinophils. The true prevalence in the United States is unknown although incidence is believed to be increasing.[43] Male gender (3:1 male/female ratio) and younger age have been reported as risk factors for the disease.[44] The pathophysiology of EE is also poorly understood but is believed to be secondary to both allergic and immunologic mechanisms. Both immunoglobulin E (IgE)-mediated and non–IgE-mediated allergic reactions have been implicated.[45] Up to 60% of patients diagnosed with EE have been noted to have concomitant food, inhalant, and seasonal allergies.[43] Furthermore, GERD and environmental allergens have been postulated to play a role in the pathophysiology of EE.

Patients typically present with complaints of dysphagia, more commonly to solids, and food impaction. Other symptoms may include GERD, diarrhea, weight loss, chest pain, and abdominal pain. Children may present with difficulty feeding, vomiting, and regurgitation. Diagnosis is made with a combination of endoscopy and biopsy. Suggestive endoscopic findings include esophageal rings, raised white specks, longitudinal furrows, whitish exudates, and extremely friable mucosa.[43] These endoscopic findings are suggestive of EE but definitive diagnosis requires biopsy. Although definitive criteria have not been established, studies indicate that multiple samples should be obtained from different esophageal locations and should contain at least 15 eosinophils per high-power field.[43] Additional diagnostic criteria include normal distal esophageal pH and no symptomatic improvement with PPIs.[46] Given the association of EE with atopic conditions such as asthma and environmental allergies, some advocate further evaluation with skin prick testing, skin patch testing, and peripheral eosinophil counts.

Treatment of EE includes dietary modifications and avoidance of suspected allergens, swallowed and inhaled topical corticosteroids, systemic corticosteroids, and possibly endoscopic dilation. Leukotriene receptor antagonists have not been shown to be effective in the treatment of EE and are not recommended.[43]

CAUSTIC INGESTIONS

Caustic injuries with strong acids and alkalis represent a true esophageal emergency, with the potential to cause severe morbidity and mortality. In 2004 the American Association of Poison Control Centers documented more than 200,000 exposures to caustic substances via household and industrial products.[47] Several factors determine the extent of esophageal injury with caustic ingestions: amount and concentration of substance ingested, substance pH, tissue contact time, and the state of the substance (solid, liquid, or gas).

Caustic injury to esophageal tissue differs with acids and alkalis. Acid exposure leads to coagulation necrosis and eschar formation. This process is believed to limit the extent to which deeper tissues are affected. In contrast, alkali ingestions result in liquefactive necrosis and saponification, leading to increased penetration and injury to deeper tissues. These classic teachings may be correct in the setting of mild acids and alkalis; however, rapid penetration into esophageal tissues has been noted with both strong bases as well as acids.[48] Initial esophageal injury occurs within minutes of exposure, may continue for hours, and leads to tissue necrosis. The initial injury is followed by a period of mucosal sloughing, bacterial invasion, and ulceration that can be complicated by esophageal perforation and can last up to 1 week. Esophageal repair begins approximately 10 days after the initial injury.[49]

After a caustic ingestion, patients may be asymptomatic or present with a variety of GI and respiratory symptoms, including dyspnea, dysphagia, odynophagia, drooling, nausea, vomiting, abdominal pain, and chest pain. Laboratory studies, radiographs, and esophagogastroduodenoscopy (EGD) are essential to the initial evaluation. Studies that have attempted to correlate a variety of laboratory values with morbidity and mortality have had mixed results; however, laboratory tests are crucial to the diagnosis and management of severe acidosis, disseminated intravascular coagulation, hemolysis, renal failure, and liver failure. Patients presenting with abdominal pain and peritoneal findings require chest and abdominal radiographs to evaluate for viscus perforation both in the abdomen and the mediastinum. Management of esophageal injury is mostly guided by EGD findings. EGD is considered safe after caustic ingestion except in the setting of known or suspected viscus perforation, when it is contraindicated. Indications for EGD after minor caustic ingestions in asymptomatic patients are controversial; however, all patients noted to have posterior pharyngeal burns, dyspnea, stridor, vomiting, chest pain, and abdominal pain should undergo endoscopy. EGD findings are used to grade the severity of injury based on the extent and depth of the burn. Endoscopic ultrasound and technetium 99m sucralfate–swallowing studies have shown potential in detecting deeper tissue injury as well as in documenting healing.[49,50]

Initial treatment of caustic ingestions should focus on airway management and hemodynamic assessment. Airway compromise should be managed by nasotracheal or endotracheal intubation and possibly with a surgical airway. Laryngoscopy can also help determine the presence of upper airway edema. Adequate intravenous (IV) access should be obtained to enable aggressive resuscitation. Use of activated charcoal is contraindicated because it does not adsorb caustic agents. Patients with evidence of viscus perforation, whether abdominal or mediastinal, require emergent surgery.

Studies in animal models indicate that early pH neutralization therapy with weak acids and bases and dilution with water or milk ingestion can decrease esophageal injury; however, no human data exist and these interventions are not recommended at this time.[51,52] There are also no data to support the use of H2 blockers and PPIs. Hence, initial ED treatment should focus on airway and hemodynamic management, pain control, and evaluation for esophageal and intestinal perforation. Once the patient has been stabilized, further management of esophageal injuries aims to prevent and treat esophageal strictures.

ESOPHAGEAL FOREIGN BODIES

Foreign bodies in the esophagus can result in dysphagia, odynophagia, and perforation; however, 80% to 90% of ingested foreign bodies traverse the GI tract spontaneously.[53] The sites at which foreign body impaction is most likely to occur correspond to the areas of anatomic narrowing of the esophageal lumen: proximally at the level of the cricopharyngeal muscle (23%–36%), in the midesophagus at the level of the aortic arch and left mainstem bronchus, and distally at the LES (38%–52%).[54,55] In adults, impaction is more likely to occur in the distal esophagus, whereas in pediatric patients most impactions occur proximally. Of esophageal foreign body ingestions, 75% to 80% occur in children, typically aged 18 to 48 months.[56] Other at-risk populations include edentulous adults, psychiatric patients, and prisoners.

The nature of the foreign bodies ingested varies significantly. Most impactions in adults result from food boluses (38%–59%) followed by bones (16%–18%), dental prostheses (2%–10%), pills (3%), coins (2%), and batteries (1%).[50,55,56] In contrast, most impactions in children are a consequence of coin ingestions. Size and shape of the ingested material determine the likelihood that the foreign body passes through the GI tract without complication. Objects less than 20 mm typically pass through the esophagus and into the stomach and generally do not require acute retrieval. Once in the stomach these smaller foreign bodies are expected to traverse the rest of the GI tract. Objects larger than 20 mm in children and 6 cm in adults that pass through the esophagus should be removed because they can become impacted at the pylorus or in the duodenum. Sharp objects such as toothpicks, safety pins, bones, and tacks are more likely to cause perforations and should be removed before they pass beyond the pylorus. Overall, less than 1% of all ingested foreign bodies result in perforation.[50]

Dysphagia, odynophagia, and chest pain are the most common presenting symptoms in adults and can be accompanied by regurgitation, drooling, and inability to tolerate secretions in cases of complete obstruction. Proximal obstructions may lead to significant dyspnea, coughing, and stridor if the trachea is compressed. Abdominal pain can result when obstructions occur in the stomach or more distally. Up to 35% of pediatric patients with ingested foreign bodies are asymptomatic,[56,57] and a high index of suspicion must be maintained, especially when the history is limited and unclear.

Initial evaluation should focus on determining the nature and location of the impacted foreign body. The ABCs of ED management are essential in these patients, and the history and physical examination must evaluate for signs and symptoms of airway compromise, hemodynamic instability, and perforation. Fiberoptic nasopharyngoscopy can be used to visualize suspected foreign bodies in the pharynx and proximal esophagus. Anteroposterior (AP) and lateral radiographs of the neck, chest, and abdomen are useful in detecting radiopaque foreign bodies but do not detect food boluses. Up to 70% of bones are not detected on radiographs because of poor calcification.[58] Symptomatic patients with negative radiographs should undergo upper endoscopy for further evaluation. Endoscopy in asymptomatic patients with negative radiographs should also be considered on a case-by-case basis depending on the nature of the ingested foreign body.

Ingested foreign bodies can be managed medically, endoscopically, and surgically. Medical therapy with IV glucagon has been shown to have variable success rates, ranging from 12% to 50%, with higher rates for distal obstructions when glucagon acts to relax the smooth muscle.[50,56,59] Typical doses range from 1 to 2 mg and can be repeated once. Nausea, vomiting, and hyperglycemia are typical side effects, and contraindications include pheochromocytoma, insulinoma, and Zollinger-Ellison syndrome. Some investigators advocate use of benzodiazepines in conjunction with glucagon because they are believed to result in striated muscle relaxation. Calcium channel blockers, nitrates, and anticholinergic medications have not been shown to be effective.[50,56] Papain, meat tenderizer, and gas-forming pellets are also not recommended because they can lead to complications of esophageal digestion, perforation, and pulmonary edema.

Use of a Foley catheter to remove foreign bodies has been successful if performed within 72 hours and in cases in which a single smooth foreign object is involved. This procedure requires sedation and should be performed under fluoroscopy in the presence of personnel with expert airway management skills. Some studies have shown the Foley catheter technique to be a more rapid and cost-effective alternative to endoscopy.[56] Endoscopy with both flexible and rigid endoscopes has become the gold standard for foreign body retrieval and should be the modality of choice if available. Several different retrieval techniques are described, with success rates approaching 100%. Difficulties arise with small and sharp foreign objects, and surgery may be required in such cases. All sharp objects and button batteries lodged in the esophagus should be removed as soon as possible. Perforation rates with sharp objects can be as high as 35%, and button batteries contain alkalis that may cause esophageal corrosion, voltage burns, or pressure necrosis.[60] Small batteries that have traversed the esophagus and passed into the stomach may be managed conservatively and given a chance to pass spontaneously.

ESOPHAGEAL PERFORATION

Esophageal perforation has many associated complications that can lead to severe morbidity. Esophageal injuries can range from superficial mucosal tears to full transmural perforations. Iatrogenic causes from endoscopic procedures or surgery account for most esophageal perforations.[56,61] Other causes include Boerhaave syndrome, trauma, foreign bodies, pills, infections, and caustic ingestions. Complications of esophageal rupture are more likely to occur in the setting of complete transmural perforation. Esophageal perforations are further characterized by their onset as acute, subacute, and chronic.

Symptoms of esophageal perforation are largely dependent on the associated complications and vary based on the location of the perforation. Proximal perforations can lead to periesophageal abscess and can further spread into the posterior mediastinum through the retropharyngeal space. Patients can present with neck pain, dysphagia, odynophagia, and hoarseness, and the physical examination is often remarkable for subcutaneous air and crepitus. Thoracic perforations are more likely to lead to mediastinitis and pleural contamination, and patients often present with dysphagia, odynophagia, chest pain, back pain, dyspnea, and fever. Pneumomediastinum can often be detected on physical examination by auscultation of a crunching, rasping sound (Hamman sign). Distal esophageal perforations are more commonly associated with abdominal pain and peritoneal signs.

Boerhaave syndrome refers to spontaneous transmural esophageal rupture resulting from increased esophageal pressure from forceful vomiting. It is most commonly associated with alcohol abuse and PUD but has also occurred with seizures, heavy lifting, and laughing, in which intraabdominal pressure can be significantly increased.[62] Rupture typically occurs in the left posterolateral aspect of the distal esophagus,[63] and patients present with severe sudden onset of abdominal pain, chest pain, dyspnea, and shock.

Initial evaluation of esophageal rupture includes AP and lateral radiographs of the neck, chest, and abdomen to look for free air. Pneumomediastinum, pneumothorax, and pleural effusions are common in thoracic perforations. Perivertebral and abdominal free air can be seen in cases of cervical and abdominal perforations, respectively. Stable patients can be further evaluated with contrast esophagography, CT scan, and endoscopy.

Unstable patients require emergent airway stabilization and aggressive resuscitation. Adequate IV access should be obtained and shock treated with volume replacement and possibly vasopressors. Broad-spectrum antibiotics aimed at covering gram-positive, gram-negative, and anaerobic organisms should be initiated. Stable patients with contained ruptures may be managed nonoperatively with antibiotics, nil-by-mouth status, and drainage of pleural effusions. Unstable patients with large ruptures require emergent surgery to undergo primary closure, esophagectomy, exclusion and diversion, or drainage.[56] Endoscopic esophageal clipping and stenting represent alternatives to surgical management, although their role is not clearly defined. Mortality remains high both with operative and nonoperative management.

PUD

PUD has a high lifetime prevalence, ranging from 8% to 14%, and is the most common cause of upper GI bleeding. Estimated annual costs attributed to PUD surpass $9 billion.[64] Prevalence is slightly greater in men than women and in elderly patients.

Ulceration of the gastric mucosa occurs when the physiologic mechanisms meant to protect the gastric mucosa are overwhelmed by the corrosive action of gastric acid. The most established risk factors for development of PUD are *H pylori* infection and chronic NSAID use. Infection with *H pylori* leads to cytokine-mediated mucosal inflammation, hypergastrinemia, and increased acid production. NSAIDs contribute to mucosal breakdown by inhibiting the synthesis of prostaglandins that function to protect the gastric mucosa by stimulating mucus and bicarbonate secretion. Once ulcers are formed, NSAIDs impede healing by preventing hemostasis and platelet aggregation. In the past, smoking, alcohol use, and dietary factors have also been associated with increased risk of PUD; however, definitive evidence to support a direct relationship is limited.[65] On the other hand, some studies have reported that psychological stress has been shown to increase gastric acid production.[66] Inflammatory, infectious, neoplastic, and endocrine causes have also been implicated in the development of PUD.

PUD classically manifests with periodic epigastric pain that can last weeks to months and is then followed by a period of remittance. This pain is commonly referred to as dyspepsia and can be associated with nausea and vomiting. In contrast to duodenal ulcers, pain secondary to gastric ulcers is typically absent during fasting and worsens immediately after eating. Patients may also report symptoms associated with GI bleeding or anemia. Complications of PUD include GI bleeding, perforation, gastric outlet obstruction, and penetration into adjacent structures. Perforation carries the highest mortality and is most commonly seen in elderly patients with chronic NSAID use.[65] Perforations cause sudden severe abdominal pain, and patients typically present with peritoneal signs, a rigid abdomen, absent bowel sounds, and hemodynamic instability.

Diagnosis of PUD is typically made with upper GI endoscopy; however, it is not performed routinely at the time of initial presentation unless severe disease or gastric cancer is suspected. Patients are initially tested for *H pylori* infection and if positive treated accordingly. Several different assays for *H pylori* can be performed and include serology, urea breath testing, urine and fecal antigens, and endoscopic biopsy.

Treatment of PUD aims to promote ulcer healing and prevent recurrence. PPIs are the mainstay of pharmacotherapy. *H pylori* infections should be treated with a combination of PPIs, antibiotics, and a bismuth; several different regimens exist, some of which are available in combination packs to ease patient compliance. In cases of NSAID-induced PUD, offending agents must be discontinued.

ED evaluation requires a thorough history and physical examination aimed at differentiating PUD from other causes of epigastric and abdominal pain. Physicians should further investigate for signs and symptoms of GI bleeding and anemia. As with GERD, cardiac and respiratory causes should also be considered and evaluated appropriately. Laboratory testing can be helpful in excluding pancreatic and biliary causes of abdominal pain and a complete blood count, coagulation studies, and blood typing should be obtained in all patients with evidence of significant GI bleeding. Patients presenting with dyspepsia should be treated with oral or IV PPIs but may require opioid analgesics for initial pain relief. In addition, nausea should be treated with antiemetics. Patients presenting with complications of PUD such as GI bleeding or perforation require aggressive management with volume resuscitation, transfusion, and endoscopy or surgery. All stable patients can be started on a PPI and should be referred to a primary care physician for further evaluation including *H pylori* testing.

SUMMARY

Gastroesophageal disease is frequently encountered in the ED and often presents subtly with a variety of symptoms that can mimic cardiovascular and respiratory disorders. Consequently, diagnosis of gastroesophageal disorders is frequently delayed. Laboratory testing and imaging are often helpful only in critically ill patients, and emergency physicians should focus on the history to differentiate gastroesophageal disorders from cardiorespiratory disease and to guide management. Whereas unstable patients require aggressive measures and a multidisciplinary approach, ED treatment of stable patients is often limited to alleviation of symptoms. All patients should be referred for definitive evaluation and treatment.

REFERENCES

1. Lind CD. Dysphagia: evaluation and treatment. Gastroenterol Clin North Am 2003;32:553–75.
2. Cook IA, Kahrilas PJ. AGA technical review on management of oropharyngeal dysphagia. Gastroenterology 1999;116:455–78.
3. Lindgren S, Janzon L. Prevalence of swallowing complaints and clinical findings among 50–70 year old men and women in an urban population. Dysphagia 1991; 6:187–92.
4. Siebens H, Trupe E, Siebens A, et al. Correlates and consequences of eating dependency in the institutionalized elderly. J Am Geriatr Soc 1986;34:192–8.
5. Croghan JE, Burke EM, Caplan S. Pilot study of 12-month outcomes of nursing home patients with aspiration on videofluoroscopy. Dysphagia 1994;9:141–6.
6. Cook IJ. Oropharyngeal dysphagia. Gastroenterol Clin North Am 2009;38: 411–31.
7. Swann LA, Munter DW. Esophageal emergencies. Emerg Med Clin North Am 1996;14:557–70.
8. Wilcox SM, Alexander LN, Clark WS. Localization of an obstructing esophageal lesion. Is the patient accurate? Dig Dis Sci 1995;40:2192–6.
9. Mayberry JF. Epidemiology and demographics of achalasia. Gastrointest Endosc Clin N Am 2001;11:235–48.
10. Woltman TA, Pellegrini CA, Oelschlager BK. Achalasia. Surg Clin North Am 2005; 85:483–93.
11. Howard PJ, Maher L, Pryde A, et al. Five year prospective study of the incidence, clinical features, and diagnosis of achalasia in Edinburgh. Gut 1992; 33:1011–5.
12. Walzer N, Hirano I. Achalasia. Gastroenterol Clin North Am 2008;37:807–25.

13. Pasricha PJ, Rai R, Ravich WJ, et al. Botulinum toxin for achalasia: long-term outcome and predictors of response. Gastroenterology 1996;110:1410–5.
14. Annese V, Bassotti G, Coccia G, et al. A multicentre randomised study of intra-sphincteric botulinum toxin in patients with oesophageal achalasia: GISMAD Achalasia Study Group. Gut 2000;46(5):597–600.
15. Katz PO, Dalton CB, Richter JE, et al. Esophageal testing of patients with noncardiac chest pain or dysphagia. Results of three years' experience with 1,161 patients. Ann Intern Med 1987;106:593–7.
16. Pandolfino JE, Kahrilas PJ. AGA technical review on the clinical use of esophageal manometry. Gastroenterology 2005;128:209–24.
17. Grubel C, Borovicka J, Schwizer W, et al. Diffuse esophageal spasm. Am J Gastroenterol 2008;103:450–7.
18. Richter JE, Castell DO. Diffuse esophageal spasm: a reappraisal. Ann Intern Med 1984;100:242–5.
19. Spechler SJ, Castell DO. Classification of oesophageal motility abnormalities. Gut 2001;49:145–51.
20. Handa M, Mine K, Yamamoto H, et al. Antidepressant treatment of patients with diffuse esophageal spasm: a psychosomatic approach. J Clin Gastroenterol 1999;28:228–32.
21. Benjamin SB, Castell DO. The "nutcracker esophagus" and the spectrum of esophageal motor disorders. Current Concepts in Gastroenterology 1980;5:3.
22. Agrawal A, Hila A, Tutuian R, et al. Clinical relevance of the nutcracker esophagus: suggested revision of criteria for diagnosis. J Clin Gastroenterol 2006;40:504–9.
23. Ferguson DD. Evaluation and management of benign esophageal strictures. Dis Esophagus 2005;18:359–64.
24. Marks RD, Richter JE. Peptic strictures of the esophagus. Am J Gastroenterol 1993;88:1160.
25. Richter JE. Peptic strictures of the esophagus. Gastroenterol Clin North Am 1999;28:875–92.
26. Richter JE. The many manifestations of gastroesophageal reflux disease: presentation, evaluation, and treatment. Gastroenterol Clin North Am 2007;36:577–99.
27. Thomas ML, Anthony AA, Fosh BG, et al. Oesophageal diverticula. Br J Surg 2001;88:629–42.
28. Ferraro P, Duranceau A. Esophageal diverticula. Chest Surg Clin N Am 1994;4:741–67.
29. Hongo M, Nagasaki Y, Shoji T. Epidemiology of esophageal cancer: orient to occident. Effects of chronology, geography and ethnicity. J Gastroenterol Hepatol 2009;24:729–35.
30. Tomizawa Y, Wang K. Screening, surveillance, and prevention for esophageal cancer. Gastroenterol Clin North Am 2009;38:59–73.
31. Shaheen N, Ransohoff D. Gastroesophageal reflux, barrett esophagus, and esophageal cancer. JAMA 2002;287:1972–81.
32. Sampliner RE. Practice guidelines on the diagnosis, surveillance, and therapy of Barrett's esophagus. The Practice Parameters Committee of the American College of Gastroenterology. Am J Gastroenterol 1998;93:1028–32.
33. Siersema PD. Esophageal cancer. Gastroenterol Clin North Am 2008;37:943–64.
34. Dent J, El Serag HB, Wallander MA, et al. Epidemiology of gastro-oesophageal reflux disease: a systematic review. Gut 2005;54:710–71.
35. El-Serag HB. Time trends of gastroesophageal reflux disease: a systematic review. Clin Gastroenterol Hepatol 2007;5:17–26.

36. Shaheen NJ, Hansen RA, Morgan DR, et al. The burden of gastrointestinal and liver diseases, 2006. Am J Gastroenterol 2006;101:2128–38.
37. Ronkainen J, Aro P, Storskrubb T, et al. High prevalence of gastroesophageal reflux symptoms and esophagitis with or without symptoms in the general adult Swedish population: a Kalixandra study report. Scand J Gastroenterol 2005;40: 275–85.
38. Raghunath A, Hungin AP, Woolf D, et al. Prevalence of *Helicobacter pylori* in patients with gastro-esophageal reflux disease: a systematic review. BMJ 2003; 326:737–40.
39. Richter JE. Ear, nose and throat and respiratory manifestations of gastro-oesophageal reflux disease: an increasing conundrum. Eur J Gastroenterol Hepatol 2004;16:837–45.
40. Kaltenback T, Crockett S, Gerson LB. Are lifestyle measures effective in patients with gastro- esophageal reflux disease? An evidence-based approach. Arch Intern Med 2006;166:965–71.
41. Moayyedi P, Talley N. Gastroesophageal reflux disease. Lancet 2006;367: 2086–100.
42. Richter J. Diseases of the esophagus. In: Andreoli TE, Carpenter CC, Griggs RC, et al, editors. Cecil essentials of medicine. Philadelphia: WB Saunders; 2001. p. 331.
43. Prasad G, Talley N. Eosinophilic esophagitis in adults. Gastroenterol Clin North Am 2008;37:349–68.
44. Sgouros SN, Bergele C, Mantides A. Eosinophilic esophagitis in adults: a systematic review. Eur J Gastroenterol Hepatol 2006;18:211.
45. Swoger JM, Weiler CR, Arora AS. Eosinophilic esophagitis: is it all allergies? Mayo Clin Proc 2007;82:1541.
46. Furuta GT, Liacouras CA, Collins MH, et al. Eosinophilic esophagitis in children and adults: a systematic review and consensus recommendations for diagnosis and treatment. Gastroenterology 2007;133:1342.
47. Watson WA, Litovitz TL, Rodgers GC Jr, et al. 2004 Annual report of the American Association of Poison Control Centers Toxic Exposure Surveillance System. Am J Emerg Med 2005;23(5):589–666.
48. Poley JW, Steyerberg EW, Kuipers EJ, et al. Ingestion of acid and alkaline agents: outcome and prognostic value of early upper endoscopy. Gastrointest Endosc 2004;60(3):372–7.
49. Salzman M, O'Malley RN. Updates on the evaluation and management of caustic exposures. Emerg Med Clin North Am 2007;25:459–76.
50. Duncan M, Wong RK. Esophageal emergencies: things that will wake you from a sound sleep. Gastroenterol Clin North Am 2003;32:1035–52.
51. Homan CS, Singer AJ, Henry MC, et al. Thermal effects of neutralization therapy and water dilution for acute alkali exposure in canines. Acad Emerg Med 1997; 4(1):27–32.
52. Homan CS, Singer AJ, Thomajan C, et al. Thermal characteristics of neutralization therapy and water dilution for strong acid ingestion: an in-vivo canine model. Acad Emerg Med 1998;5(4):286–92.
53. Guidelines for the management of ingested foreign bodies. Gastrointest Endosc 1995;42:236–8.
54. Mosca S, Manes G, Martino R, et al. Endoscopic management of foreign bodies in the upper gastrointestinal tract: report on a series of 414 adult patients. Endoscopy 2001;33:692–6.
55. Webb W. Management of foreign bodies of the upper gastrointestinal tract: update. Gastrointest Endosc 1995;41:39–51.

56. Staack LB, Munter DW. Foreign bodies in the gastrointestinal tract. Emerg Med Clin North Am 1996;14:493–522.
57. Conners GP, Chamberlain JM, Ochsenschlager DW. Symptoms and spontaneous passage of esophageal coins. Arch Pediatr Adolesc Med 1995;149:36–9.
58. Caravati EM, Bennett DL, McElwee NE. Pediatric coin ingestion: a prospective study on the utility of routine roentgenograms. Am J Dis Child 1989;143:549–51.
59. Colon V, Grade A, Pulliam G, et al. Effect of doses of glucagons used to treat food impaction on esophageal motor function of normal subjects. Dysphagia 1999;14: 27–30.
60. Sheikh A. Button battery ingestion in children. Pediatr Emerg Care 1993;9:224–9.
61. Williamson W, Ellis H. Esophageal perforation. In: Taylor MB, editor. Gastrointestinal emergencies. 2nd edition. Baltimore (MD): Williams & Wilkins; 1997. p. 31–49.
62. Ozawa S, Kitajima M. Esophageal perforation. In: Fischer JE, editor. Master of surgery. 5th edition. Philadelphia: Lippincott Williams & Wilkins; 2007. p. 789–95.
63. Brauer RB, Liebermann-Meffert D, Stein HJ, et al. Boerhaave's syndrome: analysis of the literature and report of 18 new cases. Dis Esophagus 1997;10:64–8.
64. Saad RJ, Scheiman JM. Diagnosis and management of peptic ulcer disease. Clin Fam Pract 2004;6:569–87.
65. Del Valle J. Acid peptic disorders. In: Yamada T, Alpers DH, editors. Textbook of gastroenterology. Philadelphia: Lippincott Williams & Wilkins; 2003. p. 1322–76.
66. Levenstein S. Stress and peptic ulcer: life beyond Helicobacter. BMJ 1998;316: 538–41.

Emergencies of the Liver, Gallbladder, and Pancreas

Troy W. Privette Jr, MD[a,b,*], Matthew C. Carlisle, MD[a],
James K. Palma, MD, MPH[c]

KEYWORDS

- Hepatic encephalopathy • Alcoholic hepatitis
- Hepatorenal syndrome • Spontaneous bacterial peritonitis
- Cholecystitis • Choledocholithiasis • Cholangitis • Pancreatitis

Disorders of the liver, gallbladder, and pancreas are common causes of abdominal pain. In this article, common emergencies related to the liver, gallbladder, and pancreas are reviewed. In each section, a brief discussion of underlying cellular and pathophysiological mechanisms is followed by a review of the emergency department (ED) diagnosis and management of these diseases.

EMERGENCY DISEASES OF THE LIVER

The liver is the largest abdominal organ and performs many complex vital functions, including carbohydrate, protein, and fat metabolism; waste product metabolism and detoxification; destruction of old red blood cells; bile synthesis; and formation of plasma proteins and liver-dependent clotting factors.[1] Most food and drug products pass directly from the gastrointestinal (GI) tract to the liver via the portal venous system.[1] This process allows the liver to clear potentially toxic substances prior to circulation among the other organs of the body. In addition, the hepatocyte is responsible for the synthesis of albumin, as well as clotting factors I, II, V, VII, and X.[1] Thus, albumin levels and prothrombin times can be used as a guide to liver synthetic function.

Disclaimer: The views expressed in this article are those of the authors and do not necessarily reflect the official policy or position of the Department of the Navy, Department of Defense, nor the U.S. Government.

[a] Emergency Medicine Residency, Department of Emergency Medicine, Palmetto Health Richland, 5 Richland Medical Park, Columbia, SC 29203, USA

[b] Chest Pain Unit, Palmetto Health Richland ED, 5 Richland Medical Park, Columbia, SC 29203, USA

[c] Department of Emergency Medicine, Palmetto Health Richland, 5 Richland Medical Park, Columbia, SC 29203, USA

* Corresponding author.
E-mail address: priv@aol.com

Emerg Med Clin N Am 29 (2011) 293–317
doi:10.1016/j.emc.2011.01.008
0733-8627/11/$ – see front matter © 2011 Elsevier Inc. All rights reserved.

Liver injury is often divided into acute and chronic depending on the duration of liver dysfunction. Acute insults may be reversible with the elimination of the offending agent. However, continuous acute liver injury may lead to hepatic fibrosis, the hallmark of chronic liver injury. Progressive fibrosis leads to cirrhosis and liver failure.[2] Mitochondrial dysfunction is the central molecular event in hepatocyte injury.[2]

In the ED, liver disease primarily presents as cholestasis from biliary tract disease, hepatitis, or as a complication of chronic liver disease. With regard to hepatitis, viral infections and alcohol are the most common offending agents. Other etiological factors to consider include acetaminophen, idiosyncratic drug reactions, hepatotoxins, and autoimmune disorders.

Cholestasis and hepatocellular injury/necrosis are the most common pathologic mechanisms for liver disease in the ED. Cholestasis is simply the obstruction of bile flow within the biliary tract. The obstruction may occur as secondary to intrahepatic or extrahepatic processes. Extrahepatic obstruction is covered in the section on gallbladder pathology. Disorders resulting in intrahepatic cholestasis include infection, alcoholic liver disease, pregnancy, infiltrative diseases, sclerosing cholangitis, and primary biliary cirrhosis.

Cholestatic disorders present with variable degrees of jaundice, dark-colored urine, clay-colored stools, and pruritus. Tender hepatomegaly will often be present. A palpable gallbladder indicates extrahepatic cholestasis. Characteristic laboratory findings include significant elevations of bilirubin (total and direct fraction >50%) and alkaline phosphatase.[3] Total bilirubin levels greater than 30 mg/dL make intrahepatic causes of cholestasis more likely than extrahepatic ones. Mild elevations of aminotransferases may occur with progressive disease.[3]

Hepatocellular injury/necrosis results from infection, toxins, and autoimmune processes. The signs and symptoms include nausea, vomiting, anorexia, and fever. Tender hepatomegaly will often be present and splenomegaly may occur. Characteristic laboratory changes include a greater than fivefold increase in aminotransferase levels, mild increase in alkaline phosphatase, prolonged prothrombin time, and variable elevations in bilirubin levels.[3] Continued insults will lead to chronic liver disease, cirrhosis, and liver failure.

The pathophysiology of liver disease relates to both alterations in hepatic anatomy and loss of functioning hepatocytes. Fibrosis is the final common pathway in sustained liver injury. Viral hepatitis results in early periportal fibrosis, whereas alcoholic liver disease causes centrolobular fibrosis. Continued insults by either will lead to panlobular fibrosis, nodule formation, and cirrhosis.[4] Fibrotic changes lead to increased vascular resistance in the portal venous system, with resultant portal hypertension and splanchnic vasodilation and their sequelae.[5] Loss of functional hepatocytes in association with alterations in hepatic circulation leads to decreased protein synthesis (albumin, coagulation factors), decreased detoxification, and changes in carbohydrate and fat metabolism.[1]

Laboratory Abnormalities

Liver function tests and panels include a group of biochemical markers that reflect hepatic function, including markers for hepatocellular injury/necrosis, hepatic synthesis, catabolic activity, and cholestasis.[1] While these tests may be a guide to hepatobiliary activity, one must be aware that extrahepatic diseases can also cause abnormalities in hepatic function tests.

Laboratory tests for hepatocellular injury include aspartate aminotransferase (AST), alanine aminotransferase (ALT), and to a much lesser extent lactate dehydrogenase (LDH). In addition to the liver, AST is found in the heart, muscle, kidney, and brain.

ALT is primarily present in the liver; thus it is a more specific test of hepatic necrosis. ALT is found mostly in the cytosol whereas AST is present in the cytosol and mitochondria. This fact in part explains the increased AST/ALT ratio in alcoholic liver disease where mitochondrial damage is a key factor. In cholestatic disorders, AST increases before ALT, and the levels usually do not exceed a fivefold increase. With viral hepatitis, AST and ALT levels increase over 1 to 2 weeks to levels in the thousands, and return to normal in 6 weeks in uncomplicated cases. Ischemic hepatitis results in a rapid increase to levels greater than 10,000 IU/L [B]. LDH is found in multiple tissues and is extremely nonspecific. However, significant elevation are indicative of ischemic hepatonecrosis.[1]

Tests that evaluate the hepatic synthetic capability include albumin and prothrombin time (PT). Albumin is produced in hepatocytes, with levels decreasing in advancing disease. The half-life of serum albumin is approximately 20 days. Therefore, it is useful in subacute and chronic disease but not acute hepatocellular necrosis. One should bear in mind that albumin levels are also decreased in nephrotic syndrome, cachexia, malnutrition, malabsorption, and various other GI disorders. Coagulation factors I, II, V, VII, and X are synthesized by hepatocytes. In addition, cholestasis impairs vitamin K absorption decreasing the function of coagulation factors II, VII, IX, and X.[3] The PT can prolong in as little as 24 hours of liver disease and therefore is much more sensitive than albumin for evaluating hepatic synthetic function.[3]

Bilirubin, alkaline phosphatase, and γ-glutamyl transpeptidase (GGT) are markers for hepatobiliary dysfunction and cholestasis. Bilirubin is a product of the breakdown of heme-containing proteins. Bilirubin is insoluble. In the liver, bilirubin is conjugated to glucuronic acid. Conjugated bilirubin is water soluble and excreted into bile.[6] Direct bilirubin measures the level of conjugated bilirubin, whereas indirect bilirubin is the unconjugated fraction. Bilirubin levels are traditionally reported as total bilirubin and direct bilirubin. Direct hyperbilirubinemia indicates hepatocellular dysfunction or cholestasis.[3] Indirect hyperbilirubinemia can also be caused by liver disease but also may be due to hemolysis or hereditary diseases, most commonly Gilbert syndrome (a benign genetic defect in bilirubin conjugation).[3] Alkaline phosphatase is present in many tissues including bone, placenta, intestine, kidney, and liver. Hepatic alkaline phosphatase is produced in bile duct epithelial cells. Cholestasis stimulates increased production and release of alkaline phosphatase. The half-life of circulating alkaline phosphatase is approximately 1 week.[1] Alkaline phosphatase levels are nonspecific and need to be evaluated in context of the clinical scenario and other laboratory values. GGT is also present in biliary epithelial cells, and levels increase in cholestasis. When used in conjunction with alkaline phosphatase, GGT is useful to confirm cholestasis. GGT levels are elevated in chronic alcohol use, due to increased production and decreased clearance. Increased GGT levels are also found in chronic liver disease, on use of certain drugs (anticonvulsants, oral contraceptives), and in various nonhepatic disorders including chronic obstructive pulmonary disease, renal failure, and acute myocardial infarction.[1]

Serum ammonia levels are used in the evaluation of hepatic encephalopathy. Ammonia is a by-product of protein metabolism in the intestines and liver. Ammonia produced by the intestinal flora enters the portal venous system. In the setting of portal hypertension, portal systemic shunting occurs, allowing the ammonia to bypass the liver. The result is increased levels of ammonia crossing the blood-brain barrier. In addition to shunting, hepatic dysfunction is associated with decreased metabolism of ammonia as well as increased levels.[7]

Viral Hepatitis

Viral infections are a common cause of hepatitis. The primary pathogens are hepatitis A (HAV), B (HBV), C (HCV), D (HDV), and E (HEV). Hepatitis D is a defective virus and requires coinfection with HBV.[8] The strains differ in their route of infection and long-term course.

HAV and HEV are transmitted via the fecal-oral route, most commonly through contaminated food and water. Poor hygiene and sanitation are significant risk factors.[9] HAV is most commonly nonfatal and self limited. However, HAV infection in the setting of preexisting HCV increases the risk of fulminant hepatic failure and death.[9] HEV, similar to HAV, is usually self-limited and nonfatal. However, the clinical course is often more severe than that of HAV. HEV infection during the third trimester of pregnancy is a risk factor for acute fulminant hepatitis and death.[10] In immunosuppressed patients, HEV may progress from acute to chronic hepatitis with persistent inflammation and viremia.[9]

HBV is transmitted through exposure to contaminated blood and body fluids via parenteral or mucosal exposure. During the acute phase, the presentation ranges from asymptomatic to fulminant hepatitis. Ninety-five percent of immunocompetent adults will recover from the acute infection. HBV can seroconvert to chronic hepatitis.[11] In chronic HBV, the clinical presentation ranges from asymptomatic carrier state to cirrhosis. The risk of conversion to chronic HBV is age related and much higher when the infection occurs at a very young age.[11] Chronic HBV is a risk factor for the development of hepatocellular carcinoma.[11]

HDV is also transmitted via blood and body fluid exposure. HDV requires the presence of HBV to replicate, and is only infectious as a coinfection or superinfection on preexisting HBV. HDV portends a more severe course and an increased risk of fulminant hepatitis.[8]

HCV is contracted through blood or body fluid exposure. The acute phase is often asymptomatic or very mild. Whereas fulminant hepatitis is rare in HCV, chronic hepatitis is relatively common. Seventy percent of cases will seroconvert to chronic HCV.[12] Of those with chronic HCV, 15% to 20% will progress to cirrhosis.[13] Chronic HCV, like HBV, increases the risk of hepatocellular carcinoma.

Patients with acute hepatitis will present with varying degrees of weakness, nausea, vomiting, right upper quadrant pain, and jaundice. Diagnosis is made by obtaining hepatitis viral serology. Interpretation of hepatitis viral panels is complex. These measurements can help assess the acuity or chronicity of the infection, as well as immunosuppression. However, this assessment, requiring consideration of the patients' underlying illnesses and immune status, is beyond the scope of this article. Treatment of acute viral hepatitis in the ED is primarily symptomatic and supportive. Maintaining an adequate fluid and electrolyte balance is the goal of therapy. Admission versus outpatient care is dependent on the severity of the patient's illness, the ability to maintain adequate hydration, and the absence of complications. If discharged, these patients should be referred for follow-up to monitor recovery and to determine the need for more specific treatments (antiviral, interferon).

Alcoholic Liver Disease

Alcoholic liver disease is a significant source of morbidity and mortality in the United States and worldwide. Alcoholism and its effects rank fifth on the global burden of disease by the World Health Organization.[14] Alcoholic liver disease includes the entire spectrum from alcoholic hepatic steatosis (fatty liver), to alcoholic hepatitis, to fibrosis and cirrhosis. The morbidity and mortality is related to the degree of hepatic fibrosis and dysfunction, and its sequelae.

Alcoholic hepatitis

Alcoholic hepatitis is an acute inflammatory condition of the liver secondary to alcohol use and abuse. In most cases it occurs after many years of significant alcohol abuse. In its mild form the damage is reversible. However, severe cases are potentially lethal, with a mortality rate of up to 40% at 6 months.[15] The most common age group for alcoholic hepatitis is 40 to 60 years.[15] Clinically the presentation ranges from subclinical cases, with only laboratory abnormalities, to severe multisystem dysfunction.[16] The rapid onset of jaundice is a key finding in alcoholic hepatitis.[15] Other findings include right upper quadrant pain, fever, hepatomegaly, weight loss, fatigue, and anorexia. In severe cases, patients may exhibit signs of hepatic decompensation with ascites and encephalopathy.[16] On examination, jaundice and hepatic tenderness are the key findings. In addition, clinical stigmata of chronic alcohol abuse such as spider angiomata, subcutaneous ecchymosis, feminization, and palmar erythema may be present.[10]

The pathogenesis of alcoholic hepatitis is multifactorial, involving gut permeability and endotoxemia, acetaldehyde formation, oxidant stress, and poor nutrition.[16] Ingestion of ethanol alters gut permeability, allowing the absorption of endotoxin into the portal venous circulation. Once in the liver, endotoxin activates the inflammatory cascade leading to the release of inflammatory cytokines, which have local effects on the hepatocytes (injury and necrosis) as well as systemic effects such as fever, anorexia, and weight loss.[15–17] The metabolism of ethanol in the liver is an additional source of its toxicity, due to by-products of metabolism and oxidative stress.[16] The breakdown of ethanol by alcohol dehydrogenase creates excess reducing equivalents, altering the $NADH/NAD^+$ ratio, which subsequently leads to inhibition of fatty acid oxidation and promotes lipogenesis.[15] In addition, ethanol-induced alterations in enzyme activity lead to increased hepatic lipid synthesis, fatty liver, and a decreased rate of fatty acid oxidation.[18] Oxidative stress plays an important role as well. Ethanol ingestion stimulates the activity of cytochrome P450 2E1, which generates reactive oxygen radicals leading to hepatic necrosis.[15,16] Chronic alcohol abuse also impairs the regenerative capacity of the liver because inflammatory cytokines combined with poor nutrition (lack of metabolic substrates) impairs hepatic cellular replication.[16]

Laboratory findings in alcoholic hepatitis include liver function test abnormalities as well as nonhepatic laboratory changes. Liver function abnormalities include elevations of AST and ALT—up to 7 times the normal.[19] Characteristically the ratio of AST/ALT will be greater than 2:1.[20] The total serum bilirubin is usually greater than 5 mg/dL and the PT is also elevated.[15] Nonhepatic abnormalities include an elevated white blood cell (WBC) count and neutrophil count.[15] The primary management of alcoholic hepatitis is supportive, including the maintenance of fluid and electrolyte balance, glucose supplementation as needed, thiamine, and control of withdrawal symptoms. Abstinence from alcohol is the mainstay of long-term therapy. Abstinence will prevent ongoing liver injury and allow resolution of alcoholic steatosis.[21] Nutritional support is another cornerstone of therapy for alcoholic hepatitis. A large Veteran's Affairs study found a 100% prevalence of protein calorie malnutrition in these patients; and the degree of malnutrition correlated with the severity of the liver dysfunction.[19] Numerous other agents have been studied for therapy in alcoholic hepatitis. Corticosteroids have shown some benefit in control of the inflammatory cascade, and are currently indicated for severe cases.[15,21] Pentoxifylline appears to show some promise through reduction of inflammatory cytokines and decreased incidence of subsequent hepatorenal syndrome (HRS).[21] After promising early reports, randomized controlled trials of infliximab and etanercept (direct anti–tumor necrosis factor-α agents) in patients with alcoholic hepatitis found them to be associated with increased rates of serious infection and death.[15,21]

Complications of Chronic Liver Disease

In chronic liver disease, complications occur increasingly with rising portal venous pressures and diminishing hepatic metabolic activity. This section focuses on those complications that may present to the ED including HRS, ascites, spontaneous bacterial peritonitis (SBP), and hepatic encephalopathy (HE). Esophageal variceal bleeds are covered in the article elsewhere in this issue on GI hemorrhage.

Hepatorenal syndrome

Renal failure is a common complication in patients with liver disease. HRS is the cause in a specific subset of these patients. The combination of liver disease and renal failure portends a poor prognosis and is associated with increased mortality.[22] HRS is the most common fatal complication of cirrhosis.[23]

HRS is defined as acute or subacute renal failure in the presence of advanced liver disease and structurally normal kidneys. It is a functional renal failure secondary to severe renal vasoconstriction.[23] The systemic vascular resistance is markedly reduced, leading to low arterial pressures and subsequent renal vascular constriction.[24] While this most commonly occurs in patients with cirrhosis and ascites, it can occur in alcoholic hepatitis and in the setting of acute fulminant hepatic failure.[24] Renal vasoconstriction is the hallmark event in the pathophysiology of HRS. Several theories exist to explain this phenomenon. However, the resulting final common pathway is vasoconstrictor activation, which leads to sodium retention and ascites, water retention and hyponatremia, and renal vasoconstriction and HRS.[25]

The diagnosis of HRS is complex and is beyond the scope of ED evaluation and management of liver failure patients, because it requires proof that the renal impairment is not due to volume status, shock, infection, nephrotoxic drugs, or acute tubular necrosis.[26] However, the diagnosis should be suspected in any patient with chronic liver disease and an elevated creatinine.

HRS is classified as type 1 and type 2. Type 1 HRS is characterized by a severe and rapidly progressive renal failure with a doubling of the serum creatinine to greater than 2.5 mg/dL in less than 2 weeks. Type 1 HRS usually develops in the face of an acute precipitant, with SBP the most common insult.[27] Type 1 HRS is rapidly progressive, and has an extremely high mortality with a median survival of 1 to 2 weeks.[23] Type 2 HRS is characterized by a slow and gradual increase in serum creatinine with no precipitating events. Refractory ascites is the dominant clinical feature.[27] It is important clinically to distinguish between types 1 and 2 HRS, because type 1 is an indication for evaluation for liver transplantation.[23]

The mainstay of ED management of HRS is supportive, although the only definitive therapy is transplantation.[28] Early therapy should be aimed at correcting any precipitating events such as SBP, infection, and GI bleeding. In type 1 HRS, the underlying precipitating event should be treated aggressively. Early antibiotic support is indicated, because infectious processes are the most common precipitating events.[23] Diuretics should be discontinued and the intravascular volume should be assessed. Early volume expansion with albumin may improve the renal blood flow.[23]

Spontaneous bacterial peritonitis

Cirrhosis leads to portal hypertension through the obstruction of portal blood flow. This process stimulates a cascade of events, leading to activation of the renin-angiotensin-aldosterone axis, sodium and water retention, and the development of ascites due to overflow of hepatic lymphocytic fluid into the peritoneal cavity. In addition, increased hepatic sinusoidal hydrostatic pressure and decreased plasma oncotic pressure lead to the excess production of hepatic lymphatic fluid, which ultimately leaks into the peritoneal cavity forming ascites.[29] SBP is an infection of ascitic fluid.[30]

SBP should be suspected in a patient with abdominal pain and preexisting liver disease and ascites. Fever is not always present and the abdominal pain may not be severe. Worsening ascites may be the only early symptom.[30] The patient may also have an altered mental status, GI bleeding, and azotemia.[29] The prevalence of SBP ranges from 10% to 30% in patients with preexisting ascites.[5] While SBP is readily treatable, its development increases the risk of other complications, such as type 1 HRS.

The pathogenesis of SBP involves the translocation of bacteria, most commonly from the GI tract, into the blood stream. The resulting bacteremia leads to infection of the ascitic fluid through exchange of fluids between the intravascular space and the peritoneal fluid. *Escherichia coli* is the most common pathogen isolated, with *Klebsiella pneumoniae* the second most common.[31]

The diagnosis of SBP is relatively straightforward. An abdominal paracentesis should be performed in anyone suspected of having SBP and without contraindications to the procedure. The finding of an ascitic WBC count of greater than 1000 cells/μL and a polymorphonuclear count of greater than 250 cells/μL is diagnostic. A pH of less than 7.35 in the ascitic fluid is supportive of the diagnosis. The ascitic fluid should be cultured, but a positive culture is not necessary to make the diagnosis. Approximately 30% will return a positive culture.[30]

Treatment should be started with the finding of inflammatory ascitic fluid. Third-generation cephalosporins are the treatment of choice. Regarding prevention, treatment with norfloxacin has been shown to be effective at decreasing the incidence of primary SBP as well as recurrence of SBP.[32] The most feared complication of SBP is type 1 HRS, which occurs in up to 30% of patients and carries an exceptionally high mortality. Recurrence of SBP occurs in approximately 70% of patients in 1 year. Long-term prophylaxis with fluoroquinolones has decreased this percentage, but SBP due to quinolone-resistant bacteria is on the increase.[5]

Hepatic encephalopathy

HE is a condition in which a patient with liver dysfunction and/or portal-systemic shunting displays neurologic and/or psychological abnormalities without another pathologic condition to explain the findings. HE may present in acute or chronic liver failure. HE is a key feature of fulminant hepatic failure and a is common complication of chronic liver disease. HE includes presentations ranging from mild altered mental status to coma, and neuromuscular abnormalities ranging from tremor and asterixis to decerebrate posturing.[33] The symptoms result from the inability of the liver to detoxify intestinal toxins.[33]

HE is classified into 3 types based on the underlying liver disease. Type A HE occurs in acute liver failure. Type B is caused by portosystemic shunting without intrinsic hepatocellular disease. Type C, the most common form, arises from cirrhosis-induced portal-systemic shunting, and may be persistent or episodic.[34] HE is staged using the West Haven Criteria from stage 0 to 4. Stage 0 shows no change in consciousness and behavior and no neuromuscular changes. Stage 1 involves a trivial lack of awareness with a shortened attention span, and impairment in addition and subtraction abilities. Asterixis and tremor may also begin to appear. Stage 2 involves lethargy, disorientation, and inappropriate behavior. Slurred speech and asterixis will be present as well. Stage 3 involves gross disorientation and bizarre behavior with a somnolent (but arousable) state. The patient may have muscular rigidity, and asterixis is usually absent. Stage 4 involves a comatose state that may progress to decerebrate posturing.[34]

The pathogenesis of HE is complex and multifactorial. The key feature is hepatic dysfunction (most commonly cirrhosis-induced portal-systemic shunting) or noncirrhotic portal-systemic shunting leading to the inability of the liver to clear ammonia, γ-aminobutyric acid agonists, and manganese. These substances subsequently cross the blood-brain barrier, leading to altered neurotransmission and neuronal impairment. Neurologic impairment occurs through both direct toxic effects and indirect effects through neuroinhibition. Oxidative stress and inflammatory cytokines play a role as well.[7,33,35]

The diagnosis of HE requires a thorough history as well as physical and laboratory/radiological evaluation. The diagnosis should be suspected in any patient with known liver disease who presents with altered mental status and neuromuscular abnormalities. However, a thorough evaluation is indicated to rule out other causes of the altered mental status. The differential diagnosis of HE includes, but is not limited to, metabolic encephalopathy (uremia, sepsis, hypoxia, and hypoglycemia), intracranial bleeding, cerebrovascular accident/transient ischemic attack, central nervous system infections or neoplasms, and alcohol withdrawal/intoxication states.[36] An elevated serum ammonia is typical of HE. There has been extensive controversy over the years as to whether serum ammonia levels correlated with the severity of HE; however, it appears that if drawn and analyzed appropriately, serum ammonia levels do correlate with the severity of HE.[37] Computed tomography (CT) of the head should be performed to rule out structural causes for the altered mental status, and finally the workup should include an evaluation for precipitating causes.[36]

The management of HE involves simultaneous attention to multiple goals that include general supportive care, treatment of precipitating events, inhibition of ammonia production and absorption, and avoidance of sedatives unless absolutely necessary. General supportive care entails management of the patient's fluid and electrolyte balance, protection of the airway, and cardiovascular stabilization. Treatment and correction of the precipitating events is extremely important, given that HE will not improve until the precipitant is removed. Common precipitants include gastrointestinal bleeding, infection, renal failure, and dehydration.[38] Nonabsorbable disaccharides such as lactulose and lactitol are administered to help decrease the ammonia load from the gut. These medications work by decreasing both the absorption and production of intestinal ammonia, and are considered first-line therapy for HE.[39] Antibiotics are administered in HE to decreased ammonia production by decreasing the number of urease-producing bacteria in the gut.[39] Oral neomycin has been used for many years although it is potentially ototoxic and nephrotoxic.[39] Other antibiotics studied for this purpose include metronidazole, oral vancomycin, and rifaximin.[36] Rifaximin has a favorable side effect profile compared with neomycin.[39] Finally, recurrent or intractable HE is an indication for evaluation for liver transplantation.[38]

EMERGENCY DISEASES OF THE GALLBLADDER

Biliary tract disease is one of the most common gastrointestinal disorders in the United States, ranging from asymptomatic cholelithiasis to biliary colic, cholecystitis, choledocholithiasis, cholangitis, and malignancy. With direct costs of $5.8 billion annually, biliary disease is the second most expensive digestive disease in the United States,[40] and accounts for 3% to 9% of hospital admissions for acute abdominal pain.[41] Cholecystitis is the most prevalent surgical disease in industrialized countries. An estimated 700,000 cholecystectomies are performed annually in the United States.[42] The vast majority of biliary tract disease is caused by gallstones.[42,43] Approximately 20 to 25 million Americans have gallstones,[42,44] of which 1% to 2% per year become symptomatic.[45] Thus, whereas the annual percentage of patients who develop complications is low, the incidence of acute disease is high because of the high prevalence of gallstones in the population.

Anatomy and Pathophysiology

Hepatocytes secrete bile into the bile canaliculi, which are formed by the cell walls of the hepatocytes. Bile then flows into ductules, which coalesce into successively larger ducts. The hepatic ducts course along with branches of the portal vein and hepatic artery, which together form the portal triad. The right and left hepatic ducts join to form the common hepatic duct. The cystic duct drains the gallbladder and joins the common hepatic duct to form the common bile duct. The common bile duct is usually situated anterior and to the right of the portal vein; it courses caudally behind the first portion of the duodenum, then anterior to the pancreas where it is joined by the pancreatic duct. It drains into the second part of the duodenum at the ampulla of Vater, the orifice of which is controlled by the sphincter of Oddi. Variations in hepatobiliary anatomy are common.[46]

Bile is necessary for proper digestion and absorption of dietary fats and fat-soluble vitamins, as well as the fecal excretion of excess cholesterol and the by-products of red blood cell catabolism. The gallbladder stores bile between meals and also actively concentrates it by removing water and inorganic anions (chloride, bicarbonate).[44] Gallstones are formed when cholesterol and calcium salts precipitate out of supersaturated bile. Bile stasis and a nidus for nucleation/crystallization are also factors.[44] Although most gallstones are composed primarily of cholesterol (cholesterol stones), pigmented stones can also occur. Brown pigmented stones are more common in Asians and with bacterial contamination of the biliary tree, whereas black stones are associated with hemolytic disorders, cirrhosis, cystic fibrosis, and ileal disease.[44] Historically in the United States, up to 10% to 25% of stones were pigmented[47]; however, the percentage of cholesterol stones seems to be increasing as obesity becomes more common.[44,48] Biliary sludge is a viscous mixture of small cholesterol or calcium bilirubinate crystals that have begun to precipitate; it can lead to the same symptoms and complications as gallstones.

Gallstones become symptomatic when they cause obstruction of the biliary system. When the gallbladder contracts against an obstructing gallstone (typically lodged in the gallbladder neck), biliary colic ensues. If the obstruction is relieved, the pain resolves. Prolonged obstruction leads to increased intraluminal pressure, wall edema, and an acute inflammatory response.[49] If the obstruction continues, the gallbladder wall becomes ischemic and further inflammatory mediators are released. Secondary bacterial infection may result in formation of an abscess or empyema within the gallbladder. Perforation may lead to diffuse peritonitis. Gas-forming organisms may lead to emphysematous cholecystitis.

Bacteria are cultured from the bile of patients undergoing cholecystectomy for uncomplicated gallstone disease in 13% to 32% of patients, and in 41% to 54% of those with acute cholecystitis; healthy individuals do not have bacterial isolates.[50] It is more common to find bacteria in pigment-stone–containing bile than in cholesterol-stone–containing bile (82% vs 26% in one study).[51] Bacteria are more commonly found in the bile of those with biliary obstruction, acute cholecystitis, common duct stones, cholangitis, and nonfunctioning gallbladders; in males, the elderly, and those with biliary stents.[52] Typical bacterial isolates include enterobacteriaceae (68%), enterococci (14%), bacteroides (10%), and *Clostridium* species (7%).[53]

Risk factors for cholesterol gallstones are listed in **Box 1**.[44,54,55] Age and gender are the most important risk factors for development of gallstone disease. Gallstones are rare in children, but may be associated with congenital anomalies, Down syndrome, and hemolytic diseases (such as sickle cell disease). By the fifth decade of life, approximately 15% of women have gallstones, increasing to approximately 40% by the ninth decade[47]; the incidence of gallstones increases by 1% to 3% per year in adulthood,[44,54] depending on risk factors. The female to male ratio of gallstones is approximately 4:1 in those younger than 40 years, and 2:1 in older age groups.[54] More females develop gallstones, so the overall incidence of cholecystitis is higher in females (the overall female to male ratio is 3:1), but a higher percentage of men with gallstones develop cholecystitis.[42]

Patients with previously asymptomatic gallstones have an annual risk of approximately 1% for biliary colic, 0.3% for acute cholecystitis, 0.2% for symptomatic choledocholithiasis, and 0.04% to 0.2% for gallstone pancreatitis.[55–57] After the first episode of symptoms, the rate of both recurrent symptoms and complications increase, with 1% to 3% per year developing complications.[45]

Clinical Presentation

A wide range of symptoms has been attributed to gallstones. The term "colic," applied to pain due to biliary disease, can be misleading because it is not paroxysmal, but rather a steady pain that lasts from 15 minutes to more than 12 hours per episode. Colic is perceived in the mid-epigastric region as often as the right upper quadrant. It is typically described as sharp and crampy, and may be precipitated by fatty food intake. It may radiate to the right shoulder or scapula. Associated symptoms may include nausea, vomiting, chills, bloating, belching, acid regurgitation, flatulence,

---

Box 1
Risk factors for cholesterol gallstones

Increasing age

Female gender

Obesity

Pregnancy and parity

Rapid weight loss (>1.5 kg/wk)

Family history and genetic factors

Ethnicity (increased in Native Americans and Hispanics; decreased in African Americans)

Diet (high calorie count, total fat, cholesterol, and refined carbohydrates promotes gallstones, whereas dietary fiber, vitamin C, and moderate alcohol intake protect against stones)

Ileal disease (such as Crohn disease or previous ileal resection)

Total parenteral nutrition

Hypertriglyceridemia

Low level of high-density lipoprotein cholesterol

Diabetes mellitus

Certain drugs (estrogens, clofibrate, octreotide, ceftriaxone)

constipation, and/or diarrhea. Patients frequently have had previous episodes of similar symptoms.[58-60]

In a prospective cohort study of 233 patients with abdominal symptoms that were suspicious for biliary tract disease, neither classic biliary colic nor any of the described atypical symptoms were sufficiently sensitive or specific to diagnose gallstones. The likelihood ratio for gallstones when biliary pain was present was only 1.34 (95% confidence interval [CI] 1.05–1.71).[58] A meta-analysis of 24 publications found similarly poor predictive value for abdominal symptoms. The symptom of biliary colic had an odds ratio of only 2.6 (95% CI 2.4–2.9) in predicting gallstones.[59] It is important to be aware that upper abdominal pain has test characteristics similar to right upper quadrant pain,[41] so isolated epigastric pain, rather than excluding biliary tract disease, is actually consistent with it. Approximately half of patients who develop acute cholecystitis have a history of biliary colic.[56,61]

Physical examination may elicit localized right upper quadrant tenderness, but examination will be normal between episodes of biliary colic. Murphy's sign refers to pain during right upper quadrant palpation during inspiration; as the gallbladder descends into the examiner's palpating hand, there is sudden inspiratory arrest. Among 100 ED patients with suspected acute cholecystitis (all of whom underwent hepatobiliary scintigraphy, with 53 positive studies), the presence of Murphy's sign had a sensitivity of 97.2% and specificity of 48.3%.[62] A meta-analysis that included data on 565 patients found a positive likelihood ratio of 2.8 (95% CI 0.8–8.6) and negative likelihood ratio of 0.5 (95% CI 0.2–1.0).[41] In elderly patients Murphy's sign is less reliable; the sensitivity has been reported as only 48% with specificity of 79%.[63]

Courvoisier's sign refers to a palpable gallbladder in a jaundiced patient. In a case series published in 1890, Courvoisier noted that gallstones rarely lead to persistent gallbladder dilation because they cause obstruction that is intermittent.[64] Conversely, the gradual, progressive obstruction caused by malignancy frequently leads to gallbladder dilation. Although cancer of the head of the pancreas is classically associated with Courvoisier gallbladder, there are several other nonmalignant causes.[64]

No historical features, signs, or symptoms are adequate to rule in or rule out symptomatic cholelithiasis or cholecystitis. After history and physical examination, the differential diagnosis may still be broad and may include acute coronary syndrome, pneumonia, gastritis, peptic ulcer disease, esophageal spasm, pancreatitis, hepatitis, urolithiasis, pyelonephritis, or appendicitis, among others.

Laboratory Evaluation

Laboratory studies are typically normal with episodes of uncomplicated symptomatic cholelithiasis (biliary colic). With acute cholecystitis, there is no single or combination of laboratory abnormalities that has either positive or negative likelihood ratios of sufficient magnitude to rule in or rule out cholecystitis.[41] There may be a leukocytosis with left shift, though the WBC count is usually normal. Alkaline phosphatase, liver transaminases, and bilirubin may be normal or mildly elevated. Bile flow is generally not obstructed in acute cholecystitis, so a high bilirubin should prompt consideration of choledocholithiasis. Mirizzi syndrome, when a gallstone impacted in the gallbladder neck or cystic duct compresses the common hepatic duct, can also result in various degrees of biliary obstruction.[65] Other laboratory values are nonspecific, but can be useful in ruling out other diagnostic considerations in the differential diagnosis.

Certain clinical and laboratory findings may suggest that acute cholecystitis is more likely than simple biliary colic: history of pain for more than 6 hours, more severe symptoms (pain, nausea, vomiting), pain more localized to the right upper quadrant, fever, Murphy's sign, leukocytosis, elevated liver enzymes (with greater elevation of alkaline phosphatase than transaminases), and hyperbilirubinemia.[41,66] However, because no combination of clinical or laboratory parameters are reliable for the diagnosis of acute biliary disease,[41,62] the physician's judgment will be the driving force behind decisions to pursue imaging studies. One estimate is that the physician's gestalt (after considering clinical and laboratory findings) has a positive likelihood ratio of 25 to 30.[41] Typical imaging studies include ultrasonography, hepatobiliary iminodiacetic acid (HIDA) scan, or CT.

Diagnostic Imaging Evaluation

Ultrasonography

Ultrasonography of the right upper quadrant should generally be the first-line imaging modality when considering biliary disease. Ultrasonography is considered the most appropriate initial diagnostic imaging study for right upper quadrant pain by the American College of Radiology (ACR).[67] Focused emergency ultrasonography performed by emergency physicians (EPs) is rapid and accurate not only for biliary disease, but also excludes other life-threatening processes such as abdominal aortic aneurysm. Even if used as a screening test with the plan to pursue a formal study regardless of findings, EP-performed ultrasonography may allow earlier interventions (analgesics, antibiotics, surgical consultation) and guide subsequent radiologist-interpreted imaging (eg, the choice of abdominal CT versus ultrasonography performed in the radiology department).

Gallstones appear as bright echogenic foci in the gallbladder lumen; they cast a posterior shadow and are gravity dependent (ie, move with changes in patient position) (**Fig. 1**). EPs in a wide range of settings have high rates of gallstone identification, with sensitivity of 88% to 96% and specificity of 78% to 96% when compared with radiology department ultrasonography.[68–71] Minimal training to ensure competence includes at least 25 documented and reviewed cases.[72] False-negative results may occur more frequently with small stones (<1–3 mm), artifact from bowel, and gallstones impacted in the gallbladder neck or cystic duct.[73] Smaller stones may be better visualized with higher frequencies or harmonic imaging. Imaging from different acoustic windows (subcostal, intercostal, and right flank), patient positions (recumbent, decubitus, sitting), and with inspiration if gallstones are suspected but not initially

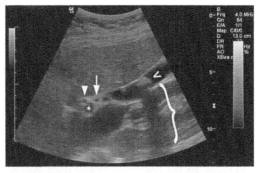

Fig. 1. In this case of uncomplicated biliary colic, the gallbladder wall is thin. The large stone (*open arrowhead*) has prominent posterior shadowing (*bracket*). The portal triad can be located by its position as the "point" of the "exclamation point" formed by the long view of the gallbladder. The classic "Mickey Mouse" transverse view of the portal triad shows the portal vein (*asterisk*), hepatic artery (*arrow*), and common bile duct (*arrowhead*). These structures were verified in real time by using color flow, which demonstrated flow in the artery and vein, but no flow in the bile duct. (*Courtesy of* Jeremy Smith, MD.)

appreciated.[73] Higher-quality ultrasound machines may improve diagnostic accuracy of EPs.[70] Given their high prevalence, identification of gallstones does not mean that they are the cause of the patient's symptoms, so this finding should be correlated with the overall clinical picture.

A sonographic Murphy sign is elicited when maximal tenderness exists when probe pressure is applied directly onto the sonographically visualized gallbladder. Compared with other ultrasonographic findings, it is technically simple to elicit and has high sensitivity in the hands of EPs. In a study of 109 right upper quadrant ultrasonographic examinations performed by EPs, the presence of gallstones and a positive sonographic Murphy sign had a sensitivity of 75% and specificity of 55% for acute cholecystitis.[70] In this study, sensitivity of sonographic Murphy sign in studies performed by technicians and radiologists was lower (45%), but specificity was higher (81%). In another study involving 116 patients using the criterion of both gallstones and sonographic Murphy sign being present, EP-performed ultrasonography was 91% sensitive and 66% specific for acute cholecystitis.[71] Sonographic Murphy sign may not be present in patients with diabetes, gangrenous cholecystitis, or perforation.[74]

Additional sonographic features of acute cholecystitis include gallbladder wall thickening and pericholecystic fluid. These secondary findings are inconsistently detected by EPs, although accuracy likely improves with greater training and experience.[70] Gallbladder wall thickness should be measured at the anterior wall in the transverse plane to avoid edge artifact, posterior acoustic enhancement, or tangent effect. Normal thickness is less than 3 mm; 50% of patients with acute cholecystitis have wall thickening.[74] Conversely, about 50% of patients with wall thickening have a nonsurgical condition such as liver disease, congestive heart failure, renal disease, or the normal contraction seen in a postprandial state.[75]

Gallbladder sludge appears as low-amplitude echoes in the dependent portion of the gallbladder without acoustic shadowing. Occasionally the gallbladder will be completely filled with gallstones, leading to the WES (wall-echo-shadow) sign, in which the gallbladder wall is seen immediately anterior to bright echoes from multiple stones with strong posterior acoustic shadowing (**Fig. 2**).[75] Although rare, gas in the lumen or wall of the gallbladder is an important finding, indicating emphysematous cholecystitis (**Fig. 3**); in this situation, CT may provide additional information. Overall, the ability of EP-performed ultrasonography to diagnose acute cholecystitis is comparably accurate to formal ultrasonography.[76] The radiology literature reports sensitivities ranging from 84% to 98% and specificities ranging from 90% to 99%.[76]

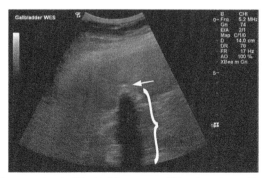

Fig. 2. A gallbladder completely filled with stones will lead to the wall-echo-shadow (WES) sign, in which the gallbladder wall (*arrow*) is seen immediately anterior to bright echoes from multiple stones with strong posterior acoustic shadowing (*bracket*).

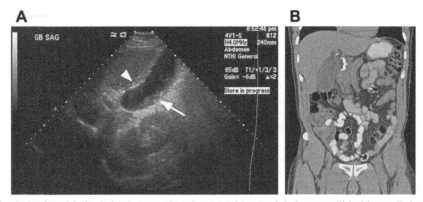

Fig. 3. In this elderly diabetic man, the ultrasound image (*A*) shows gallbladder wall thickening (measured as 7 mm). There are nondependent hyperechoic areas with comet-tail artifacts extending down from the anterior gallbladder wall (*arrowhead*), which indicate air due to emphysematous cholecystitis. There are also small gallstones and sludge (*arrow*), which do not have posterior shadowing. Computed tomography (*B*) verifies the thickened wall with tiny bubbles of gas in the gallbladder lumen and wall (*bracket*), distinguishing this from calcification. Even in this early, subtle case, the hospital course was complicated, which is typical of the high morbidity and mortality associated with emphysematous cholecystitis. (*Courtesy of* Rob Ferre, MD.)

Plain film radiography and CT

Plain radiographs have limited utility in biliary disease, except for evaluating associated ileus or identifying free air associated with emphysematous cholecystitis or perforation. Approximately 20% of gallstones are radiopaque,[42] but a much lower proportion will be seen on plain radiographs. CT scan of the abdomen is much less sensitive than ultrasonography for biliary tract disease, is more expensive, mandates patient movement out of the ED, and exposes the patient to radiation and (for best detail) contrast. The sensitivity of CT for gallstones is approximately 75%.[77] Compared with ultrasonography, one study found CT to have a sensitivity of only 39% and specificity of 93% for acute biliary disease.[78] CT may have a role in biliary disease when ultrasonographic findings are equivocal, or when the complications of perforation or emphysematous cholecystitis are suspected. With equivocal clinical findings and a broader differential diagnosis, the information provided by CT regarding alternative diagnoses may make it a preferable initial imaging modality.

Nuclear medicine hepatobiliary evaluation

Radionuclide cholescintigraphy scans, such as the HIDA scan, can be used when ultrasonographic findings are equivocal, as they have a higher sensitivity (90%–100%) and specificity (85%–90%) for cholecystitis.[62] Cholescintigraphy gives little information about nonobstructing cholelithiasis, and will therefore miss cases of resolved biliary colic after an obstructing stone has spontaneously dislodged from the gallbladder neck.[43] The ACR appropriateness criteria suggest cholescintigraphy as the initial imaging study for suspected acalculous cholecystitis, although this recommendation may be moot because the diagnosis is almost never entertained without a prior ultrasonogram showing gallbladder wall abnormalities and the absence of gallstones.[67] The limited availability and typical delays in obtaining cholescintigraphy render it of only marginal use in the ED.

The study is done after intravenous administration of technetium-labeled derivatives of iminodiacetic acid. These markers are taken up by hepatocytes and are excreted into the biliary tree. The gallbladder is normally visualized within 30 minutes of injection and the small bowel within 60 minutes. Nonfilling of the gallbladder is highly suggestive of acute cholecystitis in the proper clinical setting, but nonfilling alone is a nonspecific finding that could also be related to prolonged fasting or severe liver disease.[79] False positives may occur with high bilirubin levels and severe intercurrent illnesses.[67] Scintigraphy is expensive, takes up to 4 hours to complete, and cannot contribute to the diagnosis if the etiology does not concern the biliary tract.

Abdominal magnetic resonance imaging has high diagnostic accuracy for biliary pathology, but the lack of availability, high cost, and time involved limit its use in ED patients. Endoscopic retrograde cholangiopancreatography (ERCP) is useful in the diagnosis and treatment of bile duct obstruction, but is not typically performed in the ED. The diagnostic accuracy of magnetic resonance cholangiopancreatography reaches similar diagnostic accuracy as ERCP, but does not allow for intervention.

Treatment

During the course of ED diagnostic studies, resuscitative care, volume repletion, antiemetics, analgesics, and bowel rest are indicated. If uncomplicated symptomatic cholelithiasis is diagnosed, referral for scheduled routine cholecystectomy is indicated. Prescriptions for antiemetics and opioid analgesic are typically provided. Nonsteroidal anti-inflammatory drugs (specifically diclofenac and indomethacin) not only ameliorate pain, but may also prevent progression of disease to acute cholecystitis.[43,80] Diet and nutritional approaches, bile acids to dissolve stones, and lithotripsy can be considered in patients who refuse surgery, but these are not therapeutic options in the ED, and there are high recurrence rates.[81] As previously noted, expectant management of symptomatic gallstones leads to complicated disease (such as acute cholecystitis or pancreatitis) in 1% to 3% of patients per year.[56,61] However, because the symptoms of biliary colic are so varied and inconsistent, the EP may not be certain whether the patient's gallstones are an incidental finding or are actually responsible for his or her abdominal symptoms. One literature review found the pooled relief rate of cholecystectomy for "biliary pain" to be 92%, but broader symptomatic indications for cholecystectomy led to much lower corresponding symptom relief rates.[82] Thus, decisions regarding immediate versus outpatient surgical evaluation versus expectant management with follow-up with a primary physician require clinical judgment on a case-by-case basis. Incidentally discovered asymptomatic gallstones are not an indication for cholecystectomy, as the procedure does not improve outcome and has associated morbidity and even mortality.[56]

In addition to the supportive care described, the initial management of acute cholecystitis includes hospital admission and early surgical consultation. Although cholecystitis is predominantly an inflammatory disease, it may be difficult to determine when secondary bacterial infection has occurred, therefore antibiotics should be considered. Typical regimens include ampicillin with gentamycin, ampicillin-sulbactam, piperacillin-tazobactam, a third- or fourth-generation cephalosporin, or a third-generation fluoroquinolone.[42] More severe disease should prompt a broader spectrum of antibiotic coverage.[50,83] Aside from findings on imaging studies, risk factors for development of complicated disease include advanced age, male sex, diabetes, fever, palpable gallbladder, elevated alkaline phosphatase, and leukocytosis.[84,85]

Cholecystectomy is the definitive treatment, and should be performed within the first 24 to 48 hours of admission in most cases. The practice of delayed cholecystectomy 4 to 8 weeks after acute inflammation ("cooling off" period) is no longer recommended. Delayed cholecystectomy does not reduce the conversion rate from laparoscopic to open surgery, is associated with an increase in overall hospital stay, and 20% to 30% of such patients re-present and require emergency surgery.[42,86] Earlier surgical intervention within 12 to 24 hours should be considered in immunocompromised, elderly, male, diabetic, and febrile patients, as they may have rapid disease progression and greater risk of complications (such as gangrene, emphysematous cholecystitis, empyema, or rupture).[42,43]

Complications and Special Considerations

The primary cause of cholecystitis is gallstones, but other causes may include primary tumors of the gallbladder or common duct, metastatic lesions, benign gallbladder polyps, parasites, periportal lymph nodes, or foreign bodies (such as bullets or fish bones).[42,87] Acute acalculous cholecystitis accounts for 5% to 14% of acute cholecystitis cases.[66] Rarely diagnosed in ED patients, it is seen most commonly as a complication in patients admitted to intensive care units.[66] Other risk factors for acalculous cholecystitis include old age, male gender, diabetes, immunosuppression, vascular disease, prolonged fasting, total parenteral nutrition, acute renal failure, and childbirth.[42,43] Symptoms may be the same as calculous cholecystitis; however, fever may be the only symptom, and up to 75% of cases do not have right upper quadrant pain.[43] Sonographic features are the same as for acute calculous cholecystitis, except that no gallstones are identified (sludge may be present) and sensitivity is lower (29%–92%).[43] A combination of ultrasonography, scintigraphy, and CT may be required to establish the diagnosis. Definitive treatment is cholecystectomy, although critically ill patients may not tolerate the surgical procedure, so percutaneous cholecystostomy may be used as a temporizing measure.

The gallbladder may fistulize with bowel, allowing gallstones to pass directly into the gastrointestinal tract. A large gallstone (usually >2.5 cm) may cause a mechanical obstruction (termed gallstone ileus), typically at the ileocecal junction.[65] Invasion of the gallbladder by gas-forming organisms leads to emphysematous cholecystitis. The gas in the gallbladder lumen or wall may be seen on ultrasonography, CT, or occasionally plain abdominal radiographs. Although classically associated with mortality of 15% or higher, more sensitive ultrasonographic and CT studies now make the diagnosis earlier in the disease process and improve outcomes.[88] Biliary tract gas is a marker of severe disease and should prompt aggressive resuscitative care, broad-spectrum antibiotics, and early surgical intervention.

Approximately 10% to 15% of those with gallstones also have common bile duct stones,[55] which may be asymptomatic, present with the same biliary pain as cholelithiasis, or cause symptoms related to cholestasis.[89] Ductal stones can recur even after cholecystectomy, or may represent retained/residual stones that were not previously identified. Stones in the common bile duct lead to elevations of alkaline phosphatase and GGT levels in more than 90% of patients.[55] Ultrasonography is only 25% to 60% sensitive for detecting bile duct stones, but is very specific (95%–100%).[55] Biliary duct dilation in the presence of gallstones is highly suggestive, but an acutely obstructed bile duct may not be dilated. CT also has low sensitivity (71%–75%) in detecting bile duct stones, but is useful for detecting biliary dilation and excluding other causes (such as a mass lesion) or complications (such as liver abscess).[55] Because of procedure-related risks, ERCP is reserved for those patients at high risk of having bile duct stones and who require therapeutic intervention. Because of the high risk of severe complications such as cholangitis or pancreatitis, therapy for bile duct stones is generally indicated regardless of symptoms.[55,89]

The most common cause of cholangitis in the United States is choledocholithiasis secondary to cholelithiasis; malignant obstruction rarely causes cholangitis unless a biliary procedure has been performed.[43,55] Charcot's triad of right upper quadrant pain, jaundice, and fever is found in 50% to 70% of cases of acute cholangitis. Reynolds' pentad occurs when mental status changes and hypotension are also present (<30% of cases) with more severe disease.[43,55] In addition to hyperbilirubinemia, leukocytosis is common, and liver transaminases and alkaline phosphatase are elevated. Pancreatic enzyme elevation suggests that bile duct stones caused the cholangitis.[43,55] Resuscitative care, correction of fluid and electrolyte deficits, correction of coagulopathy (frequently present because of vitamin K deficiency related to prolonged jaundice, or thrombocytopenia from sepsis), and broad-spectrum antibiotics are indicated. ERCP is usually the preferred method of biliary decompression, which is required within 24 to 48 hours (or sooner for more severe disease).

EMERGENCY DISEASES OF THE PANCREAS

The pancreas is a retroperitoneal organ that provides both exocrine and endocrine functions, and is divided anatomically into 3 parts. The head is the widest part; located on the right in the curve of the duodenum. The body and tail of the pancreas extend to the left, with the body lying posterior to the stomach and the tail extending to the gastric surface of the spleen and kidney. The tail is in contact with the left colic flexure. The organ is loosely composed of alveolar cells without a distinct capsule. The blood supply is provided by the superior pancreaticoduodenal artery from the celiac trunk and the inferior pancreaticoduodenal artery from the superior mesenteric artery.[90] The endocrine functions of the pancreas are performed by the islets of Langerhans: clusters of cells made up of alpha, beta, and delta cells that produce insulin, glucagon, and somatostatin. The pancreas receives branches of the vagus nerve that help regulate its exocrine functions. Pancreatic amylase, lipase, and proteolytic enzymes are created in the acinar cells and secreted first into the pancreatic duct, and ultimately into the duodenum. The most important of these include trypsinogen, chymotrypsinogen, and procarboxypeptidase, which are cleaved to their active forms inside the duodenum. Acute pancreatitis is an inflammatory condition of the pancreas. Recurrent episodes of acute pancreatitis can lead to chronic pancreatitis and pancreatic dysfunction. Because of the lack of a distinct capsule, injury to the pancreas can cause leakage of pancreatic enzymes into the abdomen, damaging the surrounding organs.[91]

Epidemiology

Acute pancreatitis is commonly encountered in the ED, with an estimated incidence of 17 cases per year per 100,000 people. The number of cases appears to be rising according to several studies. One report that reviewed all discharge diagnoses of acute pancreatitis over a 6-year period in the United States from 1997 to 2003 showed an increase of 30%.[92] The investigators noted that the increase may have been secondary to better screening and detection, but there was an increased number of admissions for alcohol abuse and cholecystitis over this time period as well.[92] Patients between the ages of 18 and 64 years account for more than 70% of admissions. Pancreatitis in patients younger than 18 years is exceedingly rare (1.6%). Disease prevalence is equal in women and men (49% and 51%, respectively).[92,93]

Risk Factors

Chronic alcohol use and cholelithiasis account for more than 90% of episodes of acute pancreatitis. Worldwide, gallstones account for the majority of cases, but in the United States the incidence of gallstone and alcoholic pancreatitis is almost equal.[93] In the coming years, there may be a shift toward gallstone disease as the population becomes increasingly obese. The greatest incidence of alcoholic pancreatitis is between the ages of 45 and 55 years, as it generally takes greater than 10 years of drinking 4 to 5 alcoholic drinks per night to develop pancreatitis. In the younger patient populations, systemic diseases such as cystic fibrosis and hemolytic uremic syndrome are the main pathological conditions. Trauma is a rare cause of pancreatitis, and is seen in about 0.2% of abdominal trauma.[94] Other rare causes include scorpion stings and gila monster bites. The most common infectious causes are mumps and Coxsackie B viruses. Other infectious causes include herpes simplex, varicella zoster, *Mycoplasma*, and *Salmonella typhosa*. Ischemia is a rare cause of pancreatitis, because it has a rich blood supply and generally is secondary to some other systemic condition (such as hypotension, vasculitis, or hypercoagulable disorder). Other risk factors include anatomic abnormalities, autoimmune diseases (lupus), hypercalcemia and hyperparathyroidism, hypertriglyceridemia, hypothermia, drug reactions (such as to tetracycline, valproic acid, metronidazole, thiazides), and postprocedural (ERCP or Whipple procedure) occurrence.[94,95]

Pathophysiology

Whether due to biliary tract obstruction (choledocholithiasis) or pancreatic toxins (alcohol, drugs, and scorpion venom), the central pathophysiologic event in acute pancreatitis is thought to be the premature activation of digestive zymogens within the pancreas. Protective mechanisms normally help to inactivate trypsin and prevent premature activation of the zymogens produced inside the pancreas. In pathologic states, buildup of toxic metabolites and activated trypsin overwhelm these protective mechanisms, causing these and other enzymes (such as chymotrypsinogen and pro-carboxypeptidase) to be activated within the pancreas.[96] This injury releases inflammatory cytokines that can cause systemic inflammatory response syndrome (SIRS) in 10% to 15% of patients, worsening pancreatic damage and causing multiorgan failure by hypoperfusion.[95] Only 10% of alcoholics develop pancreatitis, and it is unclear why the protective mechanisms fail in these individuals, It is suspected that genetic deficiencies in antitrypsin enzymes may be to blame.[97] In obstructive pathologies such as cholelithiasis, bile refluxes into the pancreatic duct, causing edema and buildup of proteolytic enzymes.[94]

Clinical Findings

By far the most common finding in acute pancreatitis is abdominal pain, which can be found in up to 95% of patients and is generally described as a boring pain located in the upper abdomen, radiating in a band-like pain pattern around to the back.[94] The pain is often constant, maximal at onset, and worse with food or drink. It generally lasts for several days and is often associated with nausea and vomiting. The severity of the pain does not correlate with the severity of disease. Patients may also experience dyspnea due to diaphragmatic irritation, pleural effusion, or in severe cases, impaired oxygenation and respiratory function from acute respiratory distress syndrome (ARDS).

Physical examination findings may vary, but in general, increasingly severe pancreatitis is reflected by increasingly pronounced physical findings. In mild disease, the vital signs may be normal or minimally elevated. Abdominal tenderness is generally mild to moderate and is located in the mid-epigastric region. Peritoneal signs will not be present in early disease so that the patient may be actively writhing on the stretcher, similar to patients with renal colic. Bowel sounds may be normal or hypoactive. In moderate disease, the vital signs will become increasingly abnormal with progressive tachycardia and tachypnea. A low-grade fever may develop (50% of cases). Abdominal tenderness usually becomes increasingly severe. As peripancreatic inflammation progresses, the patient will often lie still with abdominal guarding to minimize peritoneal motion, and may adopt a fetal position to decrease pancreatic stretch. Bowel sounds will often become hypoactive secondary to an ileus. Breath sounds may be decreased in the bases, due to pleural effusions (most commonly on the left). In severe pancreatitis, tachycardia, tachypnea, and hypotension are typical. Peritoneal signs may not develop until late in the course. Crackles and hypoxia may be present, due to ARDS. Cutaneous findings are rare in acute pancreatitis (1.2% in one study[98]), but they portend a complicated hospital course and poor prognosis because they signal the presence of necrosis and hemorrhage.[94] The Grey-Turner sign is ecchymosis located on the flanks, and indicates retroperitoneal bleeding. Ecchymosis located along the inguinal ligament, a finding known as Fox's sign, also indicates retroperitoneal hemorrhage. Cullen's sign, ecchymosis located around the umbilicus, is a sign of intra-abdominal bleeding. Livedo reticularis on the abdomen, chest, or thighs, termed Walzel's sign, is caused by trypsin damage to the subcutaneous veins.[97] None of these signs are specific for pancreatitis, but if found in conjunction with the diagnosis of pancreatitis have been shown to have increased mortality. Cullen's sign and the Grey-Turner sign also occur in intra-abdominal and retroperitoneal bleeding due to any cause, such as ectopic pregnancy and ruptured aortic aneurysm. Thus these alternative diagnoses should also be considered if these findings are encountered.[98]

Diagnostic Testing and Imaging

There is no definitive test for the diagnosis of acute pancreatitis. The diagnosis requires a combination of history, physical examination, diagnostic laboratory studies, and imaging. Traditionally the diagnostic test of choice for acute pancreatitis was serum amylase. Levels above 3 times normal are more specific for the diagnosis of acute pancreatitis. However, amylase is elevated in a variety of conditions, such as pregnancy, renal failure, and esophageal perforation, and can be nondiagnostically elevated in up to 30% of acute pancreatitis cases.[95] Serum lipase has become the primary diagnostic test for acute pancreatitis. It has a sensitivity of 85% to 100% and is more specific than amylase.[99] Other pancreatic enzymes, such as phospholipase A, trypsin, trypsinogen-2, and carboxyl ester lipase, have been evaluated for use in diagnosis, but they have not been proved to be more sensitive or specific than serum amylase and lipase. Leukocytosis is common in acute pancreatitis secondary to the inflammatory cytokines produced, and is rarely indicative of an infectious cause of the disease.[94] AST and ALT may be mildly elevated in alcoholic pancreatitis, but ALT elevations of greater than 150 units/L have been shown to favor the diagnosis of gallstone pancreatitis, with a positive predictive value of 95% in some studied populations.[100]

Though not necessary for the diagnosis, imaging can help to differentiate pancreatitis from other diagnoses and help evaluate for complications of acute pancreatitis. The obstruction series (flat and upright abdominal radiographs with an upright chest film) may occasionally identify a localized ileus or sentinel loop, pleural effusion, pancreatic calcifications, or a calcified gallbladder, but has very low sensitivity and rarely alters the clinical decision regarding whether to obtain a CT if it is available. Due to its retroperitoneal location, ultrasound imaging is rarely helpful in the evaluation of the pancreas, but may be useful in revealing a gallbladder with stones, especially if these are numerous and small (more likely to cause common bile duct obstruction). If visualized, the pancreas may show increased echogenicity, enlargement, or peripancreatic fluid.[101]

CT with both intravenous and oral contrast is the best modality for evaluating pancreatitis and its complications. Routine CT use is not recommended for evaluation of mild episodes of pancreatitis. However, it should be considered for those with moderate or severe pancreatitis or in those for whom another diagnosis (such as aortic aneurysm) is considered. In acute pancreatitis, the gland may appear normal in mild disease. As the severity increases, the pancreas loses its distinct appearance and becomes hazier in appearance. Fluid collections and fat stranding may be seen as severity increases further. CT may also be helpful in visualizing complications such as pancreatic necrosis and pancreatic pseudocyst.[101]

Mortality and Complications

Overall mortality from pancreatitis is relatively low at approximately 5%, but those with severe pancreatitis can have mortality as high as 25%.[95] The problem is in distinguishing low-risk and high-risk patients. Several risk assessment scores have been developed for this purpose including Ranson's criteria, APACHE II, Imrie score, and CT severity index.[102] These scores may be used in conjunction with clinical judgment to help aid in disposition.

Pancreatic necrosis is an important complication of pancreatitis. It carries a mortality of approximately 30% and is responsible for 50% of all deaths from pancreatitis.[103] Necrosis is diagnosed on CT by decreased enhancement of the pancreas, and may require percutaneous drainage or laparotomy.

Hemorrhagic pancreatitis is caused by erosion of vasculature by proteolytic enzymes, which can lead to SIRS, diffuse intravascular coagulation, and profound shock. Cullen's sign and the Grey-Turner sign may herald the presence of this process. Pancreatic pseudocysts are collections of pancreatic enzymes and other debris encapsulated within granulation and scar tissue. Pseudocysts form in approximately 5% to 40% of pancreatitis patients and can be devastating if they rupture. Diagnosis is by CT or abdominal ultrasonography. If the pseudocyst persists past 4 weeks, percutaneous or endoscopic drainage may be required.[104]

Chronic pancreatitis should be suspected in anyone with recurrent episodes of pancreatitis or epigastric pain. It is most common in patients with a history of alcoholic pancreatitis, and is caused by progressively worsening necrosis, fibrosis, calcification of the pancreas, and destruction of the endocrine and exocrine glands leading to chronic pain, malabsorption, weight loss, steatorrhea, and diabetes mellitus. Chronic pancreatitis is part of a spectrum of disease and is often difficult to diagnose, as serum markers can be normal from chronic destruction of pancreatic tissue.[105]

Treatment

The mainstay of treatment for acute pancreatitis is supportive care. As always, the ABCs (airway, breathing, circulation) receive priority. Patients with SIRS may develop altered mental status and ARDS from circulating cytokines, requiring supplemental oxygen or even intubation. Patients suffering from acute pancreatitis are generally intravascularly depleted and require aggressive intravenous hydration.[94] Urine output should be monitored. Pain, nausea, and vomiting should be controlled.[102] Oral intake should be withheld in the acute setting to provide a "rest period" for the pancreas.[95] Routine use of antibiotics in pancreatitis is not recommended without a clear infectious cause.[103] Surgical intervention may be necessary, so early consultation is advised in the management of severe pancreatitis.[103] Initial ERCP is not currently recommended for all patients suspected of having gallstone pancreatitis, but those with signs of cholangitis or worsening jaundice may benefit from early treatment.[95]

All patients with new-onset pancreatitis should be admitted for further observation and determination of the underlying cause. If pain cannot be controlled with oral pain medications or if oral hydration is unsuccessful, the patient should be admitted for parenteral treatment. Placement in the intensive care unit should be considered in patients with hypotension or hypoxia following aggressive resuscitation. Some patients with recurrent pancreatitis can be safely discharged home in the absence of clinical findings to suggest severe disease.

SUMMARY

Disorders related to the hepatobiliary system and pancreas are common, and EPs should be familiar with their evaluation and management. While much of the care of liver disease is chronic, it is important to bear in mind that acute and life-threatening complications can occur. Hepatic decompensation is often due to an acute precipitant that needs to be identified and treated expeditiously. Biliary disease is highly prevalent. History, physical examination, and laboratory studies can narrow the differential diagnosis, but appropriate imaging studies are necessary for diagnosis. Although most cases are not life threatening, severe complications can occur and progress rapidly, requiring prompt diagnosis and treatment. Finally, although most of the cases of pancreatitis in the ED are not severe, the EP should be alert to the possible presence of hemorrhagic and necrotizing pancreatitis, as well as pancreatic pseudocyst.

REFERENCES

1. Giannini EG, Testa R, Savarino V. Liver enzyme alteration: a guide for clinicians. CMAJ 2005;172(3):367–79.
2. Malhi H, Gores G. Cellular and molecular mechanisms of liver injury. Gastroenterology 2008;134:1641–54.
3. Kamath PS. Clinical approach to the patient with abnormal liver test results. Mayo Clin Proc 1996;71:1089–95.
4. Friedman SL. The cellular basis of hepatic fibrosis. N Engl J Med 1993;328: 1828–35.
5. Gines P, Cardenas A, Arroyo V, et al. Management of cirrhosis and ascites. N Engl J Med 2004;350(16):1646–54.
6. Green RM, Flamm S. AGA technical review on the evaluation of liver chemistry tests. Gastroenterology 2002;123:1367–84.
7. Gerber T, Schomerus H. Hepatic encephalopathy in liver cirrhosis. Drugs 2000; 60(6):1353–70.
8. Najm W. Viral hepatitis: how to manage type C and D infections. Geriatrics 1997; 52(5):28–37.
9. Bernal W, Auzinger G, Dhawan A, et al. Acute liver failure. Lancet 2010;376: 190–201.
10. Lefton HB, Rosa A, Cohen M. Diagnosis and epidemiology of cirrhosis. Med Clin North Am 2009;93:787–99.
11. Liaw Y, Chu C. Hepatitis B virus infection. Lancet 2009;373:582–92.
12. Poynard T, Yuen M, Ratzui V, et al. Viral hepatitis C. Lancet 2003;362:2095–100.
13. Alter MJ, Margolis HS, Krawczynski K, et al. The natural history of community-acquired hepatitis C in the United States. The Sentinel Counties Chronic non-A, non-B Hepatitis Study Team. N Engl J Med 1992;327:1899–905.
14. Johnson B, Rosenthal N, Capece JA, et al. Improvement of physical health and quality of life of alcohol-dependent individuals with topiramate treatment. Arch Intern Med 2008;168(11):1188–99.

15. Lucey MR, Mathurin P. Alcoholic hepatitis. N Engl J Med 2009;360:2758–69.
16. Haber PS, Warner R, Seth D, et al. Pathogenesis and management of alcoholic hepatitis. J Gastroenterol Hepatol 2003;18(12):1332–44.
17. De Alwis NMW, Day CP. Genetics of alcoholic liver disease and nonalcoholic fatty liver disease. Semin Liver Dis 2007;27(1):44–54.
18. You M, Matsumoto M, Pacold CM, et al. The role of AMP-activated protein kinase in the action of ethanol in the liver. Gastroenterology 2004;127:1798–808.
19. McCullough AJ, O'Connor JFB. Alcoholic liver disease: proposed recommendations for the American College of Gastroenterology. Am J Gastroenterol 1998; I93(11):2022–36.
20. Sorbi D, Boynton J, Lindor KD. The ratio of aspartate aminotransferase to alanine aminotransferase: potential value in differentiating nonalcoholic steatohepatitis from alcoholic liver disease. Am J Gastroenterol 1999;94:1018–22.
21. Bergheim I, McClain CJ, Arteel GE. Treatment of alcoholic liver disease. Dig Dis 2005;23(3–4):275–84.
22. Mackelaite L, Alsauskas ZC, Fanganna K. Renal failure in patients with cirrhosis. Med Clin North Am 2009;93:855–69.
23. Munoz SJ. The hepatorenal syndrome. Med Clin North Am 2008;92:813–37.
24. Gines P, Guevara M, Arroyo V, et al. Hepatorenal syndrome. Lancet 2003;362: 1819–27.
25. Guevara M, Gines P. Hepatorenal syndrome. Dig Dis 2005;23:47–55.
26. Arroyo V, Terra C, Gines P. New treatments of hepatorenal syndrome. Semin Liver Dis 2006;26(3):254–64.
27. Arroyo V, Fernandez J, Gines P. Pathogenesis and treatment of hepatorenal syndrome. Semin Liver Dis 2008;28(1):81–95.
28. Salerno F, Gerbes A, Gines P, et al. Diagnosis, prevention and treatment of hepatorenal syndrome in cirrhosis. Postgrad Med J 2008;84:662–70.
29. Hou W, Sanyal A. Ascites: diagnosis and management. Med Clin North Am 2009;93:801–17.
30. Lata J, Stiburek O, Kopacova M. Spontaneous bacterial peritonitis: a severe complication of liver cirrhosis. World J Gastroenterol 2009;15(44):5505–10.
31. Tamaskar I, Ravakhah K. Spontaneous bacterial peritonitis with Pasteurella multocida in cirrhosis: case report and review of literature. South Med J 2004;97(11):1113–5.
32. Fernandez J, Navasa M, Planas R, et al. Primary prophylaxis of spontaneous bacterial peritonitis delays hepatorenal syndrome and improves survival in cirrhosis. Gastroenterology 2007;133:818–24.
33. Abou-Assi S, Vlahcevic ZR. Hepatic encephalopathy metabolic consequence of cirrhosis often is reversible. Postgrad Med 2001;109(2):52–70.
34. Ferenci P, Lockwood A, Mullen K, et al. Hepatic encephalopathy—definition, nomenclature, diagnosis, and quantification: final report of the working party at the 11th World Congresses of Gastroenterology, Vienna, 1998. Hepatology 2002;35(3):716–21.
35. Vaquero J, Polson J, Chung C, et al. Infection and the progression of hepatic encephalopathy in acute liver failure. Gastroenterology 2003;125:755–64.
36. Munoz SJ. Hepatic encephalopathy. Med Clin North Am 2008;92:795–812.
37. Ong JP, Aggarwal A, Krieger D, et al. Correlation between ammonia levels and the severity of hepatic encephalopathy. Am J Med 2003;115:188–93.
38. O'Leary JG, Lepe R, Davis GL. Indications for liver transplantation. Gastroenterology 2008;134:1764–76.
39. Sundaram V, Shaikh O. Hepatic encephalopathy: pathophysiology and emerging therapies. Med Clin North Am 2009;93:819–36.

40. Sandler RS. The burden of selected digestive diseases in the United States. Gastroenterology 2002;122:1500–11.
41. Trowbridge RL, Rutkowski NK, Shojania KG. Does this patient have acute cholecystitis? JAMA 2003;289:80–6.
42. Elwood DR. Cholecystitis. Surg Clin North Am 2008;88:1241–52.
43. Yusoff IF, Barkun JS, Barkun AN. Diagnosis and management of cholecystitis and cholangitis. Gastroenterol Clin North Am 2003;32:1145–68.
44. Lambou-Gianoukos S, Heller SJ. Lithogenesis and bile metabolism. Surg Clin North Am 2008;88:1175–94.
45. Friedman GD. Natural history of asymptomatic and symptomatic gallstones. Am J Surg 1993;165:399–404.
46. Vakili K, Pomfret EA. Biliary anatomy and embryology. Surg Clin North Am 2008; 88:1159–74.
47. Moscati RM. Cholelithiasis, cholecystitis, and pancreatitis. Emerg Med Clin North Am 1996;14:719–37.
48. Schafmayer C, Hartleb J, Tepel J, et al. Predictors of gallstone composition in 1025 symptomatic gallstones from Northern Germany. BMC Gastroenterol 2006;6:36.
49. Indar AA, Beckingham IJ. Acute cholecystitis. BMJ 2002;325:639–43.
50. Yoshida M, Takada T, Kawarada Y, et al. Antimicrobial therapy for acute cholecystitis: Tokyo guidelines. J Hepatobiliary Pancreat Surg 2007;14:83–90.
51. Abeysuriva V, Deen KI, Wijesuriya T, et al. Microbiology of gallbladder bile in uncomplicated symptomatic cholelithiasis. Hepatobiliary Pancreat Dis Int 2008;7:633–7.
52. Morris-Stiff GJ, O'Donohue P, Ogunbiyi S, et al. Microbiological assessment of bile during cholecystectomy: is all bile infected? HPB (Oxford) 2007;9:225–8.
53. Gilbert DN, Moellering RC, Eliopoulos GM, et al. The Sanford guide to antimicrobial therapy. 39th edition. Sperryville (VA): Antimicrobial Therapy, Inc; 2008. p. 15.
54. Yoo E, Lee S. The prevalence and risk factors for gallstone disease. Clin Chem Lab Med 2009;47:795–807.
55. Attasaranya S, Fogel EL, Lehman GA. Choledocholithiasis, ascending cholangitis, and gallstone pancreatitis. Med Clin North Am 2008;92:925–60.
56. Besselink MG, Venneman NG, Go PM, et al. Is complicated gallstone disease preceded by biliary colic? J Gastrointest Surg 2009;13:312–7.
57. Venneman NG, vanErpecum KJ. Gallstone disease: primary and secondary prevention. Best Pract Res Clin Gastroenterol 2006;20(6):1063–73.
58. Berger MY, olde Hartman TC, van der Velden JJ, et al. Is biliary pain exclusively related to gallbladder stones? A controlled prospective study. Br J Gen Pract 2004;54:574–9.
59. Berger MY. Abdominal symptoms: do they predict gallstones? A systematic review. Scand J Gastroenterol 2000;35:70–6.
60. Traverso LW. Clinical manifestations and impact of gallstone disease. Am J Surg 1993;165:405–9.
61. Glasgow RE, Cho M, Hutter MM, et al. The spectrum and cost of complicated gallstone disease in California. Arch Surg 2000;135:1021–7.
62. Singer AJ, McCracken G, Henry MC, et al. Correlation among clinical, laboratory, and hepatobiliary scanning findings in patients with suspected acute cholecystitis. Ann Emerg Med 1996;28:267–72.
63. Adedeji OA, McAdam WA. Murphy's sign, acute cholecystitis and elderly people. J R Coll Surg Edinb 1996;41:88–9.
64. Fitzgerald JE, White MJ, Lobo DN. Courvoisier's gallbladder: law or sign? World J Surg 2009;33:886–91.

65. Zaliekas J, Munson JL. Complications of gallstones: the Mirizzi syndrome, gall-stone ileus, gallstone pancreatitis, complications of "lost" gallstones. Surg Clin North Am 2008;88:1345–68.
66. Newton E, Mandavia S. Surgical complications of selected gastrointestinal emergencies: pitfalls in management of the acute abdomen. Emerg Med Clin North Am 2003;21:873–907.
67. American College of Radiology Appropriateness Criteria, last review date. 2007. Available at: http://www.acr.org/SecondaryMainMenuCategories/quality_safety/app_criteria/pdf/ExpertPanelonGastrointestinalImaging/RightUpperQuadrantPainDoc13.aspx. Accessed on January 23, 2009.
68. Miller AH, Pepe PE, Brockman CR, et al. ED ultrasound in hepatobiliary disease. J Emerg Med 2005;30:69–74.
69. Larson JL, Fox JC, Scruggs W, et al. An analysis of emergency department bedside ultrasound in the diagnosis of cholelithiasis [abstract]. Ann Emerg Med 2008;51:545.
70. Kendall JL, Shimp RJ. Performance and interpretation of focused right upper quadrant ultrasound by emergency physicians. J Emerg Med 2001;21:7–13.
71. Rosen CL, Brown DF, Chang Y, et al. Ultrasonography by emergency physicians in patients with suspected cholecystitis. Am J Emerg Med 2001;19:32–6.
72. Jang T, Aubin B, Naunheim R. Minimum training for right upper quadrant ultra-sonography. Am J Emerg Med 2004;22:439–43.
73. Rubins DJ. Hepatobiliary imaging and its pitfalls. Radiol Clin North Am 2004;42:257–78.
74. Rubins DJ. Ultrasound imaging of the biliary tract. Ultrasound Clin 2007;2:391–413.
75. Spence SC, Teichgraeber D, Chandrasekhar C. Emergency right upper quad-rant sonography. J Ultrasound Med 2009;28:479–96.
76. Shah K, Wolfe RE. Hepatobiliary ultrasound. Emerg Med Clin North Am 2004;22:661–73.
77. Gore RM, Yaghmai V, Newmark GM, et al. Imaging benign and malignant disease of the gallbladder. Radiol Clin North Am 2002;40:1307–23.
78. Harvey RT, Miller WT. Acute biliary disease: initial CT and follow-up US versus initial US and follow-up CT. Radiology 1999;213:831–6.
79. Wald C, Scholz FJ, Pinkus E, et al. An update on biliary imaging. Surg Clin North Am 2008;88:1195–220.
80. Akriviadis EA, Hatzigavriel M, Kapnias D, et al. Treatment of biliary colic with di-clofenac: a randomized, double-blind, placebo-controlled study. Gastroenter-ology 1997;113:225–31.
81. Gaby AR. Nutritional approaches to prevention and treatment of gallstones. Al-tern Med Rev 2009;14:258–67.
82. Berger MY, olde Hartman TC, Bohnen AM. Abdominal symptoms: do they disappear after cholecystectomy? Surg Endosc 2003;17:1723–8.
83. Solomonkin JS, Mazuski JE, Bradley JS, et al. Diagnosis and management of complicated intra-abdominal infection in adults and children: guidelines by the Surgical Infection Society and the Infectious Diseases Society of America. Clin Infect Dis 2010;50:133–64.
84. Gallili O, Eldar S, Matter I, et al. The effect of bactibilia on the course and outcome of laparoscopic cholecystectomy. Eur J Clin Microbiol Infect Dis 2008;27:797–803.
85. Bedirli A, Sakrak O, Sozuer EM, et al. Factors effecting the complications in the natural history of acute cholecystitis. Hepatogastroenterology 2001;48:1275–8.

86. Flasar MH, Goldberg E. Acute abdominal pain. Med Clin North Am 2006;90: 481–503.
87. Kunizaki M, Kusano H, Azuma K, et al. Cholecystitis caused by a fish bone. Am J Surg 2009;198:e20–2.
88. Gill KS, Chapman AH, Weston MJ. The changing face of emphysematous cholecystitis. Br J Radiol 1997;70:986–91.
89. Caddy GR, Tham TC. Gallstone disease: symptoms, diagnosis and endoscopic management of common bile duct stones. Best Pract Res Clin Gastroenterol 2006;20:1085–101.
90. Gray Henry. The pancreas, anatomy of the human body. Philadelphia: Lea & Febiger; 1918. Bartleby.com, 2000. p. 929–32.
91. Sherwood L. The digestive system, human physiology; from cells to systems. 4th edition. Pacific Grove (CA): Brooks/Cole; 2001. p. 584–87.
92. Brown A, Young B, Morton J, et al. Are health related outcomes in acute pancreatitis improving? An analysis of National Trends in the U.S. from 1997 to 2003. JOP 2008;9:408–14.
93. Lowenfels AB, Maisonneuve P, Sullivan T. The changing character of acute pancreatitis: epidemiology, etiology, and prognosis. Curr Gastroenterol Rep 2009;11:97–103.
94. Cappell MS. Acute pancreatitis: etiology, clinical presentation, diagnosis, and therapy. Med Clin North Am 2008;92:889–923.
95. Mitchell RM, Byrne MF, Baillie J. Pancreatitis. Lancet 2003;361:1447–55.
96. Halangk W, Lerch MM. Early events in acute pancreatitis. Gastroenterol Clin North Am 2004;33:717–31.
97. Behrman SW, Fowler ES. Pathophysiology of chronic pancreatitis. Surg Clin North Am 2007;87:1309–24.
98. Lankisch PG, Weber-Dany B, Maisonneuve P, et al. Skin signs in acute pancreatitis: frequency and implications for prognosis. J Intern Med 2009;265: 299–301.
99. Agarwal N, Pitchumoni CS, Sivaprasad AV. Evaluating tests for acute pancreatitis. Am J Gastroenterol 1990;85(4):356–66.
100. Tenner S, Dubner H, Steinberg W. Predicting gallstone pancreatitis with laboratory parameters: a meta-analysis. Am J Gastroenterol 1994;89:1863–6.
101. Kim DH, Pickhardt PJ. Radiologic assessment of acute and chronic pancreatitis. Surg Clin North Am 2007;87:1341–58.
102. Carroll JK, Herrick B, Gibson T, et al. Acute pancreatitis: diagnosis, prognosis, and treatment. Am Fam Physician 2007;75:1513–20.
103. Bakker OJ, van Santvoort HC, Besselink MG, et al. Prevention, detection, and management of infected necrosis in severe acute pancreatitis. Curr Gastroenterol Rep 2009;11:104–10.
104. Habashi S, Draganov PV. Pancreatic pseudocyst. World J Gastroenterol 2009; 15:38–47.
105. Nair RJ, Lawler L, Miller MR. Chronic pancreatitis. Am Fam Physician 2007;76: 1679–88, 1693–4.

Bowel Obstruction and Hernia

Geoffrey E. Hayden, MD[a],*, Kevin L. Sprouse, DO[b]

KEYWORDS

• Obstruction • Ileus • Hernia

BOWEL OBSTRUCTION

Bowel obstruction accounts for more than 15% of admissions from the emergency department (ED) for abdominal pain.[1] Intestinal obstructions (85% small bowel, 15% large bowel obstructions) generated more than 320,000 hospitalizations in the United States in 2007 alone, with 3.4 billion dollars spent on diagnosis and management.[2,3] At least 30,000 deaths per year are attributed to bowel obstruction. Delayed diagnosis and misdiagnosis of both small bowel and colonic obstruction are common and lead to increased morbidity and mortality.[4] The elderly are particularly at risk, because bowel obstruction is a common cause of abdominal pain (12%–25%), with a mortality of 7% to 14%.[5,6] A thorough understanding of these complex gastrointestinal pathologies is essential for the emergency physician. This article focuses on bowel obstruction in the adult patient. Pediatric gastrointestinal disorders are addressed in a separate article by Marin and Alpern elsewhere in this issue.

SMALL BOWEL OBSTRUCTION
Background

Small bowel obstructions (SBO) are responsible for approximately 4% of all ED visits for abdominal pain. These cases account for around 20% of all surgical admissions.[7,8] Although hernias were historically the most common cause for SBO, and continue to be a primary cause in some developing countries, postoperative adhesions now account for more than 75% of all obstructive events in the United States.[9,10] There are a variety of other causes of SBO (**Table 1**). Although the overall mortality for patients with SBO is less than 3%, it is much higher in the elderly.[11] When strangulation complicates SBO, mortality increases to 30%.[12]

The authors have no financial disclosures.
a Department of Emergency Medicine, Vanderbilt University Medical Center, Nashville, TN, USA
b Department of Emergency Medicine, New York Methodist Hospital, 506 6th Street, Brooklyn, NY 11215, USA
* Corresponding author. 358 Martello Drive, Charleston, SC 29412.
E-mail address: geoffhayden@gmail.com

Emerg Med Clin N Am 29 (2011) 319–345
doi:10.1016/j.emc.2011.01.004
0733-8627/11/$ – see front matter © 2011 Elsevier Inc. All rights reserved.

Table 1
Common causes of bowel obstruction, ileus, and colonic pseudo-obstruction

Small Bowel Obstruction (%)	Large Bowel Obstruction (%)	Adynamic Ileus	Acute Colonic Pseudo-obstruction (%)
Intestinal adhesions (75)	Malignancy (60)	Postoperative state	Postoperative state (23)
Hernias (15)	Volvulus (10–15)	Pharmacologic agents	Cardiopulmonary
Malignancy (5–10)	Diverticulitis (10)	(opioids,	disease (10–18)
Other (eg, Crohn	Other (eg,	anticholinergics,	Nonoperative
disease, volvulus,	incarcerated hernia,	antihistamines,	trauma (11)
gallstone)	fecal impaction,	psychotropic	Infections (10)
	adhesions)	medications,	Other (drugs such as
		calcium channel	opioids and
		blockers)	antidepressants,
		Infections (especially	neurologic disease,
		pneumonia)	metabolic disorders,
		Neurologic disorders	malignancy,
		Abdominal or skeletal	intra-abdominal
		trauma	disorders, obstetric
			disorders,
			retroperitoneal
			disorders)

Data from Refs.[4,72,88,126,127]

Pathophysiology

In general, SBOs are categorized on the ability of fluid or gas to travel through the site of obstruction. From a physiologic perspective, there is either no passage (complete obstruction) or some passage (partial obstruction) of enteric contents past an obstruction. More precise classification is typically based on radiologic criteria. In complete obstruction, there is no passage of contrast. In low-grade partial SBO, there is minimal delay, whereas in high-grade partial SBO there is stasis or moderate delay of contrast passage.[13] In simple terms, an occlusion of the small bowel results in the accumulation of bowel fluids and the production of gas from bacterial overgrowth. As the disease process progresses, bowel dilatation leads to increased intraluminal pressure. The feared consequences of this sequence are mucosal ischemia and, eventually, necrosis and perforation. Closed-loop obstructions, commonly caused by an incarcerated hernia or twisting of a loop of bowel, are particularly at risk. Strangulation denotes compromise in the vascular supply, either because of twisting of the mesentery or bowel, or simply from increased bowel wall transmural pressures.[13]

Clinical Features

Although the classic presentation of a complete SBO may be quickly recognized, partial SBO remains a diagnostic challenge. Decreased passage of flatus and/or stool, nausea and vomiting, abdominal distention with tympany to percussion, paroxysms of abdominal pain occurring every 4 to 5 minutes, dehydration, and tachycardia are all commonly described. Patients may initially experience colicky pain and high-pitched, hyperactive bowel sounds, but the clinical presentation may then progress to more continuous pain and hypoactive bowel sounds because of bowel fatigue. However, these various signs and symptoms are nonspecific and not reliably observed.[14] Patients with obstruction may even continue to pass stool. Classically, distention tends to be more pronounced in distal, compared with proximal, obstructions. Moreover, complete obstruction is often more sudden in onset, with a more severe and rapid course than a partial obstruction. Mild, generalized tenderness is common in SBO. It may be alleviated by vomiting. In patients with a suspicion for obstruction, localized tenderness or peritoneal signs indicate intestinal ischemia or necrosis until proved otherwise. Pain that is constant and out of proportion to findings on physical examination is a commonly described feature of both closed-loop obstructions and bowel ischemia.

Laboratory Tests

Laboratory tests are both insensitive and nonspecific, and they do not improve diagnosis or predict the need for an operation.[15] Leukocytosis is common and electrolyte abnormalities are sometimes observed. However, no laboratory test reliably detects obstruction, intestinal ischemia, or the need for operative management.[4,15,16] Serum creatinine kinase, amylase, and lactate are generally increased only late in the course of bowel obstruction.

Imaging

Because of the limitations of the clinical evaluation and laboratory assessment of bowel obstruction, imaging plays a vital role in diagnosis. A common theme to all of the imaging modalities is a high sensitivity and specificity in cases of complete or high-grade SBO, but less reliability in cases of low-grade partial SBO. Abdominal radiographs (AXR), computed tomography (CT), ultrasound, small bowel contrast studies, and magnetic resonance imaging (MRI) each contribute to the diagnosis of bowel obstruction. An ideal imaging study would define the degree of obstruction (complete, high grade, or low grade), the location (proximal vs distal), the cause, and the specific complications.

The classic findings on AXR are distended small bowel (>3 cm in diameter), air-fluid levels, and a paucity of colonic or rectal gas (**Table 2**, **Fig. 1**). Differential air-fluid levels are more specific for SBO than for other types of obstruction. Dilated bowel loops that are stacked one under the other are described as having a stepladder appearance. Overall, AXR are diagnostic in 30% to 70% of cases of SBO, with a specificity of approximately 50%.[17,18] The cause of obstruction is rarely shown. There tends to be poor interobserver agreement in terms of the degree and location of obstruction, and discrepancies commonly exist on radiographic interpretations between emergency physicians and radiologists.[19,20] In cases of proven SBO, AXR are interpreted as definite SBO in 50% of cases, probable SBO in 30%, and normal or nonspecific in 20%.[15] AXR may also appear normal in cases of closed-loop or strangulated obstructions.[21] Conversely, functional obstructions (eg, adynamic ileus) can have similar radiographic findings to SBO. Multiple gas-filled or fluid-filled loops of dilated small bowel, with little colonic gas, may also be observed in appendicitis, diverticulitis, or even mesenteric ischemia.[22]

Because of the low sensitivity of plain films in partial SBO, as well as a need for more accurate information regarding the level and cause of the obstruction, CT of the abdomen and pelvis plays an increasingly central role in diagnosis (see **Table 2**). Some investigators advocate omitting AXR and using CT as the first-line imaging modality. When the clinical picture is highly suggestive of complete SBO, AXR have comparable sensitivity with CT[17] and may quickly confirm the diagnosis and expedite surgical disposition. However, if the clinical picture is equivocal and the AXR is likely to be nondiagnostic, CT may be a reasonable initial choice. The American College of Radiology (ACR) has proposed that CT with intravenous (IV) contrast is the most appropriate imaging modality even when complete or high-grade SBO is suspected.[23] However, oral contrast material is not required in these cases because the intraluminal

Table 2
Radiographic findings for abdominal disorders

	Abdominal Radiographs	Computed Tomography
Small bowel obstruction	Distended small bowel (>3 cm in diameter), air-fluid levels (differential or step-laddering early, string of pearls late), paucity of colonic or rectal gas	Dilated proximal small bowel loops (>3 cm) and collapsed distal small bowel ± a transition zone; small bowel feces sign; absence of distal contrast; bowel wall thickening (late)
Large bowel obstruction	Dilated colon (>5 cm), disproportionate distention of the cecum (>10 cm) if competent ileocecal valve	Dilated colon and disproportionate cecal distention, with collapsed distal colon or rectum
Colonic volvulus	Sigmoid: coffee bean appearance to dilated, doubled-back bowel segment, proximal large bowel dilated Cecal: kidney bean shape of single dilated segment of cecum, distal large bowel collapsed, small bowel dilatation	Sigmoid: entire colon (especially sigmoid) markedly dilated, whirl sign at site of torsion Cecal: very dilated cecum with bird's beak or whirl sign (from twisted bowel and mesentery)
Ischemia/infarction	May see ileus or obstruction; thumbprinting or thickening of bowel wall, air in bowel wall (pneumatosis) or portal venous gas	Bowel wall thickening >5 mm, diminished or absent bowel wall enhancement, mesenteric fluid, air in bowel wall (pneumatosis) or portal venous gas; bowel wall edema (target sign)
Adynamic ileus	Distention of both small and large bowel loops, without a transition zone	Distention of both small and large bowel loops, without a transition zone
Acute colonic pseudo-obstruction	Extensive colonic distention (± small bowel), especially in the transverse colon, without a transition point (gas and stool in rectum)	Extensive colonic distention (± small bowel), especially in the transverse colon, without a transition point (gas and stool in rectum)

Data from Schwartz DT. Abdominal radiology. In: Schwartz D, editor. Emergency radiology: case studies. New York: McGraw-Hill; 2008. p. 147–87; and Stoker J, van Randen A, Lameris W, et al. Imaging patients with acute abdominal pain. Radiology 2009;253(1):31–46.

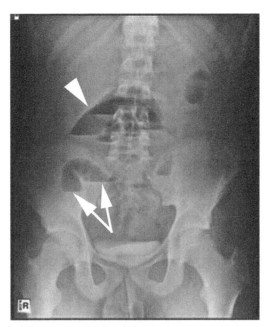

Fig. 1. Small bowel obstruction. Upright abdominal radiograph showing dilated loops of small bowel in the upper abdomen (*arrowhead*) with differential air-fluid levels (*arrows*) in the right lower quadrant. Note the paucity of colonic air. (*Courtesy of* C.E. Smith, MD, Vanderbilt University, Nashville, TN.)

fluid in distended bowel loops acts as a natural contrast agent.[24] Intravenous contrast improves the diagnosis of strangulation, ischemia, and other vascular pathologies such as superior mesenteric artery occlusion or superior mesenteric vein thrombus.[4] Positive oral contrast (standard water-soluble contrast) or neutral (water) contrast may play a role in the evaluation of partial small bowel obstructions and is recommended by the ACR. The decision to add oral contrast should be determined on a case-by-case basis, with due consideration of ED throughput, the patient's clinical condition, patient tolerance of the contrast, and the potential for added benefit with an oral contrast agent in identifying alternative diagnoses. A recent study, which addressed the value of nonenhanced (no IV, no oral contrast) CT in evaluating SBO, found a comparable accuracy between nonenhanced and enhanced CT.[25]

Findings on CT that are consistent with SBO include dilated small bowel loops proximal to collapsed loops distally (see **Table 2**). A transition zone is often identified, and a small bowel feces sign is highly specific (**Figs. 2–5**). The small bowel feces sign derives from the inspissated debris in the dilated, obstructed small bowel; it has the appearance of colonic fecal material. Overall, CT has a sensitivity of 64% to 94% and specificity of 79% to 95% in the detection of SBO, with an accuracy of 67% to 95%.[17,26,27] It provides information regarding the degree of obstruction (low grade vs high grade), proximal or distal location, and the specific cause of the obstruction. In particular, CT identifies closed-loop obstructions that have a high risk of ischemia and mandate surgery. CT is also beneficial in distinguishing SBO from other abdominal disorders such as inflammatory bowel disease, appendicitis, diverticulitis, and ileus.[28] Although CT is accurate in the diagnosis of complete and high-grade obstruction, it is only around 50% sensitive for low-grade partial obstructions.[29]

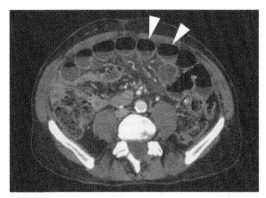

Fig. 2. Small bowel obstruction. Axial CT image showing multiple dilated loops of small bowel with air-fluid levels, as noted by arrowheads. (*Courtesy of* C.E. Smith, MD, Vanderbilt University, Nashville, TN.)

Regarding CT detection of ischemia and strangulation, a meta-analysis reported 83% sensitivity (63%–100%) and 92% specificity (61%–100%) in detecting intestinal ischemia.[30] However, one prospective study by Sheedy and colleagues[31] reported a much lower sensitivity (52%) in the detection of ischemia; the cause of this discrepancy is unclear. The most common CT findings suggestive of ischemia and/or infarction include bowel wall thickening and diminished or absent bowel wall enhancement by IV contrast (see **Table 2; Fig. 6**). It is possible that modern multidetector CT (MDCT) with coronal reformations may significantly improve diagnostic certainty in the identification or exclusion of SBO, as well as the specific cause and level of the obstruction.[32]

Abdominal ultrasound is commonly performed outside the United States for assessment of SBO. It is also recommended for this purpose by the ACR. When studied, ultrasound has been shown to have similar sensitivity and greater specificity compared with plain films.[33–35] Several factors argue for the superiority of CT, including the operator dependency of ultrasound, the logistical challenges of

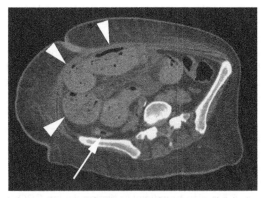

Fig. 3. Small bowel feces sign. Axial CT image showing multiple loops of small bowel distended with partially digested food holding the bowel gas in suspension in a manner normally seen only in the colon (*arrowheads*). Note the collapsed large bowel (*arrow*). (*Courtesy of* C.E. Smith, MD, Vanderbilt University, Nashville, TN.)

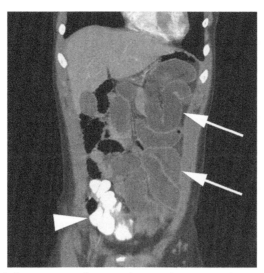

Fig. 4. Small bowel obstruction. Reformatted coronal CT image depicting numerous fluid-distended loops of small bowel (*arrows*). Note the contrast in the large bowel of the right lower quadrant from a previous enema (*arrowhead*). (*Courtesy of* C.E. Smith, MD, Vanderbilt University, Nashville, TN.)

around-the-clock sonographic assessment, limited experience with abdominal sonography in bowel evaluation, and interobserver variability in the interpretation of ultrasound images of the small bowel.[22]

The literature regarding MRI in the diagnosis of SBO is limited. One study reported a high sensitivity (95%), specificity (100%), and accuracy (71%).[36] In general, there is increasing evidence to suggest that MRI can reliably identify SBO and provide information regarding location and cause. The ACR recommends MRI only in particular circumstances, including pregnant patients with concern for SBO.[23]

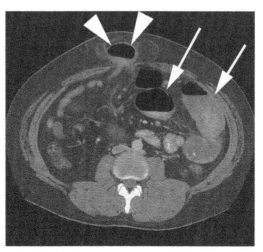

Fig. 5. Incarcerated hernia and small bowel obstruction. Axial CT image showing distended loops of small bowel (*arrows*) proximal to a ventral hernia (*arrowhead*). (*Courtesy of* C.E. Smith, MD, Vanderbilt University, Nashville, TN.)

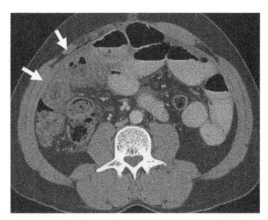

Fig. 6. Small bowel obstruction with resulting ischemia, target sign. Note the marked bowel wall thickening and target appearance (*arrows*) in this patient with ischemic small bowel. (*From* Schwartz DT. Abdominal radiology. In: Schwartz D, editor. Emergency radiology: case studies. New York: McGraw-Hill; 2008. p. 161; with permission.)

A few other diagnostic modalities, although rarely a consideration in the ED, deserve mention. Small bowel follow-through (SBFT), conventional enteroclysis, and CT enteroclysis have all been described in the subacute setting and may have particular value in patients who fail to improve after conservative management.

SBFT with barium or water-soluble contrast allows visualization of dilated loops of bowel, while identifying a transition point as defined by barium. Because SBFT is time consuming and the volume of contrast is not well tolerated by patients, it has been largely supplanted by CT in the United States.[7] Enteroclysis involves intubation of the small bowel through the stomach (often under conscious sedation), allowing infusion of enteral contrast directly into the jejunum. This technique is only applicable to the subacute setting, because it is time-intensive and resource-intensive, although when used appropriately has been reported by 1 author to have 100% sensitivity, 88% specificity, and 86% accuracy in determining the cause of obstruction.[18] With the advent of MDCT, CT enteroclysis is increasingly used for the nonemergent evaluation of SBO. It is both more sensitive (89%) and more specific (100%) than CT regarding partial SBO.[37] Similar to conventional enteroclysis, this modality necessitates intubation of the descending duodenum under fluoroscopy, infusion of enteric contrast material, and an abdominopelvic CT.[38]

Management and Disposition

Most surgeons support conservative therapy for SBO in the absence of peritonitis or strangulation. Success rates with nonoperative management range from 43% to 73%.[39–41] Of those successfully treated, more than 80% have substantial improvement within 48 hours. In partial SBO, strangulation only occurs in a minority of cases (3%–5%) that are managed conservatively.[40]

Conservative management includes intravenous resuscitation, decompression, and bowel rest. Rehydration is essential, because liters of gastrointestinal secretions can accumulate during an obstructive episode. Nasogastric tube decompression remains a mainstay of therapy, with no added benefit from long intestinal tubes.[42] There are no data to support or refute the administration of antibiotics in SBO, although they are often given before surgery.

Although conservative management is common practice, several studies do suggest that a nonsurgical approach renders a greater risk of recurrent obstruction.[10,41,43] Nonetheless, recurrence is common with or without surgical intervention, and further surgeries lead to additional adhesion formation. Adhesive SBO has been shown to recur in 19% to 53% of cases.[43,44] Recurrence also becomes more likely with each subsequent SBO episode.[43]

With complete obstruction, the failure rate of conservative management is higher, and subsequent complications more severe. The dictum "never let the sun rise or set on a small bowel obstruction" continues to have some validity. Although 35% to 50% of those with high-grade and complete obstruction may resolve with fluid resuscitation and bowel decompression alone, many advocate early surgical intervention owing to the high failure rate of conservative management.[45,46] Around 30% of patients with complete SBO require bowel resection because of compromise of the small intestine.[46] Of all patients admitted to the ED with SBO, an estimated one-quarter undergo surgery.[47] Other causes of SBO, including impacted gallstones, bezoars, food, or other foreign bodies, are generally managed endoscopically or surgically.

The frequency of strangulation is largely dependent on the degree of obstruction. Strangulation is less often observed in nonoperative, partial obstructions (typically ≤10%). Conversely, retrospective studies of obstructions requiring surgery, in particular high-grade or complete obstructions, report strangulated bowel in 25% to 45% of cases. When looking at all surgeries for SBO, nonviable strangulation (necrotic bowel) is found in 13% to 16% of cases. Strangulation risk is also known to increase with patient age.[40,43,48,49] The rapid identification of strangulation is essential, because delayed surgery (>24 hours after the onset of symptoms of strangulation) increases mortality threefold.[48] Clearly, patients with fever and peritonitis require early operative intervention, because this is suggestive of ischemia and strangulation. In cases in which the CT is negative but the clinical examination is concerning, surgical consultation is warranted because of the false-negative rate of CT.

The admission service is also important in the management of SBO. One study showed a higher mortality when patients with SBO were admitted to a medical, rather than a surgical, service. This increased mortality was attributed to delays in surgical disposition.[50] Bowel obstructions are most appropriately admitted to a surgical service.

LARGE BOWEL OBSTRUCTION
Background

Large bowel obstruction (LBO) occurs much less frequently than SBO, although it is disproportionately more common in the elderly. Around 60% of LBOs are caused by neoplasm. Of all patients diagnosed with primary colorectal cancer, 15% to 20% initially present with a malignant bowel obstruction (MBO).[51–53] Colonic volvulus, involving either the sigmoid or cecum, is responsible for an additional 5% to 15% of cases of LBO.[54,55] Volvulus, which most commonly occurs in the sigmoid or cecum, is typically a disease of older patients, although it may affect all ages. Sigmoid volvulus is often observed in debilitated, institutionalized patients; diet and constipation may contribute. Cecal volvulus is attributed to a congenital defect in the mesentery that allows for increased bowel motility and occasionally torsion.[56] Another 10% of LBO cases are related to strictures from chronic diverticular disease (see **Table 1**). LBO carries a higher morbidity and mortality than SBO because of an older patient population and a variety of underlying medical conditions. Overall in-hospital mortality is approximately 10%, with poorer outcomes observed in those with renal failure, peritonitis, proximal colonic ischemia, and infarction.[57]

Pathophysiology

The ileocecal valve plays an important role in colonic obstruction. If the valve is competent, then fluid and gas necessarily accumulate in the cecum, resulting in a functional closed-loop obstruction. The cecum rapidly dilates, producing further wall tension because of a larger radius (Laplace law).[4] Eventually, acute dilatation may result in wall ischemia and perforation. Regardless of the ileocecal valve, volvulus is of particular concern because it creates a closed-loop segment of bowel that can quickly become ischemic and perforate.

MBO may result from external, intramural, or intraluminal compression. Tumor infiltration of the mesentery, muscle, and nerves may cause bowel dysmotility, further contributing to obstructive findings.[58]

Clinical Features

LBO commonly presents with abdominal pain, distention, and progressive obstipation. However, these features are nonspecific, and clinical diagnosis is difficult because the onset of symptoms is frequently gradual, especially with MBO. With continued colonic absorption of nutrients, water, and electrolytes, LBO may be tolerated for days to weeks before the patient seeks medical care. Because of vascular effects, volvulus may present more acutely with pain, abdominal distention, and occasionally shock. Important elements in the history include the patient's bowel habits, recent weight loss, rectal bleeding, history of inflammatory bowel disease, and prior obstruction.[59] Diarrhea is common, because there may be overflow from bacterial liquefaction of blocked fecal material. In contrast with the early onset of vomiting after oral intake in SBO, patients with LBO may never develop vomiting if the ileocecal valve is competent.[58] Marked abdominal pain or fever is suggestive of underlying ischemia, perforation, or peritonitis. Rectal examination may identify bleeding, a mass (malignancy), or a large volume of stool suggesting fecal impaction.

Laboratory Studies

Similar to small bowel obstruction, laboratory studies in LBO are generally unhelpful. A significantly increased white blood cell count may be concerning for ischemia or perforation, and electrolyte abnormalities may be present because of vomiting or poor oral intake.[56]

Imaging

The reliability of abdominal radiographs in the evaluation LBO is poorly studied. One retrospective study described abdominal plain films as 84% sensitive and 72% specific in the diagnosis of LBO.[60] However, another study reported that one-third of patients diagnosed with LBO based on clinical assessment and AXR had no obstruction. Conversely, up to 20% of patients initially believed to have pseudo-obstruction were then shown to have a mechanical LBO.[61] There is also poor interobserver agreement in AXR of large bowel obstructions.[19] Radiographs provide limited information regarding the underlying disease process. Moreover, the sensitivity of AXR for volvulus has been reported as less than 50%.[62] LBO presents radiographically as marked colonic dilatation, with disproportionate distention of the cecum (>10 cm diameter) if the ileocecal valve is competent. Volvulus has several unique radiographic findings, as described in **Table 2** and **Fig. 7**.

CT remains the imaging modality of choice for LBO in most circumstances (see **Table 2**). It provides further information regarding the cause of obstruction, allows for tumor staging in malignant obstruction, and facilitates management decisions.

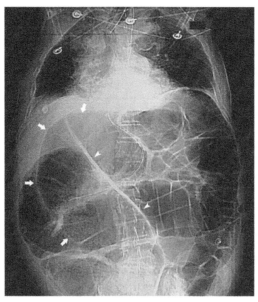

Fig. 7. Sigmoid volvulus. Abdominal CT scout image of a sigmoid volvulus. Note the coffee bean appearance (*arrows*) of the dilated, doubled-back bowel segment. Arrowheads show apposed walls of the volvulus. (*From* Schwartz DT. Abdominal radiology. In: Schwartz D, editor. Emergency radiology: case studies. New York: McGraw-Hill; 2008. p. 170; with permission.)

Sensitivity and specificity are approximately 90%,[63] and intravenous contrast with or without oral contrast is recommended. Historically, contrast enema has been used to confirm LBO or volvulus, and may still have a role when CT is equivocal.

Management and Disposition

A variety of techniques are advocated in the management of LBO. The first step is volume resuscitation and correction of electrolyte abnormalities. The urgency for decompression of the bowel depends on the clinical context (eg, fever, shock, perito-nitis) and the degree and duration of cecal distention. Patients with free perforation, peritonitis, and sepsis are immediate surgical candidates. A more stable patient with massive colonic dilatation (>12–13 cm), particularly of prolonged duration, is also considered at risk for complications.[64,65]

In MBO, colonic stenting has increased in popularity, either as a staging procedure for surgical management, or, in some cases, as definitive therapy.[66] When emergency surgery is required, postoperative mortality is high (10%–40%), with complication rates ranging from 27% to 90%.[67,68] LBO caused by diverticulitis is initially managed medically, with antibiotics, bowel rest, and percutaneous drainage.

Sigmoid volvulus without strangulation or peritonitis may be managed with endo-scopic decompression (sigmoidoscopy) and derotation. Success rates range from 70% to 90%.[69,70] However, recurrence is common and elective sigmoid resection is usually performed.[69] Cecal volvulus is treated surgically.

Adynamic Ileus

Around $1.5 billion is spent each year on the evaluation and management of adynamic ileus.[71] Ileus results in significant morbidity, resource use, and prolonged hospital course.[72,73] It is loosely defined as impairment in the transit of intestinal material, in the absence of mechanical obstruction. Ileus is most commonly observed in the postoperative patient, in whom a variety of neuronal pathways and inflammatory mediators are initiated because of intestinal handling, surgical incisions, and spillage of intestinal material.[72] These pathways lead to inhibition of bowel motility. Classically, the small intestine recovers first (0–24 hours), followed by the stomach (24–48 hours), and eventually the large bowel (48–72 hours).[74] Some variants of ileus result in more prolonged dysmotility. As noted in **Table 1**, several other disease states and various pharmacologic agents may contribute to the development of ileus.[72]

The clinical presentation of ileus is marked by abdominal distention and diffuse, mild pain. Nausea and vomiting are common, and the patient may report a lack of flatus or stool. Hypoactive or absent bowel sounds may be observed. In contrast with postoperative SBO, patients with ileus tend to have gastrointestinal symptoms immediately after surgery. Patients with SBO generally have an asymptomatic period after surgery, followed by progressive distention and obstipation.[72] Clinically, adynamic ileus is frequently difficult to differentiate from small and LBO.

Abdominal radiographs may show distention of both small and large bowel loops (see **Table 2**; **Fig. 8**). If clinical uncertainty exists, CT with intravenous contrast is recommended to rule out an evolving small or LBO.[22]

Management of ileus is supportive. For hospitalized patients, early postoperative enteral feeding has been shown to be safe and, in some studies, to shorten hospital stay.[75,76] Gum chewing has been shown to have variable efficacy.[77,78] Although early ambulation may have other benefits after surgery, it does not affect the course of an ileus. Nasogastric decompression is generally not recommended.[79,80] No specific pharmacotherapy has been definitively (and consistently) proved to treat ileus in the ED.

Acute Colonic Pseudo-obstruction

Acute colonic pseudo-obstruction (ACPO), also known as Ogilvie syndrome, represents severely impaired bowel motility, resulting in massive dilatation of the colon. Similar to ileus, no mechanical obstruction is identified. However, rather than an adynamic process, there is diffuse incoordination and attenuation of colonic muscle

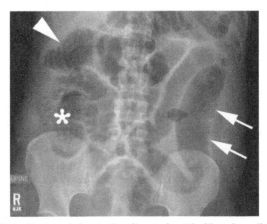

Fig. 8. Adynamic ileus. Supine abdominal radiograph with dilated small (*arrows*) and large bowel (*arrowhead*) loops in a patient with ileus. Note the stool in the right colon (*asterisk*). (*Courtesy of* C.E. Smith, MD, Vanderbilt University, Nashville, TN.)

contractions.[72] Diagnostic uncertainty often causes delays and contributes to the high morbidity and mortality associated with ACPO.[65] Studies report that, in up to 20% to 35% of patients, ACPO may be incorrectly identified as a mechanical obstruction based on clinical features and abdominal radiographs.[61,81]

The precise mechanism by which patients develop ACPO is unclear. It is believed that a variety of autonomic abnormalities produce hypotonic bowel, accumulation of gas and stool, and colonic distention.[82] Underlying medical illnesses are observed in more than 90% of cases (see **Table 1**). ACPO tends to occur in elderly and chronically debilitated patients, especially those who are hospitalized or institutionalized.[83] Delayed diagnosis and grave complications such as ischemia and perforation result in an operative mortality of more than 25%.[72,83]

The classic presentation for ACPO involves impressive abdominal distention with only mild, diffuse tenderness, and little systemic toxicity. Although about half of patients may not pass flatus or stool, some may have diarrhea. Nausea and vomiting are frequent. On physical examination, distention is observed and bowel sounds are variable. The differential diagnosis includes mechanical obstruction and toxic megacolon caused by *Clostridium difficile* infection.[84] Toxic megacolon also involves marked colonic distention, although it is accompanied by systemic signs of toxicity. It typically occurs in the context of ulcerative colitis or an infectious colitis (eg, *C difficile*). Differentiation between ACPO and toxic megacolon by abdominal radiography is challenging. On CT, findings for toxic megacolon include characteristic bowel wall edema and thickening, hemorrhage, and areas of ulceration.[85]

The radiographic appearance of ACPO is notable for massive colonic dilatation without bowel wall thickening (see **Table 2**; **Fig. 9**). Classically, an air-filled, dilated

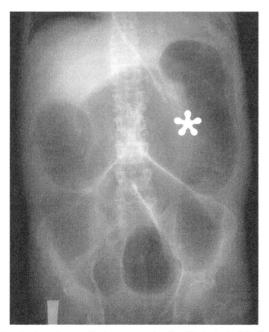

Fig. 9. ACPO. Abdominal radiograph shows markedly dilated air-filled colon (*asterisk*) in a patient in a nursing home. (*From* Schwartz DT. Abdominal radiology. In: Schwartz D, editor. Emergency radiology: case studies. New York: McGraw-Hill; 2008. p. 183; with permission.)

colon extending to the rectosigmoid region supports a diagnosis of ACPO as opposed to LBO.[72] Most patients are also found to have small bowel dilatation.[83] The ideal imaging modality remains CT of the abdomen and pelvis with contrast, which is more than 90% sensitive and specific for ACPO.[63,86]

Management of ACPO is generally supportive, because 75% of cases resolve spontaneously within several days.[72] Hydration, discontinuing any offending drugs, and correcting electrolytes are all recommended measures. Although a rectal tube may help decompress an air-filled sigmoid colon, it does little to address more proximal distention. Ambulation may be helpful. Laxatives are not considered effective or recommended.

Lack of resolution of pseudo-obstruction after 48 to 72 hours, or a cecal diameter greater than 12 cm, may necessitate more aggressive management.[82,83] The preferred pharmacologic therapy, in the inpatient setting, is neostigmine.[87] Colonoscopic decompression is the next step and is successful in 70% to 80% of cases.[83,88,89] On occasion, because of colonic ischemia or perforation, surgery becomes necessary. Perforation is estimated to occur in 3% to 20% of cases, with mortality reaching 40% to 50%.[83,90] Overall, most deaths associated with ACPO are related to underlying medical conditions, rather than direct sequelae of the colonic distention.

Abdominal Hernias

Hernias have been a subject of discussion for thousands of years. There are descriptions of hernia management from Babylon in 1700 BC and ancient Egypt in 1500 BC.[91,92] However, the definition of hernia has generally remained the same: an extrusion of intra-abdominal contents through the wall of the abdomen. These contents may consist of bowel, mesentery, or simply an empty sac. Herniorrhaphy is the most common general surgery procedure in the United States, although most hernias require neither urgent nor emergent surgical treatment.

Abdominal hernias have variable frequency, and are described in terms of their anatomic location and cause (**Table 3**). Inguinal hernias comprise more than 75% of all abdominal hernias.[93] Hernias also occur at several other sites on the abdomen, including the umbilicus, epigastrium, lateral abdomen, and even the lumbar region. They may present asymptomatically or as surgical emergencies. In this article, groin hernias (indirect inguinal, direct inguinal, and femoral) serve as the template for describing clinical presentations, imaging techniques, and the identification of incarceration and strangulation. The specific epidemiology, pathophysiology, and anatomy of other clinically relevant abdominal hernias are discussed later.

Table 3 Data on abdominal hernias, incarceration, and strangulation		
	Percentage of all Hernia Surgeries	Percentage of Incarcerated Hernias that Strangulate
Inguinal	66–75	29
Umbilical	15	60
Incisional	9	50
Femoral	3	46
Other (eg, epigastric, spigelian)	<5	No data

Data from Refs.[94,108,119,122,123]

Background

The true incidence of abdominal and groin hernias is difficult to estimate, because many are asymptomatic and often remain undiagnosed. In the United States, almost $6 billion is spent annually on patients with a diagnosis of abdominal hernia, with more than 180,000 admissions, a median 3-day hospital stay, and a 1% in-hospital mortality.[2] There are more than 1 million herniorrhaphy procedures performed each year for abdominal wall hernias; more than 75% involve inguinal hernias.[94] Men have a 27% lifetime chance of undergoing inguinal herniorrhaphy, compared with 3% for women.[95] This translates to more than 770,000 surgeries for inguinal hernias each year (2003), at a cost of roughly $2.5 billion.[94] Most (90%) surgeries occur in the outpatient setting, and 90% are performed on men. Umbilical hernias account for approximately 175,000 annual repairs, whereas femoral hernia repairs account for another 30,000 procedures annually.[94,96]

In addition to a male predominance, identified risk factors include increased age, family history, and connective tissues disorders. The literature is conflicting regarding chronic obstructive pulmonary disease, chronic cough, and strenuous activity and manual labor as other risk factors. Obesity seems to lower inguinal hernia risk, although this finding may be partly the result of a higher missed diagnosis rate in patients with higher body mass indices.[93,97,98]

Pathophysiology

Because intra-abdominal contents extrude through a defect in the abdominal wall, symptoms often depend on the reducibility of the hernia. If the contents return freely to their original location, mild symptoms such as a bulge or minimal discomfort will often occur. If the extruded contents cannot be reduced, the hernia is described as incarcerated. An incarcerated hernia may continue to cause no symptoms other than a local bulge if the contents are well perfused, and passage of bowel contents is uninterrupted. With any degree of ischemia or obstruction, the hernia is said to be strangulated. Pain may arise from both the contents of the hernia and the surrounding abdominal wall tissue. Strangulation may ultimately progress to infarction and eventual organ death.

Indirect inguinal hernias are the most common type of hernia, and they occur when abdominal contents follow the course of the inguinal canal to exit the abdominal cavity (**Fig. 10**). The inguinal canal is a cone-shaped opening, approximately 4 to 6 cm in length, originating intra-abdominally where the spermatic cord (or the round ligament in women) passes through the transversalis fascia at the internal inguinal ring.[99] Indirect herniation is most often caused by the presence of a patent processus vaginalis in men, which allows abdominal contents to pass through the canal into the scrotum. Normally, the processus vaginalis closes between weeks 36 and 40 of fetal development, but, in roughly 12% of adults, patency is maintained.[100] Most indirect inguinal hernias in male patients are observed during the first year of life, or after the age of 55 years.[101]

A direct inguinal hernia violates the wall of the inguinal canal and passes directly through the fascial and muscular structures of the abdominal wall (see **Fig. 10**). The hernia originates at the Hesselbach triangle, which is bordered by the inferior epigastric vessels superiorly and laterally, the rectus sheath medially, and the inguinal ligament laterally. This anatomic triangle lies medial to the internal inguinal ring and the origin of indirect inguinal hernias. A patient with both a direct and indirect inguinal hernia is said to have a pantaloon, or combined hernia, named for the anatomic appearance of 2 legs of a pair of trousers.

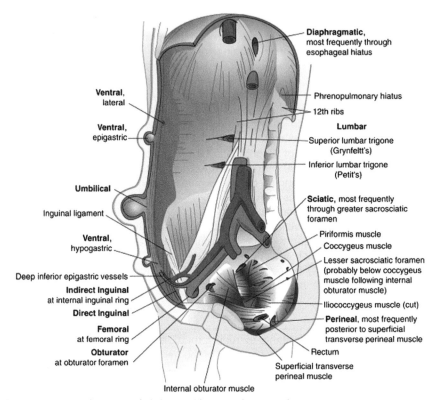

Fig. 10. Anatomic location of abdominal hernias. (*From* Malangoni MA, Rosen MJ. Hernias. In: Townsend CM, Beauchamp RD, Evers BM, et al. editors. Sabiston textbook of surgery. 18th edition. Philadelphia: Saunders Elsevier; 2007. p. 1156. Chapter 44; with permission.)

The third type of groin hernia is a femoral hernia. A femoral hernia occurs when abdominal contents pass through the femoral canal, inferior to the inguinal ligament and medial to the femoral vein (see **Fig. 10**). In most studies, these occur more often in women than in men, although the most common hernia overall in women remains the indirect inguinal hernia.[102] Femoral herniorrhaphies tend to be emergent operative cases; there is a greater incidence of strangulation, presumably because of the small, inflexible femoral ring.[96,99,103]

Clinical Features

Groin hernias are primarily diagnosed clinically after a thorough history and physical examination. Most patients with a groin hernia present to the ED with an asymptomatic bulge, or with mild tenderness to the affected area. Actions that increase intra-abdominal pressure often exacerbate symptoms. The patient is best examined while standing so that the increased intra-abdominal pressure will make the hernia as pronounced as possible. The patient should be fully exposed and, in male patients, the examiner should place a finger in the scrotum pointed toward the external inguinal ring. The examination is often more challenging in women, because of a narrower external ring. A Valsalva maneuver may cause extrusion of the hernia contents, with palpation of the hernia at the fingertip or finger pad. Examination of the contralateral side should also be performed. Significant tenderness, discoloration of the site, or

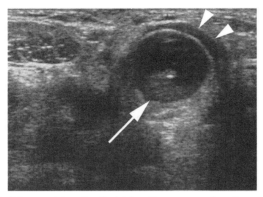

Fig. 11. Incarcerated femoral hernia. Bedside ultrasonography of a right inguinal mass, notable for an incarcerated loop of bowel (*arrow*) in the femoral canal. Rim of fluid (*arrowheads*) likely caused by acute inflammation/edema from strangulated bowel. (*Courtesy of* Anthony J. Dean, MD, Hospital of the University of Pennsylvania, Philadelphia, PA.)

generalized abdominal pain may indicate ischemia or obstruction. Differentiation of direct from indirect hernias by physical examination alone is difficult.[104] However, for the emergency physician, this distinction is of little clinical importance, because the 2 are treated similarly in the ED. The examination is also limited in the presence of an obese patient or a small hernia, and up to one-third of hernias may be present in completely asymptomatic patients. Based on one study, the overall sensitivity and specificity of the clinical examination for hernia identification were 75% and 96%, respectively.[105]

Imaging

When diagnostic uncertainty remains after the physical examination, imaging may be indicated. Ultrasound is the most common diagnostic tool, and has a high degree of accuracy (**Figs. 11** and **12**). Improved yield is obtained with a dynamic scanning technique, incorporating lying and standing, and Valsalva maneuvers. The classic criterion

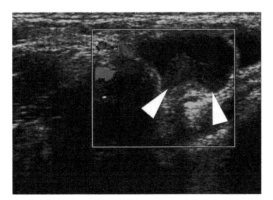

Fig. 12. Incarcerated femoral hernia. Bedside ultrasonography of a right inguinal mass, notable for an incarcerated loop of bowel (*arrowheads*) in the femoral canal. Doppler color flow shows increased vascularity in the inflamed surrounding soft tissues. (*Courtesy of* Anthony J. Dean, MD, Hospital of the University of Pennsylvania, Philadelphia, PA.)

for hernia includes a hernial sac containing omentum or bowel, especially with a cough or Valsalva maneuver.[106] Sensitivity and specificity of groin ultrasound for all hernias are 92% to 100%, although determination of direct versus indirect inguinal hernia is less precise on ultrasound.[105,106] Ultrasound is also helpful in the identification of incarceration, alternate diagnoses, and postoperative seromas, hematomas, or abscesses.

MRI has a comparable sensitivity, specificity, and accuracy compared with ultrasound.[106] However, cost and access issues limit its applicability in the ED. CT (with intravenous contrast, ± oral contrast) is not a routine imaging modality for hernias, but may be helpful in ruling out alternative diagnoses, diagnosing hernias in unusual locations, and identifying complications of strangulated hernias.

Management and Disposition

When an easily reducible, asymptomatic inguinal hernia has been identified, the patient may be safely discharged for outpatient surgical follow-up. Emergent surgery is generally not warranted. The risk of strangulation for inguinal hernias is highest soon after the initial diagnosis, but studies have shown that outpatient management of asymptomatic inguinal hernias is appropriate and safe.[101,107] This strategy does not apply if a femoral hernia is diagnosed, owing to the higher rate of strangulation.[101] Femoral hernias should be repaired expeditiously when detected, even if asymptomatic; as many as 40% are strangulated on initial ED presentation.[103]

The first consideration for the emergency physician is whether or not a hernia is the source of the patient's symptoms. A broad differential diagnosis exists for groin masses, including lymphadenopathy, hematoma, infection, thrombosis, malignancy, testicular process (eg, torsion, spermatic corditis), and femoral artery aneurysm or pseudoaneurysm.[99] The next determination pertains to the reducibility of a hernia. As noted earlier, uncomplicated, easily reduced hernias are quickly dispositioned to home. If the hernia is incarcerated, a determination must be made regarding evidence of strangulation, which can cause pain, discoloration, nausea, vomiting, abdominal distention, fever, bowel obstruction, and/or shock. In general, hernias with small defects (typically femoral, small indirect inguinal, and abdominal wall hernias) are more likely to cause incarceration and strangulation.[99] No specific laboratory test can reliably differentiate a reducible, incarcerated, or strangulated hernia.[101]

When an inguinal hernia does not reduce spontaneously, the physician must decide whether an attempt at manual reduction should be made. A gentle attempt at reduction of an acute hernia is reasonable. When strangulation is suspected, the hernia should not be reduced in the ED. Such a procedure would risk giving the appearance of curing the patient's disease while introducing necrotic bowel into the abdominal cavity, with consequent peritonitis and perforation. Although differentiation between strangulated and nonstrangulated bowel may seem difficult, the physician is usually accurate in determining whether or not to attempt reduction of the hernia.[108]

A successful reduction requires adequate preparation and appropriate positioning. For reduction of an inguinal hernia, the patient should be placed in a Trendelenburg position. Having the patient bend the knees relaxes the abdominal musculature. Gravity assists in pulling the contents of the hernia back into the abdomen. The patient can be left in this position with a cold compress on the hernia, and many spontaneously reduce as swelling decreases. If reduction does not occur spontaneously, gentle and steady pressure should be applied while using one hand to direct the most proximal component of the hernia through the defect in the abdominal wall. Sufficient analgesia and sedation should be administered during the procedure.[109]

In addition to the possibility of introducing necrotic bowel into the abdominal cavity, potential complications of hernia reduction include bowel injury from overly aggressive reduction attempts and displacement of bowel to a preperitoneal location. In the latter circumstance, the hernia sac, although still extraintestinal, may no longer be palpable, which places the patient at increased risk of delayed management and bowel ischemia.[109]

If reduction cannot be achieved, or strangulation is suspected, immediate surgical consultation should be obtained. In addition, resuscitation and electrolyte replacement may be needed. Antibiotics, although commonly administered, are of no proven benefit in the treatment of incarcerated or strangulated hernia. In general, older age, longer duration of hernia, and longer duration of irreducibility are considered risk factors for acute hernia complications.[110] Although risk of death is small, hernia was listed as the underlying cause of death for 1595 deaths in the United States in 2002.[111] Expedited diagnosis and management of uncomplicated hernias is important, because higher morbidity and mortality are observed after emergent hernia repair.[112,113]

Specific surgical options for groin hernias are numerous and beyond the scope of this article. After surgery, patients may present with a variety of pain complaints (radiation into the flank, leg, thigh, or genital areas), which is likely related to nerve injury or tissue adherence to the mesh.[99] Urinary retention is also reported in 0.2% of patients after hernia repair with local anesthetics and up to 13% of cases under general anesthesia.[114]

Ventral Hernias

Ventral hernias occur when intra-abdominal contents violate the anterior wall of the abdomen. The location and cause of the ventral hernia informs its classification as either umbilical, incisional, epigastric, or spigelian.

Umbilical hernias occur in both children and adults, but the cause differs for each group. In children, umbilical hernias form when the umbilical ring fails to close at birth. This failure occurs frequently and is seen more commonly in children of African descent.[115] These hernias, which rarely incarcerate, usually resolve spontaneously in the first 2 years of life. Surgical repair is generally not recommended until the child is approximately 3 to 4 years of age, although it is unclear whether the incidence of incarceration is significantly higher after this age.[116] One study reported spontaneous closure of umbilical hernias in children as old as 14 years.[115] From an emergency medicine perspective, asymptomatic children older than 3 to 4 years should be given a surgical referral.[117]

In adults, umbilical hernias occur as a result of an acquired rather than congenital defect, and are often the result of conditions that cause increased intra-abdominal pressure. These conditions include obesity, ascites, and pregnancy. Women have a threefold greater incidence of umbilical hernias than men. Elective repair is suggested for all umbilical hernias in adults, because they are much more prone to incarceration than in children[118] and account for as many as 13% of incarcerated hernias in adults.[119] When presenting to the ED, asymptomatic umbilical hernias in adults should be given a surgical referral for elective repair.

Approximately 10% to 15% of abdominal surgical procedures result in an incisional hernia.[101] Most of these present within the first year after surgery, although incisional hernias have been reported up to 10 years after surgery.[120] Herniation may occur through any type of surgical incision, including those used for introduction of trocars during laparoscopic procedures. Certain factors influence the likelihood of herniation, such as incision location and size, patient characteristics, and the emergent nature of the surgical procedure. There is a decreased incidence of herniation from incisions higher on the abdomen, and from those that are less than 1 cm or greater than 7 cm. Risk factors for poor wound healing, such as obesity, smoking, and immune compromise, can lead to an increased incidence of incisional hernia. Likewise, hernias occur more commonly after emergent abdominal surgery. As many as 15% of incisional hernias present incarcerated, and up to 2% strangulate.[121]

Epigastric hernias occur in the abdominal midline, between the umbilicus and the sternum. They occur 3 times more often in men, and account for 1.6% to 3.6% of all abdominal hernias.[122] Epigastric hernias are attributed to a combination of straining and weakening of the abdominal wall. Most occur during middle age, but there have been accounts of early-onset epigastric hernias that present in childhood.[122] The abdominal wall defect in epigastric hernias is often less than 1 cm, which accounts for a greater likelihood of incarceration. However, the herniation typically contains only omentum and rarely bowel. If symptomatic, the hernia may be repaired electively as long as there is no evidence of strangulation.

Spigelian hernias occur along the linea semilunaris at the lateral edge of the rectus abdominis and exit between the fibromuscular layers of the abdominal wall. They account for 1% to 2% of all hernias and occur more commonly in adults and in women.[123] In all age groups, the diagnosis can be difficult because the hernia contents often lie between muscle layers rather than in the subcutaneous tissue. In the ED, ultrasound can be reliably used to diagnose spigelian hernias.[124] Once diagnosed, the patient should be referred for surgical repair, because the risk of incarceration is high.

Ventral hernias that present with incarceration in the ED are appropriate for attempted reduction. As with inguinal hernias, findings suggestive of strangulation necessitate urgent surgical consultation.

Other Hernias

There are several rare abdominal hernias with which the emergency physician should be familiar. Although uncommon, these should be part of the differential diagnosis of any suspected hernia, because they are difficult to identify and may need emergent management.

In most cases of bowel herniation, an entire loop of bowl is contained within the sac. However, in the case of a Richter hernia, only a portion of the antimesenteric bowel wall is herniated. This condition can lead to a focal, noncircumferential area of bowel necrosis without bowel obstruction, which is particularly dangerous. The bowel wall may become necrotic without the patient having any of the typical signs or symptoms of a hernia.

Hernias can also occur through the obturator canal (obturator hernia) and through the sciatic foramen (sciatic hernia). Bowel obstruction, as well as local pain and swelling, may occur with either. A sciatic hernia may also be the cause of a patient's sciatica, although this is believed to be exceedingly rare. Lumbar hernias may occur when abdominal contents herniate through the lumbar triangles. When this occurs through the superior lumbar triangle, it is termed a Grynfeltt hernia. Herniation through the inferior lumbar triangle is known as a Petit hernia.[99]

Internal hernias are increasingly seen in the context of gastric bypass surgery for bariatric treatment. In this hernia subtype, bowel protrudes through a peritoneal or mesenteric space within the confines of the abdomen. They are described by location, with the most common being paraduodenal. Vague epigastric pain to periumbilical pain is common, and occasionally they may cause obstruction. As opposed to other hernias, CT is the preferred imaging modality. Management is generally surgical.[125]

SUMMARY

Intestinal obstruction and abdominal hernia are frequently encountered in the ED. SBO is the most common form of intestinal obstruction and is mainly caused by intestinal adhesions. LBO is generally caused by malignancy. Both result in nausea and vomiting, abdominal pain, and abdominal distention. However, the clinical features and laboratory workup are not adequately sensitive or specific to reliably detect either form of obstruction. CT is more sensitive than abdominal radiographs, and offers incremental information regarding the level, cause, and complications of obstruction (closed-loop obstruction and bowel ischemia). High-grade and complete SBO are generally managed operatively, whereas malignant LBO may be amenable to colonic stenting, with subsequent elective surgery. Partial SBO is often treated conservatively, whereas peritonitis requires immediate surgical evaluation and management.

Adynamic ileus, resulting from impaired bowel motility, is associated with considerable health expenditure and prolonged hospitalizations. Treatment is conservative, because no pharmacologic or decompressive intervention is effective. ACPO, or massive dilatation of the colon caused by impaired bowel motility, has a particularly high morbidity and mortality. It occurs across a wide spectrum of chronic disease and is notable for significant abdominal distention. Treatment is typically conservative, although neostigmine and/or colonoscopic decompression may be used later in the hospital course. Surgical management for ACPO, especially in the case of colonic perforation, portends a grave prognosis.

Abdominal hernias are the second leading cause of small bowel obstruction. Inguinal hernias are the most commonly encountered and are usually managed in an outpatient setting with elective surgery. Many hernias can be reduced successfully in the ED, although strangulation necessitates emergent surgical evaluation. The diagnosis is often clinical, with abdominal ultrasonography used in cases of an uncertain examination.

ACKNOWLEDGMENTS

The authors wish to thank Jose Diaz, MD, Keith Wrenn, MD, David Schwartz, MD, and C.E. Smith, MD for their assistance.

REFERENCES

1. Hayanga AJ, Bass-Wilkins K, Bulkley GB. Current management of small-bowel obstruction. Adv Surg 2005;39:1.
2. HCUPnet. Healthcare cost and utilization project. Rockville (MD): Agency for Healthcare Research and Quality; 2007. Available at: http://hcupnet.ahrq.gov/. Accessed February 25, 2010.
3. Ray NF, Denton WG, Thamer M, et al. Abdominal adhesiolysis: inpatient care and expenditures in the United States in 1994. J Am Coll Surg 1998;186(1):1–9.
4. Cappell MS, Batke M. Mechanical obstruction of the small bowel and colon. Med Clin North Am 2008;92:575–97.
5. Miettinen P, Pasanen P, Salonen A, et al. The outcome of elderly patients after operation for acute abdomen. Ann Chir Gynaecol 1996;85(1):11–5.
6. Bugliosi TF. Acute abdominal pain in the elderly. Ann Emerg Med 1990;19(12): 1383–6.
7. Maglinte DD, Balthazar EJ, Kelvin FM, et al. The role of radiology in the diagnosis of small-bowel obstruction. AJR Am J Roentgenol 1997;168(5):1171–80.

8. Welch JP. General consideration and mortality in bowel obstruction. In: Welch JP, editor. Bowel obstruction: differential diagnosis and clinical management. Philadelphia: Saunders; 1990. p. 59–95.

9. Ghosheh B, Salameh JR. Laparoscopic approach to acute small bowel obstruction: Review of 1061 cases. Surg Endosc 2007;21:1945–9.

10. Miller G, Boman J, Shrier I, et al. Etiology of small bowel obstruction. Am J Surg 2000;180:33–6.

11. Bizer LS, Leibling RW, Delany HM, et al. Small-bowel obstruction: the role of nonoperative treatment in simple intestinal obstruction and predictive criteria for strangulation obstruction. Surgery 1981;89:407–13.

12. Ellis H. The clinical significance of adhesions: focus on intestinal obstruction. Eur J Surg 1997;163(Suppl 577):5.

13. Kendrick ML. Partial small bowel obstruction: clinical issues and recent technical advances. Abdom Imaging 2009;34:329–34.

14. Sarr MG, Bulkley GB, Zuidema GD. Preoperative recognition of intestinal strangulation obstruction. Prospective evaluation of diagnostic capability. Am J Surg 1983;145:176–82.

15. Mucha P Jr. Small intestinal obstruction. Surg Clin North Am 1987;67:597–620.

16. Jancelewicz T, Vu LT, Shawo AE, et al. Predicting strangulated small bowel obstruction: an old problem revisited. J Gastrointest Surg 2009;13(1):93–9.

17. Maglinte DDT, Reyes BL, Harmon BH, et al. Reliability and the role of plain film radiography and CT in the diagnosis of small-bowel obstruction. AJR Am J Roentgenol 1996;167:1451–5.

18. Shrake PD, Rex DK, Lappas JC, et al. Radiographic evaluation of suspected small bowel obstruction. Am J Gastroenterol 1991;86:175–8.

19. Markus JB, Somers S, Franic SE, et al. Interobserver variation in the interpretation of abdominal radiographs. Radiology 1989;171(1):69–71.

20. Suh RS, Maglinte DD, Lavonas EE, et al. Emergency abdominal radiography: discrepancies of preliminary and final interpretation and management relevance. Emerg Radiol 1995;2:1–4.

21. Gough IR. Strangulating bowel obstruction with normal radiographs. Br J Surg 1978;65(6):431–4.

22. Maglinte DD, Howard TJ, Lillemoe KD, et al. Small-bowel obstruction: state-of-the-art imaging and its role in clinical management. Clin Gastroenterol Hepatol 2008;6:130–9.

23. Ros PR, Huprich JE. ACR appropriateness criteria on suspected small-bowel obstruction. J Am Coll Radiol 2006;3:838–41.

24. Nicolaou S, Kai B, Ho S, et al. Imaging of acute small-bowel obstruction. AJR Am J Roentgenol 2005;185:1036–44.

25. Atri M, McGregor C, McInnes M. Multidetector helical CT in the evaluation of acute small bowel obstruction: comparison of non-enhanced (no oral, rectal or IV contrast) and IV enhanced CT. Eur J Radiol 2009;71(1):135–40.

26. Megibow AJ, Balthazar EJ, Cho KC, et al. Bowel obstruction: evaluation with CT. Radiology 1991;180(2):313–8.

27. Obuz F, Terzi C, Sokmen S, et al. The efficacy of helical CT in the diagnosis of small bowel obstruction. Eur J Radiol 2003;48:299–304.

28. Sandrasegaran K, Maglinte DDT, Howard N, et al. The multifaceted role of radiology in small bowel obstruction. Semin Ultrasound CT MR 2003;24:319–35.

29. Maglinte DD, Gage SN, Harmon BH, et al. Obstruction of the small intestine: accuracy and role of CT in diagnosis. Radiology 1993;188:61–4.

30. Mallo RD, Salem R, Lalani T, et al. Computed tomography diagnosis of ischemia and complete obstruction in small bowel obstruction: a systematic review. J Gastrointest Surg 2005;9(5):690–4.
31. Sheedy SP, Earnest FT, Fletcher JG, et al. CT of small bowel ischemia associated with obstruction in emergency department patients: diagnostic performance evaluation. Radiology 2006;241(3):729–36.
32. Jaffe TA, Martin LC, Thomas J, et al. Small-bowel obstruction: coronal reformations from isotropic voxels at 16-section multi-detector row CT. Radiology 2006; 238(1):135–42.
33. Ko YT, Lim JH, Lee DH, et al. Small bowel obstruction: sonographic evaluation. Radiology 1993;188(3):649–53.
34. Czechowski J. Conventional radiography and ultrasonography in the diagnosis of small bowel obstruction and strangulation. Acta Radiol 1996;37:186–9.
35. Schmutz GR, Benko A, Fournier L, et al. Small bowel obstruction: role and contribution of sonography. Eur Radiol 1997;7:1054–8.
36. Beall DP, Fortman BJ, Lawler BC, et al. Imaging bowel obstruction: a comparison between fast magnetic resonance imaging and helical computed tomography. Clin Radiol 2002;57:719–24.
37. Walsh D, Bender GN, Timmons JH. Comparison of computed tomography-enteroclysis and traditional computed tomography in the setting of suspected partial small bowel obstruction. Emerg Radiol 1998;5:29–37.
38. Maglinte DD, Sandrasegaran K, Lappas JC, et al. CT enteroclysis. Radiology 2007;245(3):661–71.
39. Seror D, Feigin E, Szold A, et al. How conservatively can postoperative small bowel obstruction be treated? Am J Surg 1993;165:121–6.
40. Fevang BT, Jensen D, Svanes K, et al. Early operation or conservative management of patients with small bowel obstruction? Eur J Surg 2002;168: 475–81.
41. Williams SB, Greenspon J, Young HA, et al. Small bowel obstruction: conservative vs surgical management. Dis Colon Rectum 2005;48(6):1140–6.
42. Meissner K. Effectiveness of intestinal tube splinting: a prospective observational study. Dig Surg 2000;17:49–56.
43. Fevang BT, Fevang J, Lie SA, et al. Long-term prognosis after operation for adhesive small bowel obstruction. Ann Surg 2004;240:193–201.
44. Barkan H, Webster S, Ozeran S. Factors predicting the recurrence of adhesive small-bowel obstruction. Am J Surg 1995;170:361–5.
45. Diaz JJ, Bokhari F, Mowery NT, et al. Guidelines for management of small bowel obstruction. J Trauma 2008;64:1651–64.
46. Nauta RJ. Advanced abdominal imaging is not required to exclude strangulation if complete small bowel obstructions undergo prompt laparotomy. J Am Coll Surg 2005;200:904–11.
47. Foster NM, McGory ML, Zingmond DS, et al. Small bowel obstruction: a population- based appraisal. J Am Coll Surg 2006;203:170–6.
48. Fevang BT, Fevang J, Stangeland L, et al. Complications and death after surgical treatment of small bowel obstruction: a 35-year institutional experience. Ann Surg 2000;231(4):529–37.
49. Lo OS, Law WL, Choi HK, et al. Early outcomes of surgery for small bowel obstruction: analysis of risk factors. Langenbecks Arch Surg 2007;392: 173–8.
50. Schwab DP, Blackhurst DW, Sticca RP. Operative acute small bowel obstruction: admitting service impacts outcome. Am Surg 2001;67(11):1034–8.

51. Serpell JW, McDermott FT, Kantrivessus H, et al. Carcinomas of the colon causing intestinal occlusion. Br J Surg 1989;76:965–9.
52. Phillips KK, Hittinger R, Fry JS, et al. Malignant large bowel obstruction. Br J Surg 1985;72:296–302.
53. Umpleby HC, Williamson RC. Survival in acute obstructing colorectal carcinoma. Dis Colon Rectum 1984;27:299–304.
54. Buechter KJ, Boustany C, Caillouette R, et al. Surgical management of the acutely obstructed colon. a review of 127 cases. Am J Surg 1988;156:163–8.
55. Ballantyne GH. Review of sigmoid volvulus: clinical patterns and pathogenesis. Dis Colon Rectum 1982;25(8):823–30.
56. Peterson MA. Disorders of the large intestine. In: Marx J, Hockberger R, Walls R, editors. Rosen's emergency medicine: concepts and clinical practice. 7th edition. Philadelphia: Mosby; 2010. Chapter 93.
57. Biondo S, Pares D, Frago R, et al. Large bowel obstruction: predictive factors for postoperative mortality. Dis Colon Rectum 2004;47(11):1889–97.
58. Roeland E, Von Gunten CF. Current concepts in malignant bowel obstruction management. Curr Oncol Rep 2009;11:298–303.
59. Baron TH. Acute colonic obstruction. Gastrointest Endosc Clin N Am 2007;17: 323–39.
60. Chapman AH, McNamara M, Porter G. The acute contrast enema in suspected large bowel obstruction: value and technique. Clin Radiol 1992;46(4):273–8.
61. Koruth NM, Koruth A, Matheson NA. The place of contrast enema in the management of large bowel obstruction. J R Coll Surg Edinb 1985;30: 258–60.
62. Ballantyne GH, Brandner MD, Beart RW, et al. Volvulus of the colon: incidence and mortality. Ann Surg 1985;202(1):83–92.
63. Beattie GC, Peters RT, Guy S, et al. Computed tomography in the assessment of suspected large bowel obstruction. ANZ J Surg 2007;77(3):160–5.
64. Johnson CD, Rice RP, Kelvin FM, et al. The radiologic evaluation of gross cecal distension: emphasis on cecal ileus. AJR Am J Roentgenol 1985;145: 1211–7.
65. Saunders MD, Kimmey MB. Systematic review: acute colonic pseudo-obstruction. Aliment Pharmacol Ther 2005;22:917–25.
66. Sebastian S, Johnston S, Geoghegan T, et al. Pooled analysis of the efficacy and safety of self-expanding metal stenting in malignant colorectal obstruction. Am J Gastroenterol 2004;99:2051–7.
67. Feuer DJ, Broadley KE, Shepherd JH, et al. Systematic review of surgery in malignant bowel obstruction in advanced gynecological and gastrointestinal cancer. Gynecol Oncol 1999;75:313–22.
68. Ripamonti C. Bowel obstruction. In: Bruera E, Higginson I, Ripamonti C, et al, editors. Textbook of palliative medicine. New York: Oxford University Press; 2006. p. 587–600.
69. Grossmann EM, Longo WE, Stratton MD, et al. Sigmoid volvulus in Department of Veterans Affairs medical centers. Dis Colon Rectum 2000;43(3):414–8.
70. Lal SK, Morgenstern R, Vinjirayer EP, et al. Sigmoid volvulus an update. Gastrointest Endosc Clin N Am 2006;16(1):175–87.
71. Goldstein JL, Matuszewski KA, Delaney CP, et al. Inpatient economic burden of postoperative ileus associated with abdominal surgery in the United States. P&T 2007;32(2):82–90.
72. Batke M, Cappell MS. Adynamic ileus and acute colonic pseudo-obstruction. Med Clin North Am 2008;92:649–70, ix.

73. Iyer S, Saunders WB, Stemkowski S. Economic burden of postoperative ileus associated with colectomy in the United States. J Manag Care Pharm 2009; 15(6):485–94.

74. Condon RE, Cowles VE, Ferraz AA, et al. Human colonic smooth muscle electrical activity during and after recovery from postoperative ileus. Am J Physiol 1995;269(3 Pt 1):G408–17.

75. Minig L, Biffi R, Zanagnolo V, et al. Early oral versus "traditional" postoperative feeding in gynecologic oncology patients undergoing intestinal resection: a randomized controlled trial. Ann Surg Oncol 2009;16(6):1660–8.

76. Lewis SJ, Andersen HK, Thomas S. Early enteral nutrition within 24 h of intestinal surgery versus later commencement of feeding: a systematic review and meta-analysis. J Gastrointest Surg 2009;13:569–75.

77. Watson H, Griffiths P, Lamaparelli M, et al. Does chewing (gum) aid recovery after bowel resection? A randomised controlled trial. Colorectal Dis 2008; 10(1):6.

78. Purkayastha S, Tilney HS, Darzi AW, et al. Meta-analysis of randomized studies evaluating chewing gum to enhance postoperative recovery following colectomy. Arch Surg 2008;143(8):788–93.

79. Nelson R, Edwards S, Tse B. Prophylactic nasogastric decompression after abdominal surgery. Cochrane Database Syst Rev 2007;3:CD004929.

80. Cheatham ML, Chapman WC, Key SP, et al. A meta-analysis of selective versus routine nasogastric decompression after elective laparotomy. Ann Surg 1995; 221(5):469–76.

81. Stewart J, Finan PJ, Courtney DF, et al. Does a water soluble contrast enema assist in the management of acute large bowel obstruction: a prospective study of 117 cases. Br J Surg 1984;71:799–801.

82. De Giorgio R, Knowles CH. Acute colonic pseudo-obstruction. Br J Surg 2009; 96:229–39.

83. Vanek VW, Al-Salti M. Acute pseudo-obstruction of the colon (Ogilvie's syndrome): an analysis of 400 cases. Dis Colon Rectum 1986;29(3):203–10.

84. Sheikh RA, Yasmeen S, Pauly MP, et al. Pseudomembranous colitis without diarrhea presenting clinically as acute intestinal pseudo-obstruction. J Gastroenterol 2001;36:629–32.

85. Schwartz DT. Abdominal radiology. In: Schwartz D, editor. Emergency radiology: case studies. New York: McGraw-Hill; 2008. p. 147–87.

86. Mehta R, John A, Nair P, et al. Factors predicting successful outcome following neostigmine therapy in acute colonic pseudo-obstruction: a prospective study. J Gastroenterol Hepatol 2006;21:459–61.

87. Ponec RJ, Saunders MD, Kimmey MB. Neostigmine for the treatment of acute colonic pseudo-obstruction. N Engl J Med 1999;341(3):137–41.

88. Wegener M, Borsch G. Acute colonic pseudo-obstruction (Ogilvie's syndrome): presentation of 14 of our own cases and analysis of 1027 cases reported in the literature. Surg Endosc 1987;1(3):169–74.

89. Saunders MD. Acute colonic pseudo-obstruction. Best Pract Res Clin Gastroenterol 2007;21(4):671–87.

90. Rex DK. Colonoscopy and acute colonic pseudo-obstruction. Gastrointest Endosc Clin N Am 1997;7(3):499–508.

91. Read RC. The development of inguinal herniorrhaphy. Surg Clin North Am 1984; 64(2):185–96.

92. Matthews R, Neumayer L. Inguinal hernia in the 21st century: an evidence-based review. Curr Probl Surg 2008;45(4):261–312.

93. Ruhl CE, Everhart JE. Risk factors for inguinal hernia among adults in the US population. Am J Epidemiol 2007;165:1154–61.

94. Rutkow IM. Demographic and socioeconomic aspects of hernia repair in the United States in 2003. Surg Clin North Am 2003;83:1045–51.

95. Primatesta P, Goldacre MJ. Inguinal hernia repair: incidence of elective and emergency surgery, readmission and mortality. Int J Epidemiol 1996;25(4):835–9.

96. Russo CA, Owens P, Steiner C, et al. Ambulatory surgery in US hospitals, 2003—HCUP fact book no. 9. AHRQ; 2007. Publication No 07–0007. Available at: http://www.ahrq.gov/data/hcup/factbk9/. Accessed February 20, 2010.

97. Carbonell JF, Sanchez JL, Peris RT, et al. Risk factors associated with inguinal hernias: a case control study. Eur J Surg 1993;159:481.

98. Flich J, Alfonso JL, Delgado F, et al. Inguinal hernia and certain risk factors. Eur J Epidemiol 1992;8:277.

99. Sherman V, Macho JR, Brunicardi FC. Inguinal hernias. In: Brunicardi FC, Andersen DK, Billiar TR, et al, editors. Schwartz's principles of surgery. 9th edition. New York: McGraw-Hill Professional; 2010. p. 1305–42.

100. Van Wessem KJ, Simons MP, Plaisier PW, et al. The etiology of indirect inguinal hernias: congenital and/or acquired? Hernia 2003;7:76–9.

101. Kingsnorth A, LeBlanc K. Hernias: inguinal and incisional. Lancet 2003; 362(9395):1561–71.

102. Dahlstrand U, Woolert S, Nordin P, et al. Emergency femoral hernia repair: a study based on a national register. Ann Surg 2009;249(4):672–6.

103. Gallegos NC, Dawson J, Jarvis M, et al. Risk of strangulation in groin hernias. Br J Surg 1991;78:1171–3.

104. McIntosh A, Hutchinson A, Roberts A, et al. Evidence-based management of groin hernia in primary care—a systematic review. Fam Pract 2000;17:442–7.

105. Van den Berg JC, De Valois JC, Go PM, et al. Detection of groin hernia with physical examination, ultrasound, and MRI compared with laparoscopic findings. Invest Radiol 1999;34(12):739–43.

106. Bradley M, Morgan D, Pentlow B, et al. The groin hernia—an ultrasound diagnosis? Ann R Coll Surg Engl 2003;85:178–80.

107. Fitzgibbons RJ, Giobbie-Hurder A, Gibbs JO, et al. Watchful waiting vs repair of inguinal hernia in minimally symptomatic men: a randomized clinical trial. JAMA 2006;295(3):285–92.

108. Kauffman HM, O'Brien DP. Selective reduction of incarcerated inguinal hernia. Am J Surg 1970;119:660–73.

109. Manthey DE. Abdominal hernia reduction. In: Roberts JR, Hedges JR, editors. Clinical procedures in emergency medicine. 4th edition. Philadelphia: Saunders; 2004. p. 860–7.

110. Rai S, Chandra SS, Smile SR. A study of the risk of strangulation and obstruction in groin hernias. Aust N Z J Surg 1998;68:650–4.

111. Kochanek KD, Murphy SL, Anderson RN, et al. no. 5. Deaths: final data for 2002. National vital statistics reports, vol. 53. Hyattsville (MD): National Center for Health Statistics; 2004.

112. Henderson WG, Khuri SF, Mosca C, et al. Comparison of risk-adjusted 30-day postoperative mortality and morbidity in Department of Veterans Affairs hospitals and selected university medical centers: general surgical operations in men. J Am Coll Surg 2007;204(6):1103–14.

113. Nilsson H, Stylianidis G, Haapamaki M, et al. Mortality after groin hernia surgery. Ann Surg 2007;245(4):656–60.

114. Finley RK Jr, Miller SF, Jones LM. Elimination of urinary retention following inguinal herniorrhaphy. Am Surg 1991;57:486 [discussion: 488].
115. Meier DE, OlaOlorun DA, Omodele RA, et al. Incidence of umbilical hernia in African children: redefinition of "normal" and reevaluation of indications for repair. World J Surg 2001;25:645–8.
116. Skinner MA, Grosfeld JL. Inguinal and umbilical hernia repair in infants and children. Surg Clin North Am 1993;73(3):439–49.
117. Katz DA. Evaluation and management of inguinal and umbilical hernias. Pediatr Ann 2001;30(12):729–35.
118. Halm JA, Heisterkamp J, Veen HF. Long-term follow-up after umbilical hernia repair: are there risk factors for recurrence after simple and mesh repair. Hernia 2005;9:334–7.
119. Kulah B, Kulacoglu IH, Oruc T. Presentation and outcome of incarcerated external hernias in adults. Am J Surg 2001;181:101–4.
120. Mudge M, Hughes LE. Incisional hernia: a 10 year prospective study of incidence and attitudes. Br J Surg 1985;72:70–1.
121. Luijendijk RW, Hop WCJ, Van Den Tol MP, et al. A comparison of suture repair with mesh repair for incisional hernia. N Engl J Med 2000;343:392–8.
122. Lang B, Lau H, Lee F. Epigastric hernia and its etiology. Hernia 2002;6:148–50.
123. Skandalakis PN, Zoras O, Skandalakis JE, et al. Spigelian hernia: surgical anatomy, embryology, and technique of repair. Am Surg 2006;72(1):42–8.
124. Mufid MM, Abu-Yousef MM, Kakish ME. Spigelian hernia: diagnosis by high-resolution real-time sonography. J Ultrasound Med 1997;16(3):183–7.
125. Martin LC, Merkle EM, Thompson WM. Review of internal hernias: radiographic and clinical findings. AJR Am J Roentgenol 2006;186:703–17.
126. Holte K, Kehlet H. Postoperative ileus: a preventable event. Br J Surg 2000; 87(11):1480–93.
127. Nanni G, Garbini A, Luchetti P, et al. Ogilvie's syndrome (acute colonic pseudo-obstruction): review of the literature (October 1948 to March 1980) and report of four additional cases. Dis Colon Rectum 1982;25(2):157–66.

Appendicitis, Diverticulitis, and Colitis

Amanda E. Horn, MD*, Jacob W. Ufberg, MD

KEYWORDS

- Appendicitis • Diverticulitis • Colitis
- Inflammatory bowel disease • *Clostridium difficile*
- Emergency medicine

APPENDICITIS
Overview and Epidemiology

Appendicitis is the most common cause of abdominal pain requiring surgical intervention. The lifetime risk of appendicitis is approximately 7%, with a current incidence of 86 per 100,000 patients per year.[1] Rates of appendicitis are highest in the second decade of life, with a slightly higher incidence of appendicitis occurring in males (ratio 1.4:1).[2] Appendiceal perforation rates also vary; patients at extremes of age are more likely to have perforated at their time of diagnosis.[1] Early diagnosis of appendicitis is paramount, because patient morbidity is increased once appendicitis becomes complicated by abscess and perforation.

Pathophysiology

The appendix is located on the posteromedial surface of the cecum, approximately 3 cm from the ileocecal valve. Its length varies from 8 to 13 cm, and its anatomic location within the abdomen is variable.[3] Although the appendix has no known function, recent studies propose that it acts as a reservoir for commensal bacteria in the colon.[4]

Appendicitis occurs when the appendiceal lumen becomes obstructed by fecaliths, adhesions, enlarged lymph nodes, foreign bodies, parasites, or, less commonly, tumors.[5,6] Once obstruction occurs, the intraluminal pressure within the appendix begins to increase as mucosal secretions accumulate, leading to appendiceal distension. This distension in turn stimulates visceral afferent nerves that enter the spinal cord at the T8 to T10 level, causing dull epigastric or periumbilical pain. As obstruction continues, pressures within the appendix impede venous and lymphatic drainage, allowing bacteria and neutrophils to invade the walls of the appendix. More localized

Department of Emergency Medicine, Temple University School of Medicine, 10th Floor Jones Hall, 3401 North Broad Street, Philadelphia, PA 19140, USA
* Corresponding author.
E-mail address: aehorn@temple.edu

Emerg Med Clin N Am 29 (2011) 347–368
doi:10.1016/j.emc.2011.01.002
0733-8627/11/$ – see front matter © 2011 Elsevier Inc. All rights reserved.

pain occurs after continued inflammation within the appendiceal serosa causes irritation of local somatic fibers on the parietal peritoneum. If this process remains unchecked, the appendix becomes gangrenous and is at risk for perforation, abscess formation, and peritonitis, often within 24 to 36 hours of symptom onset.[7]

Clinical Presentation

Classically, a patient with appendicitis presents with constant pain that is poorly localized to the periumbilical or epigastric region, and is accompanied by anorexia, nausea, and vomiting. Vomiting usually begins after the abdominal pain. Illness progression leads to migration of pain to the right lower quadrant at the area of the McBurney point, and can be accompanied by low-grade fever. A meta-analysis evaluating patients with abdominal pain reported an increased likelihood of appendicitis when the patient's pain was located in the right lower quadrant, had migrated from the periumbilical region, and had been accompanied by fever.[8]

However, this classic clinical presentation is not always present, partly because of the variability of the appendiceal location within the abdomen. For example, the appendix may lie in a retrocecal, retroiliac, or pelvic location, leading to pain in the right flank, pelvis, testicle, suprapubic region, or even left lower quadrant if the appendix crosses the midline. Likewise, patients may experience dysuria, urinary frequency, diarrhea, or tenesmus depending on the location of the inflamed appendix. These varied positions of the appendix and their associated complaints can delay the early diagnosis of appendicitis and increase the risk of gangrene and perforation.[9]

Multiple physical examination findings exist to aid in the diagnosis of appendicitis. Pain with palpation is classically found at the McBurney point, located "exactly between an inch and a half and two inches from the anterior spinous process of the ileum on a straight line drawn from that process to the umbilicus."[10] A positive Rovsing sign is present when palpation of the left lower quadrant elicits tenderness in the right lower quadrant. Patients may also show rebound tenderness or guarding, which are responses to the inflamed parietal peritoneum, and, when present, have been found to be independent predictors of appendicitis.[11]

Additional signs can aid in the physical diagnosis. The psoas sign is performed either by having the patient flex at the right hip against resistance, or by extending the hip with the patient in the left lateral decubitus position, thereby irritating the iliopsoas muscle. A positive obturator sign is present when internal rotation of the flexed right hip with the knee in flexion exacerbates the patient's pain. A rectal examination is often performed, although the sensitivity and specificity of rectal tenderness for appendicitis are weak.[8]

Temperature is either normal or slightly increased early in the course of appendicitis. Patients may develop fever as the disease state progresses toward perforation and abscess formation. Therefore, temperature increase alone cannot rule in the diagnosis of appendicitis, but the presence of a fever, when taken in concert with other history and physical examination findings, such as migration of pain, can make the diagnosis more likely.[8]

Special populations

Pregnancy In theory, the gravid uterus can displace the inflamed appendix cephalad and lead to right upper quadrant or right flank discomfort. However, most pregnant women with appendicitis present with right lower quadrant pain, regardless of their stage of pregnancy.[12,13] There is a slightly higher incidence of appendicitis in the second trimester compared with the first and third.[14] Although pregnant women are not at increased risk for appendicitis compared with nongravid controls, appendicitis is the most common nonobstetric surgical emergency in pregnancy. Early recognition in the pregnant patient with appendicitis is important because complications such as peritonitis or abscess formation can affect fetal outcomes. Studies have shown high rates of fetal loss in both uncomplicated and complicated appendicitis (15% and 37%, respectively). Pregnant women are also at risk of early delivery, with some series showing rates reaching 45%, although recent data show improvement in these outcomes.[15,16]

Children Young children and the aged are also at risk for delayed diagnosis of appendicitis and its complications, and therefore a high index of suspicion is necessary when evaluating these populations. Studies have found pediatric patients to be initially misdiagnosed with gastroenteritis, urinary tract infection, otitis media, or respiratory infections, ultimately increasing perforation rates (approximately 70%–80%) and hospital lengths of stay.[17–19]

Elderly Likewise, elderly patients tend to have a delay between symptom onset and treatment of appendicitis. This delay leads to increased rates of perforation. Mortality from appendicitis in the aged increases to 4% from 0.1% for younger patients, and is particularly high in those greater than 70 years of age (32%). Reasons for delay in diagnosing this population include misdiagnosis and atypical patient presentation,[20,21] although more recent data show early computed tomography (CT) scanning and laparoscopy are improving outcomes.[22]

Immunocompromise Immunocompromised patients, such as those with acquired immune deficiency syndrome (AIDS), are also at risk for complications from appendicitis, partly because of the similar symptoms that opportunistic infections can cause in this population. Although patients with AIDS have been found to present with typical symptoms of appendicitis, these symptoms may be misattributed to opportunistic infections or other AIDS complications. However, patients with AIDS are more likely than those without the disease to be perforated at the time of surgical intervention.[23] Recent retrospective data suggest that antiretroviral therapy may play a protective role in the development of appendicitis in patients with AIDS.[24]

Diagnosis

Appendicitis should be considered in the differential diagnosis for all patients presenting with epigastric, periumbilical, or right-sided abdominal or flank pain. Although no single test is specific for appendicitis, some laboratory data may aid in the diagnosis. A urinary pregnancy test should be performed in all women of childbearing age, and pelvic examination should be performed in addition to the abdominal examination. Some women may have adnexal tenderness with inflamed pelvic appendices. A urinalysis should be performed as well, although it is important to keep in mind that hematuria or pyuria can be present in appendicitis if the inflamed appendix is in close proximity to the bladder or ureter.

Laboratory
The clinical usefulness of a white blood cell (WBC) count with differential remains uncertain. In one recent series, an increased WBC count of greater than 10,000 cells/mm^3 had a sensitivity of 76% and specificity of 52%.[25] This is similar to other data showing that leukocytosis alone is a poor predictor of appendicitis and does not distinguish between simple versus complicated cases.[26] The inflammatory marker C-reactive protein (CRP) has been shown to have both a low sensitivity and low specificity when used alone in appendicitis evaluation.[27,28] However, the combination of

leukocytosis, leftward shift, and increased CRP may be more useful than each test alone in the diagnosis of appendicitis. A recent meta-analysis showed an increased likelihood of appendicitis when 2 or more of these studies were increased and a decreased likelihood when all 3 were within normal limits.[29] Therefore, laboratory testing should be seen as an adjunct to other elements of the history and physical examination when appendicitis is suspected, but cannot definitively make the diagnosis.

Imaging

Multiple imaging studies in the evaluation of appendicitis exist, although the usefulness of each study can vary. Plain films are seldom used in the diagnosis of appendicitis; however, they can help rule out other causes of abdominal pain (volvulus, intussusception, or nephrolithiasis) and may be performed rapidly at the bedside. Signs suggestive of appendicitis on radiograph include localized paralytic ileus, gas or fecalith in the appendix, blurring in the area of the right psoas muscle, and free air, although no sign is sensitive or specific in making the diagnosis,[30] which limits the value of plain film in this disease.

Ultrasound

Ultrasound can be a useful test in the evaluation of appendicitis, particularly in children and pregnant women in whom there are particular concerns regarding ionizing radiation. The sensitivity of graded compression ultrasonography is as high as 98% (although these numbers vary widely between studies)[31] and is considered positive for appendicitis when the diameter of the appendix is greater than 6 to 7 mm (**Fig. 1**).[27,32,33] Inflammation surrounding the appendix, appendicoliths, or hyperemia of the appendiceal wall can also be visualized by ultrasound in the setting of acute appendicitis. False negatives can occur once the appendix has perforated, thus reducing the diameter of the appendix, or when the appendix is retrocecal or inflammation is confined to the tip of the appendix.[34] Another challenge in using ultrasound is that the appendix cannot always be visualized. Even using skilled sonographers, the appendix is not visualized between 25% and 35% of the time,[27,33] which can be partly caused by patient's body habitus or bowel gas overlying the appendix. The negative predictive value of a nonvisualized appendix on ultrasound is 90%.[27] Thus, although a positive ultrasound is diagnostic of appendicitis, a negative ultrasound in which the appendix is not seen cannot rule out the diagnosis of acute appendicitis, and other diagnostic tools should be used.

CT

CT has become widely used in the evaluation of suspected appendicitis. Advantages include its widespread availability as well as its capacity to detect other abdominal disorders. Disadvantages include patient radiation exposure, time delay to diagnosis if oral contrast is used, and risk of contrast-induced nephropathy or contrast reaction when intravenous contrast is used. Some investigators consider increased cost to be a disadvantage of this imaging modality, but data have suggested a decrease in the rates of unnecessary appendectomy since CT scan use has increased.[35] Findings suggestive of acute appendicitis on CT scan include an enlarged appendix with diameter greater than 6 mm, appendiceal wall thickening, and pericecal inflammation (**Fig. 2**). An appendicolith alone is not sufficient to make a radiographic diagnosis of appendicitis.[36]

Some controversy exists about the use of contrast in the evaluation of appendicitis on CT. The sensitivity (83%–97%) and specificity (93%–98%) of CT in acute appendicitis vary with the presence or absence of contrast, as well as type of contrast used.

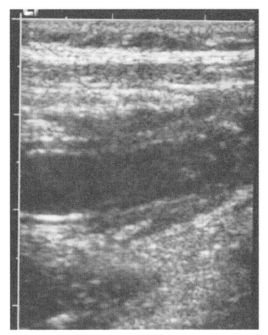

Fig. 1. Ultrasound shows an enlarged appendix with a fluid-filled lumen. (*From* Paterson A, Sweeney LE, Connoly B. Paediatric abdominal imaging. In: Grainger R, Allison D, eds. Grainger & Allison's Diagnostic Radiology: A Textbook of Medical Imaging. 5th Edition. Philadelphia: Churchill Livingston, 2008; with permission.)

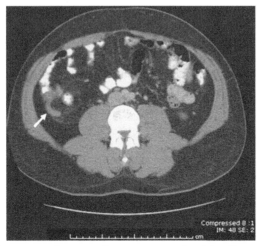

Fig. 2. Appendicitis. A CT scan shows an edematous appendix with a diameter greater than 1 cm (*arrow*), consistent with acute, uncomplicated appendicitis. (*From* Prather C. Inflammatory and anatomic diseases of the intestine, peritoneum, mesentery, and omentum. In: Goldman L, Ausiello DA, eds. Cecil medicine. 23rd edition. Philadelphia: Saunders, 2007; with permission.)

A recent review article found the sensitivity and negative predictive value of CT without oral contrast to be equal to that of CT with oral contrast; the specificity, accuracy, and positive predictive value of CT without oral contrast was superior to that of CT with oral contrast in this analysis.[37] The implication of this review may have important ramifications on emergency department (ED) length of stay and may decrease time until surgical intervention for patients. Other studies have shown the sensitivity of noncontrast scans to be greatly inferior to those using contrast.[38]

Another promising option uses rectal contrast only. In a series of 100 patients, CT with rectal contrast had a sensitivity, specificity, positive and negative predictive values, and accuracy of 98% in diagnosing acute appendicitis.[39] More recent prospective data have shown more modest outcomes for this modality, but imply that rectal contrast studies can be useful in the evaluation of acute appendicitis.[38] Perhaps the best approach to the use of contrast in patients suspected of having appendicitis should take into account the breadth of the differential diagnosis. Oral and intravenous contrast may help better delineate other causes of abdominal pain (particularly in young women) and should be considered when the diagnosis of appendicitis is uncertain. Establishing an institutional protocol with respect to contrast administration may also aid in the decision of whether contrast should be used, and by what route.

Magnetic resonance imaging
Magnetic resonance imaging (MRI) may also have a limited role in the work-up of appendicitis. Unlike CT, MRI does not expose patients to ionizing radiation. It is therefore considered safe in pregnancy. Gadolinium crosses the placenta and should therefore be avoided, particularly in the first trimester. Disadvantages include limited availability, high cost, and lengthy scan times. If obtainable, MRI may be a good second-line imaging study when a pregnant patient has an indeterminate ultrasound.[40]

Clinical scoring
Several scoring systems have been developed in an attempt to assist in the diagnosis of acute appendicitis. The most often cited is the MANTRELS score, which is a mnemonic that uses 8 different variables on a total 10-point scale.[41] These variables include migration of pain, anorexia, nausea or vomiting, tenderness in the right lower quadrant, rebound tenderness, elevation of temperature, leukocytosis, and leftward shift. The score may aid clinicians in deciding which patients can be observed and which require operative intervention. It has also been shown to be helpful in discriminating between patients who require imaging for suspected appendicitis and those who may be discharged without imaging.[42]

Treatment

Patients with appendicitis should receive intravenous hydration, symptomatic relief, and antibiotics. Electrolyte imbalances should be corrected and crystalloids administered for patients with dehydration or sepsis. Antiemetics should be considered in patients with vomiting. Narcotic pain medication can be administered to maximize patient comfort.

A recent review article confirms that antibiotics can prevent postoperative wound infection in uncomplicated appendicitis and minimize abscess formation in cases of perforation.[43] Antibiotic therapy should include coverage for enteric gram-negative organisms as well as anaerobes, and should be considered in conjunction with the consulting surgeon. Possible regimens include a second-generation or third-generation cephalosporin for uncomplicated cases. In the event of abscess formation or perforation, broader-spectrum coverage with a medication such as piperacillin-tazobactam or a 3-drug regimen including a cephalosporin and aminoglycoside along with metronidazole is warranted.[44]

A study investigating antibiotic and medical management versus appendectomy showed that, although most patients improved in the short term with medical management, greater than one-third of patients required surgery for recurrent appendicitis within a year.[45] Therefore, operative intervention remains the definitive treatment of acute appendicitis, and early surgical consultation is necessary. In cases of abscess formation at time of presentation, surgeons may opt for initial percutaneous abscess drainage initially, followed by interval appendectomy.

DIVERTICULITIS
Overview and Epidemiology

Diverticular disease is commonly seen in the adult population. The overall prevalence of diverticulosis has been reported to be roughly 27% and increases with advancing age.[46] Of those patients with symptoms from diverticular disease, 3% are less than 40 years of age, whereas each decade between the ages of 50 and 70 years accounts for approximately 25% to 30% of cases.[47] The prevalence is much higher in developed countries, and is believed to be partly the result of physical inactivity[48] and a low-fiber diet.[49] Symptomatic disease, including diverticular pain and diverticulitis, occurs in roughly 10% to 25% of patients with diverticulosis.[50]

Pathophysiology

Diverticula are small outpouchings or herniations that form at areas of weakness in the wall of the colon. In general, they are located at the vulnerable areas in which the vasa recta enters the muscularis. Except for diverticula of the cecum, which comprise all 3 layers of the colonic wall, most acquired diverticula contain mucosa and submucosa only. Diverticular disease affects the left-sided and sigmoid colon more than 90% of the time.[51] Although many causes of diverticulosis have been proposed, the exact cause of the condition is not known. Problems of colonic motility and muscular abnormalities of the colon wall are possible causes. Another hypothesis is that diverticulosis is a disorder arising from increased intraluminal pressure.[52] Although diverticulosis is largely an asymptomatic condition, these areas can perforate and become inflamed, leading to diverticulitis.

Patients can have either complicated or uncomplicated episodes of diverticulitis, which has ramifications for treatment as well as patient morbidity. Complicated cases are those in which there is perforation, obstruction, abscess, or fistula formation.[53]

Clinical Presentation

Patients with diverticulitis typically present with constant left lower quadrant or suprapubic pain. Patients may also complain of fever, malaise, constipation, diarrhea, tenesmus, and urinary symptoms if the bladder becomes irritated by the inflamed colon. On examination, patients typically have left lower-quadrant tenderness, which may be accompanied by localized guarding or rebound. At times, a palpable abdominal mass caused by an underlying abscess may be appreciated.

Patients with acute diverticulitis may also present with right-sided abdominal symptoms. This possibility applies particularly to Asian[54] and younger[55] patients, who are more likely to have proximal colonic disease. In addition, redundant sigmoid colon may be present on the right side of the abdomen, leading to right-sided symptoms in patients with distal colonic disease.

A high index of suspicion is necessary when evaluating patients who are elderly or immunocompromised. These groups may present with less-impressive symptoms and physical examination findings. As a result, they are more likely to have perforation at the time of diagnosis.[56,57]

Patients may also complain of symptoms related to fistula formation, which may occur between the bowel and bladder, leading to pneumaturia or fecaluria, or between the bowel and vagina, with women complaining of a feculent vaginal discharge. In addition, enterocolonic fistulas may occur and lead to copious diarrhea.

Diagnosis

Patients with acute diverticulitis often have an increased WBC count and may also have a leftward shift. Other laboratory abnormalities may be present in patients with vomiting and diarrhea or in those with more advanced septicemia.

Imaging options are available when the diagnosis of diverticulitis is uncertain, or if suspicion exists for complications of diverticular disease. Contrast enema has typically been considered the gold standard in diagnosis, although it is falling out of favor as a first-line study. Although contrast enema is able to diagnose diverticulitis, it is unable to assess for the presence of an abscess and cannot determine the severity of inflammation.[58] Thickened colonic folds, contrast extravasation, and localized mass effect may be seen on contrast radiography.[59] Fistula formation may also be evident. The use of non–water-soluble contrast material in colonic contrast studies can also lead to problems associated with intraperitoneal barium when perforation is present, and should therefore be avoided in patients with signs of local peritonitis on examination. If this type of imaging is used, it is best to use water-soluble contrast.

CT is the study most used for the diagnosis of diverticulitis. CT with both oral and intravenous contrast has the advantage of being able to evaluate the colonic walls as well as extraluminal areas, in addition to being able to assess for other causes of abdominal pain. The sensitivity of CT for diagnosis of diverticulitis ranges from 85% to 97%.[60] Positive findings of diverticulitis include thickening of the bowel wall and fascia, pericolic fat stranding, and local abscess formation (**Fig. 3**).[61]

Ultrasound also has a role in the radiologic evaluation of diverticulitis. Findings compatible with the disease include a thickened colon wall with protrusions consistent with diverticula. Pericolic inflammation may also be evident. Although the sensitivity of ultrasound in diverticulitis is modest (91%), its specificity was almost 100% in a study evaluating patients with right-sided abdominal pain.[62] As with the use of ultrasound for other diseases, its accuracy is highly operator dependent.

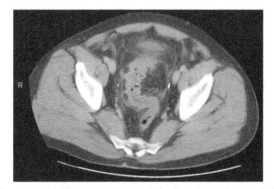

Fig. 3. CT scan of a patient with acute diverticulitis showing colon wall thickening, a mass adjacent to the sigmoid, and stranding of the fat. (*From* Brandt LJ, Feuerstat P. Intestinal ischemia. In: Feldman M, Friedman LS, Brandt LJ, eds. Sleisenger & Fordtran's gastrointestinal and liver disease. 8th edition. Philadelphia: Saunders, 2010; with permission.)

Treatment

The treatment of diverticulitis is largely dependent on the severity of illness and overall health status of the patient. Young immunocompetent patients with uncomplicated diverticulitis may be managed as outpatients with oral antibiotics. Regimens should cover both gram-negative aerobes and anaerobes, and include a combination of ciprofloxacin and metronidazole, trimethoprim-sulfamethoxazole and metronidazole, or amoxicillin-clavulanic acid alone. Patients should be instructed to follow a liquid diet with advancement to solids as tolerated after 2 to 3 days. These patients should receive prompt follow-up to assess for response to treatment, and may require hospitalization if symptoms do not improve. Surgical referral should be given to those patients experiencing a recurrence of diverticulitis. In addition, it is generally recommended that patients presenting with a first episode of diverticulitis undergo a colonoscopy about 6 weeks after the resolution of symptoms to evaluate for neoplasm and other diseases of the colon.

Patients who have failed outpatient treatment, who require intravenous analgesia, the elderly or immunocompromised, and those with complications of diverticulitis should be hospitalized. Antibiotic options include intravenous ciprofloxacin and metronidazole, or single-drug regimens of β-lactamase inhibitor combinations such as ampicillin-sulbactam or ticarcillin-clavulanate. Severe infections may necessitate the use of imipenem alone or the use of gentamicin or ciprofloxacin in combination with ampicillin and metronidazole. These patients warrant urgent surgical evaluation to determine the need for CT-guided percutaneous drainage or surgical resection.[63] In general, between 15% and 30% of patients presenting with acute diverticulitis require operative intervention. An equal number have recurrences of their disease.[64,65]

COLITIS
Inflammatory Bowel Disease

Overview and epidemiology

The term inflammatory bowel disease (IBD) refers to 2 types of chronic intestinal disorders, Crohn disease (CD) and ulcerative colitis (UC). These diseases differ in their pathophysiology, but are similar in their clinical presentation. Both diseases are characterized by a relapsing and remitting course of alimentary tract inflammation, and both diseases require intensive chronic medical management during both exacerbations and periods of remission.

IBD has a peak onset between 15 and 30 years of age, with a second small peak later in life that is more consistently seen with UC than with CD.[66] IBD affects more than 1 million Americans, with CD and UC represented roughly equally. Worldwide, IBD prevalence varies with geographic location, with higher rates occurring in more industrialized countries and lower rates occurring in Asia, Africa, and South America. IBD is more common among the Jewish population, and studies have shown higher rates in white people than African Americans and Asians.[67]

Pathophysiology

Although the exact cause of IBD remains unknown, a complex interplay of multiple factors likely contributes to the development of these diseases. At present, the best evidence points to an inflammatory response to intestinal microbes occurring in a host who is genetically susceptible to IBD.[68] Numerous environmental factors have also been shown to affect IBD. Cigarette smoking lowers the risk of UC for current smokers, but the risk for those who stop smoking is higher than for those who never smoked.[69] Conversely, smoking doubles the risk of Crohn disease.[70]

Diet, oral contraceptives, and nonsteroidal antiinflammatory agents have also been shown to influence IBD.[71]

The role of genetics in IBD is supported by twin studies that show a definite genetic predisposition that is stronger in CD than in UC.[72] It is thought that microbes also play a role, with inflammation believed to be the result of a dysfunctional response to infection. However, no particular bacterium has been identified in studies as the pathogenic cause of IBD.[71] The immune system clearly plays a significant role in IBD, and many agents used for the treatment of disease are immunosuppressive or specifically target certain aspects of immune system dysregulation.[73]

Crohn disease is characterized by involvement of any part of the gastrointestinal tract, but most frequently involves the distal small intestine and colon. The inflammation is transmural, sometimes leading to the development of fistulas, abscesses, or strictures. The mucosa often assumes a cobblestone appearance, and granulomatous disease is commonly present. The lesions may be discontinuous (skip lesions), which may help to distinguish between forms of IBD. Perianal involvement, with fistula formation and perianal abscess formation, is common in CD.

UC leads to inflammation of the mucosa and submucosa of the colon. Transmural involvement is rare, leading to little, if any, perianal disease or fistula formation. UC generally appears as a continuous lesion confined to the colon, and the absence of skip lesions can help distinguish this disease from CD. Rectal involvement is the rule, with inflammation extending a variable distance into the colon. The inflammation of UC often takes the appearance of ulceration, and cobblestoning of the mucosa is rare.

Clinical presentation

Patients with IBD typically present with diarrhea and varying amounts of crampy abdominal pain. Diarrhea in UC may be bloody and is typically frequent and small in volume. Tenesmus or fecal incontinence may also occur. These diarrheal features are also typical of CD with colonic involvement. However, in CD limited to the small intestine, stools may be less frequent and larger in volume, and tenesmus is absent. Vomiting may be present, and, if significant, should lead to the consideration of bowel obstruction.

Abdominal pain and tenderness in IBD are variable based on the anatomic location of disease. Tenderness may be isolated to the rectum or the left lower quadrant, as is often the case in UC. In other cases, it may be localized to the right lower quadrant, such as in patients with ileal CD. Pain and tenderness may be diffuse in patients with significant areas of bowel involvement. Thickened bowel loops or an abscess may lead to a palpable mass and tenderness at the affected location. Patients may present with frank peritonitis if bowel perforation has occurred.

Patients with CD are prone to fistula and abscess formation because of the transmural nature of disease. The location of fistula and abscess formation correlates with the location of disease. Patients with isolated small intestine involvement are more prone to internal fistula formation, whereas perianal disease presents more commonly in patients with ileocolic disease.[74]

Patients with IBD may present with systemic complaints, such as fever, fatigue, and weight loss. Often, symptoms are gradually progressive and, more frequently in CD, may be intermittently present for a long period of time before diagnosis. Some degree of dehydration and malnutrition may also be present.

In most cases, the severity of IBD flares can be classified as mild, moderate, or severe. Mild flares are classified as having no systemic toxicity, fewer than 4 bowel movements per day with little or no blood, and an erythrocyte sedimentation rate (ESR) of less than 20 mm/h. Severe flares are classified as having systemic toxicity, 6 or more bowel movements per day with blood, and ESR greater than 30 mm/h. Moderate flares have symptoms that are between the criteria for mild and severe.[75] Some patients may present with serious complications of IBD (see Serious Complications of IBD).

Diagnosis

Many patients present to the ED with a known diagnosis of IBD. It has previously been shown that compliance with maintenance therapy reduces the risk of acute attacks,[76] and thus patients should be queried as to medication compliance.

No specific testing routinely available in the ED can reliably diagnose IBD, and endoscopy with biopsy is generally necessary to confirm the diagnosis. Patients presenting with IBD may be anemic because of chronic disease or bloody stools. Electrolyte abnormalities may occur because of significant diarrhea or vomiting or because of malabsorption. Nonspecific markers of inflammation, such as the ESR or CRP, are frequently increased.

Plain radiography may be useful in cases in which bowel obstruction, perforation, or toxic megacolon (see Serious Complications of IBD) are suspected. However, in most IBD cases presenting to the ED, plain radiography is unlikely to be of benefit. CT may be helpful to identify extraluminal complications such as nephrolithiasis, abscess, obstruction, or perforation, but severity of disease does not otherwise correlate well with radiographic findings.

Treatment

Medical therapy in the treatment of IBD is centered on supportive care as well as a variety of antiinflammatory and immunosuppressive agents. In patients with known IBD, treatment should be decided in concert with the patient's physician, because IBD management is a chronic, ongoing process tailored on a patient-by-patient basis. Medications commonly used to treat IBD are discussed later. An ED approach to treatment of IBD follows this description.

Supportive care Dehydration and electrolyte imbalance should be treated with intravenous fluids and electrolyte supplementation as needed. Anemia caused by serious hemorrhage should be addressed with blood transfusion if necessary. Pain medications should be used as needed, but opiates are discouraged as part of the chronic management of IBD. Nonsteroidal antiinflammatory medications may exacerbate IBD and should be avoided. Antidiarrheal agents may be useful in mild IBD to decrease the number of stools and improve rectal urgency, but they should be avoided in severe disease because of the risk of precipitating toxic megacolon.

Aminosalicylates These agents are the cornerstone of therapy for UC, and although they are less effective in CD, they are also often used as maintenance therapy for patients with CD. The choice of preparation and route of these 5-aminosalicylic acid (5-ASA) derivatives is based on the location of disease. Suppositories are often useful in patients with rectal disease, and retention enemas treat the rectum and descending colon. For patients with diffuse disease, oral controlled-release formulations are most successful, sometimes in combination with suppositories or enemas.

Corticosteroids Corticosteroids are often used as first-line agents in CD, and are used in UC which is refractory to 5-ASA preparations. Oral steroids are effective in the management of mild-to-moderate exacerbations of disease, with parenteral steroids reserved for more severe disease requiring hospital admission. The typical dose of prednisone used is 40 mg/d, and therapy can be slowly tapered once symptoms begin to diminish. The many known adverse effects of long-term corticosteroid use limit the role of steroids in maintenance therapy.

Immunomodulators Azathioprine and mercaptopurine (6-MP) are immunomodulators that have been shown to be effective in CD and, to a lesser degree, in UC. These drugs are useful in patients who are refractory to corticosteroids, or to help reduce corticosteroid dependence in those who are unsuccessful in weaning from steroids.

Antibiotics Antibiotics have a limited role in UC, but have shown some usefulness in CD and in infectious complications of CD such as perianal fistula and abscess. Metronidazole and ciprofloxacin are the 2 most commonly used agents.

Anti–TNF-α antibody Infliximab is effective in managing moderate-to-severe Crohn disease, as well as in healing fistula disease associated with CD.[77] A recent Cochrane review also showed usefulness in patients with difficult-to-treat UC.[78]

Initial ED treatment of IBD Supportive therapy should be instituted as indicated for all patients. If possible, the patient's treating physician should be contacted to ensure appropriate therapy based on the type of IBD, location of disease, and previous response to therapy.

In general, first-line therapy for patients with mild-to-moderate UC should be with oral 5-ASA derivatives, whereas enemas or foams are appropriate for those with proctitis only. For those with UC who are failing several weeks of 5-ASA agents, corticosteroids are the next therapeutic step. Patients who are failing steroids may be stepped up to another therapy, but this should always be done at the discretion of the patient's gastroenterologist.

First-line therapy for mild-to-moderate CD usually involves oral corticosteroids or antibiotics. If the patient has significant abdominal pain, fever, or increased leukocyte count, an abdominal CT should be strongly considered to rule out abscess or perforation before instituting steroid therapy. To increase the likelihood of success of steroid withdrawal, 5-ASA preparations are often added, but they are not generally considered first-line therapy for CD.

Patients with severe IBD from either UC or CD should receive aggressive supportive care. Parenteral corticosteroids are often necessary, but only after suppurative disease has been ruled out (predominantly in CD). Care should be taken to ensure that no serious complications of IBD are present (see Serious Complications of IBD). Other causes of colitis should be considered, including enteric infection (especially *Clostridium difficile* infection), radiation colitis, and ischemic colitis. Appropriate consultation with a gastroenterologist should occur as soon as possible, and the patient should be admitted to the appropriate level of care based on clinical presentation.

Serious complications of IBD
Complications associated with UC Acute fulminant colitis occurs when inflammation extends beyond the colonic mucosa. Patients present with overt signs of systemic toxicity in addition to abdominal pain and bloody diarrhea. Leukocytosis and metabolic acidosis are often present.[79] Plain radiography may show an edematous colon with thumbprinting. This condition may progress to toxic megacolon. These patients require aggressive supportive care, and enteric infections should be ruled out with stool studies. Broad-spectrum antibiotics should be considered, especially if perforation is suspected, and gastroenterologic and surgical consultation should occur emergently.

Toxic megacolon results as the bowel becomes paralyzed and begins to dilate. Signs of systemic toxicity are present, and the colon is generally more than 6 cm in diameter (**Fig. 4**). When the colon reaches 12 to 15 cm, perforation is likely imminent.[79] Enteric

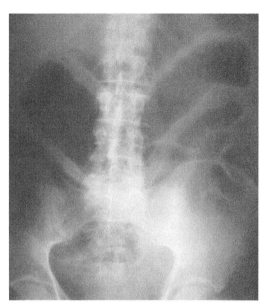

Fig. 4. Toxic megacolon. The ascending and transverse colon appears gas-filled and dilated with a thickened wall. There is an absence of haustral markings, indicating full-thickness mural inflammation. (*From* Morrison I. The plain abdominal radiograph and associated anatomy and techniques. In: Grainger R, Allison D, eds. Grainger & Allison's Diagnostic Radiology: A Textbook of Medical Imaging. 5th Edition. Philadelphia: Churchill Livingston, 2008; with permission.)

infection should be ruled out, as in fulminant colitis. Gastrointestinal decompression with a nasogastric tube should occur, and aggressive resuscitation and supportive care should be instituted. Although the initial management is often medical, surgical consultation is necessary to evaluate the need for urgent operative intervention.

Lower gastrointestinal bleeding is common in IBD, although life-threatening bleeding is uncommon. Aggressive supportive care should occur, as in other causes of lower gastrointestinal bleeding, and surgical treatment is often necessary.[79]

Complications associated with CD In patients with CD, intra-abdominal and perirectal abscesses are common. In CD, perforation often creates a walled-off abscess rather than acute peritonitis because of seepage of bacteria through sinus tracts.[79] The signs and symptoms of acute CD exacerbation may be difficult to distinguish from an intra-abdominal abscess. CT scanning is often necessary to clarify the diagnosis. Management of intra-abdominal abscess includes broad-spectrum antibiotics and early consultation for operative or percutaneous drainage.

Perirectal abscess may be treated as in patients without CD. Antibiotics should be initiated. The choice of metronidazole and ciprofloxacin is often used, because they may also aid in fistula healing, although there is no strong evidence to support this common practice.

Bowel obstruction is a common problem in CD, with the most common location being the terminal ileum. Most patients have repeated partial small bowel obstructions rather than complete obstructions, and thus may respond to supportive management with bowel rest and nasogastric suction. Surgical consultation should be requested, but most patients improve without operative intervention.[79]

Extraintestinal manifestations

Extraintestinal manifestations of IBD may occur simultaneously with flares of bowel disease, or may be temporally unrelated to the course of bowel disease. Common extraintestinal manifestations include arthritides such as ankylosing spondylitis, hepatic manifestations including hepatitis, pericholangitis, sclerosing cholangitis (UC), and gallstones or renal stones (CD). Other complications may be dermal (pyoderma gangrenosum and erythema nodosum) or ocular (uveitis and episcleritis). For reasons that are unclear, thromboembolic disease is more common in patients with IBD. Most of these thromboembolic events manifest as thrombophlebitis, lower extremity deep venous thrombosis, or pulmonary embolus.[80] Thromboembolism may also affect the portal vein, leading to variceal bleeding. Many other sites of thromboembolism can also occur, including cerebral vascular occlusions.

Disposition

Most patients with mild-to-moderate IBD exacerbation may ultimately be discharged to follow-up closely with their physician. Alterations in therapy should be discussed whenever possible with the physician managing the patient's disease. Patients with severe disease, or ill-appearing patients who are failing outpatient steroid therapy, require hospitalization. In addition to hospital admission, patients with severe complications of IBD also require emergent consultation with gastroenterology and surgery.

C difficile Colitis

Overview and epidemiology

C difficile is a highly transmissible, gram-positive, spore-forming anaerobic bacterium that colonizes about 3% of healthy adults and 16% to 35% of hospitalized patients.[81] This organism is identified as the cause in 10% to 25% of cases of antibiotic-associated diarrhea, 50% to 75% of antibiotic-associated colitis, and more than 90% of antibiotic-associated pseudomembranous colitis.[81] The epidemiology of C difficile is changing rapidly, with a recent large increase in disease frequency, severity, and rate of treatment failure.[82] This has correlated with the emergence of a new and highly virulent strain designated NAP1.

Antibiotics are the most widely recognized risk factor, and almost all cases are associated with prior use.[81] The antibiotics most commonly associated with C difficile include clindamycin, fluoroquinolones, and the third-generation cephalosporins, although any antibiotic may predispose patients to colonization. Increased duration of therapy, use of multiple agents, and broader-spectrum antibiotic use all increase the incidence, although even single perioperative doses of antibiotics have been implicated.[83,84]

Other established risk factors include hospitalization, advanced age, and severe underlying illness. Acid suppression, gastrointestinal surgery, and chemotherapy have also been implicated in C difficile–associated disease. The incidence of community-associated infection, although low, is rising, and infection may occur in the absence of risk factors.[85]

Pathophysiology

Most commonly, antibiotic exposure alters the gut flora, allowing C difficile to multiply. C difficile releases 2 toxins that cause colitis and diarrhea, an enterotoxin termed toxin A and a cytotoxin termed toxin B. In addition, the NAP1 strain produces binary toxin, which is not present in other strains. These toxins act through a variety of mechanisms to cause neutrophil activation and chemotaxis, cell retraction, apoptosis, and disruption of intercellular tight junctions. This process leads to watery diarrhea, colitis, and the formation of pseudomembranes. Severity of disease is correlated with stool toxin levels.[86]

Clinical presentation
The clinical presentation of *C difficile* colitis is highly variable. Most patients report a previous history of antibiotic exposure, and most of those either present during the course of antibiotics or within several weeks of completion. Symptoms may begin as late as months after antibiotic completion. Patients may present with diarrhea, mild colitis, pseudomembranous colitis, fulminant colitis, or toxic megacolon.

Patients with mild-to-moderate disease generally present with lower abdominal cramping and nonbloody, watery diarrhea, but lack systemic symptoms. Patients with more severe colitis present with profuse watery diarrhea that may have occult blood, crampy abdominal pain and bloating, and systemic signs and symptoms such as dehydration and fever. Patients with fulminant colitis present with severe abdominal pain, fever, diarrhea, bloating, and appear clinically ill. Physical examination findings are variable based on severity of disease, but may range from isolated mild lower abdominal tenderness to severe tenderness, peritonitis, distention, fever, and signs of shock.

Diagnosis
The gold standard test for diagnosis is the cell cytotoxicity assay. It is a sensitive assay but is labor intensive, not widely available, and results are slow to return. In clinical practice, most institutions are using commercially available enzyme immunoassay (EIA) kits. These tests are easy to use, can be batched, and results are available within hours. EIA kits may test for toxin A alone or for both toxins A and B, but testing for both toxins is preferred. EIA testing is less sensitive than the cytotoxicity assay; however, the yield may be increased by as much as 10% if serial testing is performed.[87]

Other laboratory testing may be suggestive, but not diagnostic. Fecal leukocytes are usually present and may help to distinguish between mild *C difficile* and other antibiotic-associated diarrhea. Patients with more severe disease often have a leukocytosis, which may be profound in patients with fulminant colitis. Sigmoidoscopy may also help make the diagnosis if classic pseudomembranes are visualized. When the disease is particularly severe, thickening of the wall of the colon may be seen on CT scan, but it is not diagnostic of *C difficile*. Plain radiography is not widely useful, but should be obtained if toxic megacolon or perforation is suspected.

Treatment
Whenever possible, the offending antibiotic should be stopped or, if this is not possible, switched to an agent less commonly associated with *C difficile* infection. Supportive management with fluid and electrolyte repletion should be given as indicated, and contact precautions should be instituted if infection is proved or suspected. Patients with typical symptoms and a positive EIA should receive antibiotics, and treatment may be started pending EIA results if clinical suspicion is high.

Antibiotic treatment of mild-to-moderate disease is generally with oral metronidazole or oral vancomycin. Most recommendations favor metronidazole as first-line therapy because of lower cost and similar efficacy. The recommended regimen is 500 mg 3 times daily or 250 mg 4 times daily for 14 days. If oral vancomycin is used, the dosage is 125 mg 4 times daily for 14 days. Intravenous metronidazole may be used if oral therapy cannot be given, but intravenous vancomycin has no clinical effect on *C difficile* colitis.

Relapse occurs in roughly 14% of patients after treatment.[88] Relapse does not necessarily indicate metronidazole resistance, and most patients respond to another course of metronidazole. The addition of the probiotic *Saccharomyces boulardii* to oral antibiotics has been shown to decrease the number of recurrences in patients with relapse, but it did not prove beneficial in the first episode of disease.[89]

Patients with severe C difficile disease require antibiotic therapy, aggressive supportive care, and close monitoring. The possibility of toxic megacolon should be considered. Oral vancomycin (at 500 mg 4 times daily) is preferred for severe cases, and showed a significantly higher cure rate in a head-to-head study with metronidazole.[90] Patients with ileus may benefit from the addition of intravenous metronidazole. Some severely ill patients may require surgery for toxic megacolon, perforation, necrotizing colitis, or severe disease with systemic toxicity refractory to treatment. Surgical consultation should be considered in the severely ill patient with C difficile–associated disease.

Disposition
Most patients with mild symptoms caused by C difficile infection may be discharged to home, with close follow-up with their primary care provider. If EIA results are not available at the time of discharge, appropriate follow-up of test results with appropriate treatment must be ensured. Patients with severe disease require admission to the appropriate level of inpatient care.

Ischemic Colitis

Overview and epidemiology
Intestinal ischemia is rare. However, ischemic colitis is the most frequent type of mesenteric ischemia, and predominantly affects the elderly.[91] Most patients have non-gangrenous ischemia, which is generally transient and resolves without long-term complications. Ischemic colitis may present insidiously, and often no cause is identified. In addition to age, several risk factors exist for colonic ischemia, including recent aortoiliac surgery, myocardial infarction or heart failure, extreme exercise (such as marathon running or triathlon competitions), and prothrombotic conditions.

Pathophysiology
The colon has considerable collateral blood supply, which is weakest at the splenic flexure and the rectosigmoid junction. As such, these 2 areas are at greatest risk for ischemia during systemic hypoperfusion events. Most episodes are secondary to systemic low-flow states and rarely occur as a result of large artery disease. Colonic injury from an ischemic event may be caused by either hypoxia or subsequent reperfusion injury, or both.

Clinical presentation
Manifestations of colonic ischemia are variable based on the extent and duration of the ischemic event. Patients generally present with acute onset of mild, crampy abdominal pain, usually on the left side. Rectal bleeding or bloody diarrhea are common and develop within 24 hours of the onset of pain. Ischemic colitis differs from mesenteric ischemia of the small bowel in that the pain is generally less severe and often located laterally, rectal bleeding is usually an earlier finding, and patients do not typically appear severely ill.[92] When more severe pain, peritonitis, fever, or systemic toxicity is present, colonic infarction with gangrene or perforation should be considered.

Diagnosis
No accurate laboratory markers exist to diagnose ischemic colitis. However, markers of hypoperfusion, such as the serum lactate and anion gap, may be increased in significant disease. Lower endoscopy often clarifies the diagnosis but is rarely performed in

the ED. Plain radiography may show signs of colonic dilation, but more specific signs such as thumbprinting of the bowel wall because of submucosal edema or hemorrhage were present in only 30% of patients with mesenteric infarction in one series.[93]

A CT scan with intravenous contrast is generally the first imaging test in patients presenting with suspected colonic ischemia. However, early scans may be normal, and findings such as bowel wall thickening are nonspecific. Pneumatosis may be seen in advanced disease. Angiography is rarely diagnostic. Often, blood flow has normalized at the time of the study and ischemia is rarely caused by large vessel occlusion.

Treatment

In cases of suspected nonocclusive ischemia, aggressive supportive care is the mainstay of therapy. Patients should receive intravenous fluids to improve perfusion, and cardiac status and oxygenation should be maximized. Bowel rest should be implemented, and nasogastric suction may be necessary if an ileus is present. Careful monitoring should be instituted to detect signs of clinical deterioration early.

In cases of suspected or documented infarction, aggressive supportive care is necessary, and broad-spectrum antibiotics should be initiated. A surgeon should be consulted for likely operative intervention, because bowel necrosis can lead to perforation, peritonitis, and sepsis.

Disposition

Patients with mild symptoms from a detectable, reversible cause such as extreme exercise may be managed on an outpatient basis if symptoms improve with treatment in the ED. However, the diagnosis of colonic ischemia is rarely confirmed in the ED, and disposition is generally based on the presenting clinical picture. Most patients do not ultimately require surgery, but all ill-appearing patients with suspected colonic ischemia should be hospitalized.

Radiation Proctocolitis

The gastrointestinal epithelium has a high cell turnover rate, making it susceptible to free radical injury from radiation therapy. As such, sloughed endothelium is not replaced at the normal rate, leading to ulcerations, edema, and inflammatory changes. Radiation proctocolitis can manifest either early (during or soon after completion of a course of radiation therapy), or late (usually months to years after therapy).

Acute radiation proctocolitis presents with abdominal pain, diarrhea, malaise, and bleeding. Tenesmus may be present if the rectum is involved. The diagnosis is made clinically based on the history of radiation therapy and the symptoms involved. Treatment is symptomatic, and should be decided in conjunction with the physician performing the radiation therapy.

Chronic radiation proctocolitis may present with a variety of symptoms. In patients with ulcerative disease, these include pain, bleeding, and tenesmus. In cases of stricture formation, patients may present with constipation, decreased stool caliber, or signs of partial or complete obstruction. Patients may also present with fistula disease or signs of pancolitis. Some patients with fistula disease or stricture ultimately require surgery, but this is often not performed emergently. Treatment of chronic radiation proctocolitis is symptomatic and based on the presenting clinical picture.

SUMMARY

Appendicitis, diverticulitis, and colitis are diseases that commonly present to the ED. Acute appendicitis may present classically, but often the diagnosis is difficult because of variable symptoms and examination findings, as well as the lack of a perfect laboratory or imaging test. Diverticulitis usually presents with left-sided abdominal symptoms, but right-sided disease occurs in a minority of patients and should be considered in younger patients and those of Asian descent. Colitis may be caused by IBD, infection, ischemia, or radiation therapy. The treatment of colitis varies based on its cause.

REFERENCES

1. Korner H, Sondenaa K, Soreide JA, et al. Incidence of acute nonperforated and perforated appendicitis: age-specific and sex-specific analysis. World J Surg 1997;21:313–7.
2. Addiss DG, Shaffer N, Fowler BS, et al. The epidemiology of appendicitis and appendectomy in the United States. Am J Epidemiol 1990;132:910–25.
3. Buschard K, Kjaeldfaard A. Investigation and analysis of the position, fixation, length, and embryology of the vermiform appendix. Acta Chir Scand 1973;139: 293–8.
4. Bollinger R, Barbas A, Bush E, et al. Biofilms in the large bowel suggest an apparent function of the human vermiform appendix. J Theor Biol 2007;249:826.
5. Collins DC. 71,000 human appendix specimens. A final report summarizing forty years of study. Am J Proctol 1963;14:365–81.
6. Hadl H, Quah H, Maw A. A missing tongue stud: an unusual appendicular foreign body. Int Surg 2006;91:87.
7. Bickell NA, Aufses AH, Rojas M, et al. How time affects the risk of rupture in appendicitis. J Am Coll Surg 2006;202(3):401–6.
8. Wagner JM, McKinney WP, Carpenter JL. Does this patient have appendicitis? JAMA 1996;276:1592.
9. Guidry SP, Poole GV. The anatomy of appendicitis. Am Surg 1994;60(10):68–71.
10. McBurney C. Experience with early operative interference in cases of disease of the vermiform appendix. NY Med J 1889;50:676.
11. Andersson RE, Hugander AP, Ghazi SH, et al. Diagnostic value of disease history, clinical presentation, and inflammatory parameters of appendicitis. World J Surg 1999;23:133–40.
12. Mourad J, Elliott JP, Erickson L, et al. Appendicitis in pregnancy: new information that contradicts long-held clinical beliefs. Am J Obstet Gynecol 2000;182:1027–9.
13. Hadjati H, Kazerooni T. Location of the appendix in the gravid patient: a re-evaluation of the established concept. Int J Gynaecol Obstet 2003;81:245–7.
14. Andersson RE, Lambe M. Incidence of appendicitis during pregnancy. Int J Epidemiol 2001;30:1281–5.
15. McGory ML, Zingmond DS, Tillou A, et al. Negative appendectomy in pregnant women is associated with a substantial risk of fetal loss. J Am Coll Surg 2007; 205(4):534–40.
16. Cohen-Kerem R, Railton C, Oren D, et al. Pregnancy outcome following non-obstetric surgical intervention. Am J Surg 2005;190(3):467–73.
17. Rappaport WD, Peterson M, Stanton C. Factors responsible for the high perforation rate seen in early childhood appendicitis. Am Surg 1989;55:602.
18. Golladay ES, Sarrett JR. Delayed diagnosis in pediatric appendicitis. South Med J 1988;81:38–42.
19. Cappendijk VC, Hazebroek FWJ. The impact of diagnostic delay on the course of acute appendicitis. Arch Dis Child 2000;83:64–6.
20. Kraemer M, Franke C, Ohmann C, et al. Acute appendicitis in late adulthood: incidence, presentation, and outcome. Results of a prospective multicenter acute abdominal pain study and a review of the literature. Arch Surg 2000;385:470–81.

21. Franz MG, Norman J. Increased morbidity of appendicitis with advancing age. Am Surg 1995;61(1):40–4.
22. Paranjape C, Dalia S, Pan J, et al. Appendicitis in the elderly: a change in the laparoscopic era. Surg Endosc 2007;21(5):198–201.
23. Flum DR, Steinberg SD, Sarkis AY, et al. Appendicitis in patients with acquired immunodeficiency syndrome. J Am Coll Surg 1997;184(5):481–6.
24. Crum-Cianflone N, Weekes J, Bavaro M. Appendicitis in HIV-infected patients during the era of highly active antiretroviral therapy. HIV Med 2008;9(6):421–6.
25. Cardall T, Glasser J, Guss D. Clinical value of the total white blood cell count and temperature in the evaluation of patients with suspected appendicitis. Acad Emerg Med 2004;11(10):1021–7.
26. Coleman C, Thompson JE, Bennion RS, et al. White blood cell count is a poor predictor of severity of disease in the diagnosis of appendicitis. Am Surg 1998; 64(10):983–5.
27. Kessler N, Cyteval C, Gallix B, et al. Appendicitis: evaluation of sensitivity, specificity, and predictive values of US, Doppler US, and laboratory findings. Radiology 2004;230:472–8.
28. Johansson EP, Rydh A, Riklund KA. Ultrasound, computed tomography, and laboratory findings in the diagnosis of appendicitis. Acta Radiol 2007;48:267–73.
29. Andersson RE. Meta-analysis of the clinical and laboratory diagnosis of appendicitis. Br J Surg 2004;91:28–37.
30. Rao PM, Rhea JT, Rao JA. Plain abdominal radiography in clinically suspected appendicitis: diagnostic yield, resource use, and comparison with CT. Am J Emerg Med 1999;17(4):325–8.
31. Terasawa T, Blackmore C, Bent S, et al. Systematic review: computed tomography and ultrasonography to detect acute appendicitis in adults and adolescents. Ann Intern Med 2004;141(7):537–46.
32. Jeffrey RB, Laing FC, Townsend MD. Acute appendicitis: sonographic criteria based on 250 cases. Radiology 1998;167:327–9.
33. Retenbacher T, Hollerweger A, Macheiner P, et al. Outer diameter of the vermiform appendix as a sign of acute appendicitis: evaluation at US. Radiology 2001;218:757–62.
34. Jeffrey RB, Jain KA, Nghiem HV. Sonographic diagnosis of acute appendicitis: interpretive pitfalls. Am J Roentgenol 1994;162:55–9.
35. Rao PM, Rhea JT, Novelline RA, et al. Effect of computed tomography of the appendix on treatment of patients and use of hospital resources. N Engl J Med 1998;338:141–6.
36. Lane ML, Liu DM, Huynh MD, et al. Suspected acute appendicitis: nonenhanced helical CT in 300 consecutive patients. Radiology 1999;213:341–6.
37. Anderson BA, Salem L, Flum DR. A systematic review of whether oral contrast is necessary for the computed tomography diagnosis of appendicitis in adults. Am J Surg 2005;190:474–8.
38. Hershko DD, Awad N, Fischer D, et al. Focused helical CT using rectal contrast material only as the preferred technique for the diagnosis of suspected acute appendicitis: a prospective, randomized, controlled study comparing three different techniques. Dis Colon Rectum 2007;50:107.
39. Rao PM, Rhea JT, Novelline RA. Helical CT combined with contrast material administered only through the colon for imaging of suspected appendicitis. Am J Roentgenol 1997;169(5):1275–80.
40. Pedrosa I, Levine D, Eyvazzadeh AD, et al. MR imaging evaluation of acute appendicitis in pregnancy. Radiology 2006;238:891–9.

41. Alvarado A. A practical score for the early diagnosis of acute appendicitis. Ann Emerg Med 1986;15(5):557–64.
42. McKay R, Shepherd J. The use of the clinical scoring system by Alvarado in the decision to perform computed tomography for acute appendicitis in the ED. Am J Emerg Med 2007;25(5):489–93.
43. Andersen BR, Kallehave FL, Andersen HK. Antibiotics versus placebo for prevention of postoperative infection after appendectomy. Cochrane Database Syst Rev 2003;2:CD001439, 1–73.
44. Dominguez EP, Sweeney JF, Choi YU. Diagnosis and management of diverticulitis and appendicitis. Gastroenterol Clin North Am 2006;35:367–91.
45. Eriksson S, Granstrom L. Randomized controlled trial of appendectomy versus antibiotic therapy for acute appendicitis. Br J Surg 1995;82(2):166–9.
46. Loffeld RJ, Van Der Putten AB. Diverticular disease of the colon and concomitant abnormalities in patients undergoing endoscopic evaluation of the large bowel. Colorectal Dis 2002;4:189–92.
47. Parks TG. Natural history of diverticular disease of the colon: a review of 521 cases. Br Med J 1969;4:639–42.
48. Aldoori WH, Giovannucci EL, Rimm EB, et al. Prospective study of physical activity and the risk of symptomatic diverticular disease in men. Gut 1995;36: 276–82.
49. Aldoori WH, Giovannucci EL, Rockett HR, et al. A prospective study of dietary fiber types and symptomatic diverticular disease in men. J Nutr 1998;128: 714–9.
50. Farrell RJ, Farrell JJ, Morrin MM. Diverticular disease in the elderly. Gastroenterol Clin 2001;30(2):475–96.
51. Stollman NH, Raskin JB. Diverticular disease of the colon. Lancet 2004;363: 631–9.
52. Mimura A, Emanuel A, Kamm A. Pathophysiology of diverticular disease. Best Pract Res Clin Gastroenterol 2002;16(4):563–76.
53. Touzios JG, Dozois EJ. Diverticulosis and acute diverticulitis. Gastroenterol Clin North Am 2009;38(3):513–25.
54. Sugahara K, Mutu T, Morioka Y, et al. Diverticular disease of the colon in Japan: a review of 615 cases. Dis Colon Rectum 1984;27:531–7.
55. Reisman Y, Ziv Y, Kravrovitc D, et al. Diverticulitis: the effect of age and location on the course of disease. Int J Colorectal Dis 1999;14(4–5):250–4.
56. Ferzoco LB, Raptopoulos V, Sileu W. Acute diverticulitis. N Engl J Med 1998;338: 1521–6.
57. Tyau ES, Prystowsky JB, Joehl RJ, et al. Acute diverticulitis. A complicated problem in the immunocompromised patient. Arch Surg 1991;126(7):855–8.
58. Halligan S, Saunders B. Imaging diverticular disease. Best Pract Res Clin Gastroenterol 2002;16:595.
59. Johnson CD, Barker ME, Rice RP. Diagnosis of acute colonic diverticulitis: comparison of barium enema and CT. AJR Am J Roentgenol 1987;148:541.
60. Ambrosetti P, Grossholz M, Becker C, et al. Computed tomography in acute left colonic diverticulitis. Br J Surg 1997;84:532–4.
61. Shen SH, Chen JD, Tiu CM, et al. Colonic diverticulitis diagnosed by computed tomography in the ED. Am J Emerg Med 2002;20:551–7.
62. Chou YH, Chiou HJ, Tiu CM, et al. Sonography of acute right side colonic diverticulitis. Am J Surg 2001;181:122–7.
63. Kaiser AM, Jiang JK, Lake JP, et al. The management of complicated diverticulitis and the role of computed tomography. Am J Gastroenterol 2002;100:910–7.

64. Mueller MH, Glatzle J, Kasparek MS, et al. Long-term outcome of conservative treatment in patients with diverticulitis of the sigmoid colon. Eur J Gastroenterol Hepatol 2005;17:649–54.
65. Sarin S, Boulos PB. Long-term outcome of patients presenting with acute complications of diverticular disease. Ann R Coll Surg Engl 1994;76:117–20.
66. Sandler R, Loftus E Jr. Epidemiology of inflammatory bowel disease. In: Sartor R, Sandborn W, editors. Kirsner's inflammatory bowel diseases. 6th edition. Philadelphia: Saunders; 2004. p. 245–62.
67. Ahmad T, Satsangi J, McGovern D, et al. Review article: the genetics of inflammatory bowel disease. Aliment Pharmacol Ther 2001;15:731–48.
68. Abraham C, Cho JH. Inflammatory bowel disease. N Engl J Med 2009;361: 2066–78.
69. Franceschi S, Panza E, Vecchia C, et al. Nonspecific inflammatory bowel disease and smoking. Am J Epidemiol 1987;125:445–52.
70. Lindberg E, Tysk C, Andersson K, et al. Smoking and inflammatory bowel disease. A case control study. Gut 1988;29:352–7.
71. Thoreson R, Cullen JJ. Pathophysiology of inflammatory bowel disease: an overview. Surg Clin North Am 2007;87:575–85.
72. Halme L, Paavola-Sakki P, Turunen U, et al. Family and twin studies in inflammatory bowel disease. World J Gastroenterol 2006;12:3668–72.
73. Tamboli CP. Current medical therapy for chronic inflammatory bowel diseases. Surg Clin North Am 2007;87:697–725.
74. Farmer RG, Hawk WA, Turnbull RB Jr. Clinical patterns in Crohn's disease: a statistical study of 615 cases. Gastroenterology 1975;68:627–35.
75. Stenson WF. Inflammatory bowel disease. In: Goldman L, Ausiello D, editors. Cecil medicine. 23rd edition. Philadelphia: Saunders Elsevier; 2008. p. 1042–9.
76. Hanauer SB, Present DH. The state of the art in the management of inflammatory bowel disease. Rev Gastroenterol Disord 2003;3:81–92.
77. Hanauer SB, Feagan BG, Lichtenstein GR, et al. Maintenance infliximab for Crohn's disease: the ACCENT 1 randomized trial. Lancet 2002;359:1541–9.
78. Lawson MM, Thomas AG, Akobeng AK. Tumour necrosis factor blocking agents for induction of remission in ulcerative colitis. Cochrane Database Syst Rev 2006; 3:CD005112.
79. Cheung O, Regueiro MD. Inflammatory bowel disease emergencies. Gastroenterol Clin North Am 2003;32:1269–88.
80. Yassinger S, Adelman R, Cantor D, et al. Association of inflammatory bowel disease and large vascular lesions. Gastroenterology 1976;71:844–6.
81. Aslam S, Musher DM. An update on diagnosis, treatment, and prevention of *Clostridium difficile*-associated disease. Gastroenterol Clin North Am 2006;35: 315–35.
82. Bartlett JG. Narrative review: the new epidemic of *Clostridium difficile*-associated enteric disease. Ann Intern Med 2006;145:758–64.
83. Bignardi GE. Risk factors for *Clostridium difficile* infection. J Hosp Infect 1998;40:1–15.
84. Carignan A, Allard C, Pepin J, et al. Risk of *Clostridium difficile* infection after perioperative antibacterial prophylaxis before and during an outbreak of infection due to a hypervirulent strain. Clin Infect Dis 2008;46:1838–43.
85. Centers for Disease Control and Prevention (CDC). Surveillance for community-associated *Clostridium difficile*—Connecticut 2006. MMWR Morb Mortal Wkly Rep 2008;57:340–3.
86. Akerlund T, Svenungsson B, Lagergren A, et al. Correlation of disease severity with fecal toxin levels in patients with *Clostridium difficile*-associated diarrhea

and distribution of PCR ribotypes and toxin yields in vitro of corresponding isolates. J Clin Microbiol 2006;44:353–8.

87. Manabe YC, Vinetz JM, Moore RD, et al. *Clostridium difficile* colitis: an efficient clinical approach to diagnosis. Ann Intern Med 1995;123:835–40.

88. Bartlett JG, Tedesco FJ, Shull S, et al. Symptomatic relapse after oral vancomycin therapy of antibiotic-associated pseudomembranous colitis. Gastroenterology 1980;78:431–4.

89. McFarland LV, Surawicz CM, Greenberg RN, et al. A randomized placebo-controlled trial of *Saccharomyces boulardii* in combination with standard antibiotics for *Clostridium difficile* disease. JAMA 1994;271:1913–8.

90. Zar FA, Bakkanagari SR, Moorthi KM, et al. A comparison of vancomycin and metronidazole for the treatment of *Clostridium difficile*-associated diarrhea, stratified by disease severity. Clin Infect Dis 2007;45:302–7.

91. Higgins PD, Davis KJ, Laine L. Systematic review: the epidemiology of ischaemic colitis. Aliment Pharmacol Ther 2004;19:729–38.

92. Reinus JF, Brandt LJ, Boley SJ. Ischemic diseases of the bowel. Gastroenterol Clin North Am 1990;19:319–43.

93. Smerud MJ, Johnson CD, Stephens DH. Diagnosis of bowel infarction: a comparison of plain films and CT scans in 23 cases. Am J Roentgenol 1990;154:99–103.

Foreign Bodies in the Gastrointestinal Tract and Anorectal Emergencies

Kenton L. Anderson, MD[a],*, Anthony J. Dean, MD[b]

KEYWORDS

• Foreign bodies • Gastrointestinal tract • Endoscopic surgery
• Anorectal emergency

FOREIGN BODIES IN THE GASTROINTESTINAL TRACT

In the United States, 1500 people die each year due to ingested foreign bodies (FBs).[1] Eighty percent of FB ingestions occur in young children who swallow small objects such as coins, toys, crayons, and ballpoint pen caps.[2,3] Accidental FBs in adults tend to be caused by meat and bones. The remaining cases are found primarily among edentulous adults, prisoners, and psychiatric patients, who often intentionally ingest objects such as toothbrushes, spoons, and razor blades; and who are also more likely to recurrently ingest FBs.[4–8] Wearing dentures is a significant risk factor in FB ingestion.[9,10] Dentures eliminate the tactile sensitivity of the palate so that small objects or incompletely masticated food boluses are inadvertently swallowed. Of the FBs brought to the attention of physicians (probably a small minority of all ingestions), 80% to 90% will pass through the gastrointestinal (GI) tract spontaneously; however, 10% to 20% will require endoscopic removal, and about 1% will require surgery.[11,12]

The GI tract can be divided into several regions in which presentation, clinical findings, and management of FBs is distinct. These regions include the oropharynx, esophagus, stomach and duodenum, small and large intestine, and rectum. In this article the relevant anatomy, clinical features, and management strategies for impacted FBs in each of these regions are discussed.

[a] Department of Emergency Medicine, Wilford Hall Medical Center, 2200 Bergquist Drive, Lackland AFB, San Antonio, TX 78236, USA
[b] Division of Emergency Ultrasonography, Department of Emergency Medicine, University of Pennsylvania Medical Center, 3400 Spruce Street, Philadelphia, PA 19104, USA
* Corresponding author.
E-mail address: kentonlanderson@gmail.com

Emerg Med Clin N Am 29 (2011) 369–400
doi:10.1016/j.emc.2011.01.009
0733-8627/11/$ – see front matter © 2011 Published by Elsevier Inc.

emed.theclinics.com

OROPHARYNGEAL FOREIGN BODIES

Most ingested FBs do not become impacted in the oropharynx. The most common exceptions are fish or chicken bones (**Fig. 1**), although any sharp or irregular object may become impacted.[13–16] These objects most often lodge in the soft tissue at the base of the tongue, but may also be found in other areas such as the tonsil or piriform sinus.[13] Minor lacerations and abrasions are common and self-limited. If the patient is drooling or is unable to tolerate oral intake of liquids, the clinician should be concerned about complete obstruction. Rarely, patients may also present with airway compromise. An unremoved FB may serve as a nidus for infection such as a retropharyngeal abscess, usually weeks later.[17]

Patients usually know exactly when the object became impacted. Typically they present to the Emergency Department (ED) with a FB sensation and odynophagia several hours after ingestion, and they may have attempted one or more home remedies such as drinking fluid, eating bread, or trying to grasp the object with their own fingers. Due to the sensory innervation by the vagus and glossopharyngeal nerves, patients are able to accurately lateralize and determine the level of a FB in this region (**Fig. 2**).[18] With larger objects the patient may also be drooling, retching, or vomiting.

Management of an oropharyngeal FB begins with an attempt at direct visualization. If this is possible, the FB can usually be removed using forceps or a hemostat. However, most FBs will have passed beyond the level of direct visualization and will require indirect laryngoscopy or fiberoptic nasopharyngoscopy. If an FB is identified, yet attempts at removal are unsuccessful, an ear/nose/throat consultation should be made.

More commonly, no FB can be identified. Indeed, less than 25% of patients with FB sensation after eating fish or chicken actually have an FB located by endoscopy.[19–21] Despite this low rate, endoscopy within 24 hours rather than imaging studies is the next logical step, because radiography alters management extremely rarely (in only 1.5% [4 of 267] in one series).[5,16,20,22,23]

If imaging modalities are indicated because of the ingestion of a radiopaque object, plain films are usually the first step.[13,16,24–26] Most radiopaque objects such as metal

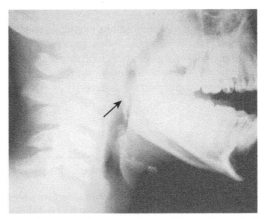

Fig. 1. A lateral neck radiograph demonstrating a chicken bone lodged in the pharynx with associated soft tissue swelling. The arrow identifies the bone. Plain radiography has poor diagnostic accuracy in identifying bones in the pharynx and esophagus. (*From* Munter DW. Esophageal foreign bodies. In: Roberts JR, Hedges JR, eds. Clinical Procedures in Emergency Medicine, 5th ed. Philadelphia: Elsevier, 2010; with permission.)

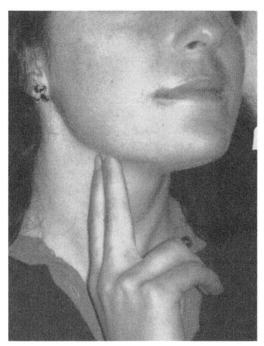

Fig. 2. Due to the innervation of the oropharynx and proximal esophagus, patients are able to correctly localize foreign bodies when they become lodged in these proximal areas of the GI tract. (*From* Munter DW. Esophageal foreign bodies. In: Roberts JR, Hedges JR, eds. Clinical Procedures in Emergency Medicine, 5th ed. Philadelphia: Elsevier, 2010; with permission.)

or glass should be visible. The visibility of fish bone depends on the fish species, location, and orientation; however, the majority are not seen on plain films, with much higher success in the hypopharynx than oropharynx.[13,19,25,27]

If plain films do not successfully locate an FB, an esophagogram with diluted barium or gastrografin can be performed in an attempt to outline the object.[22,23,28] Further radiographs with barium-impregnated cotton balls and xeroradiography may be useful.[5,23,29] Finally, computed tomography (CT) may identify fish or chicken bones missed on plain film.[13,19,30,31]

With the limited availability of prompt endoscopy at many times and in many EDs, there is likely to be a continued role for imaging studies in the initial assessment of these patients, even though most patients who present with an FB sensation will have no definitive findings at the conclusion of an extensive radiologic workup. At this point, because lacerations and abrasions may also cause an FB sensation and most serious complications are delayed, patients with a negative evaluation may be discharged home with strict return instructions and referral for endoscopy.[5]

ESOPHAGEAL FOREIGN BODIES
Overview

The esophagus is a common site for impaction of FBs that are accidentally or purposefully swallowed. Most patients will present with minor irritation and an FB sensation, others will have more severe symptoms, and rarely the impacted FB may result in a life-threatening airway obstruction. The mucosa of the esophagus does not tolerate retained FBs well. Over time edema, necrosis, then infection or perforation occur. Some retained FBs may become less symptomatic over time; however, retained esophageal FBs should be removed expeditiously, as prolonged impaction frequently results in severe complications. With the exception of distal esophageal coins (see later discussion), allowing entrapped foreign objects to pass spontaneously or dissolve in minimally symptomatic patients is not recommended.

Anatomy

The esophagus is a muscular tube that is continuous with the hypopharynx proximally and extends 18 to 25 cm distally to the gastroesophageal junction. It is divided anatomically into thirds: the proximal third consists of striated (voluntary) muscle, the distal third consists of smooth (involuntary) muscle, and the middle third is a mixture of the two. The proximal third has both somatic motor and sensory innervation through branches of the recurrent laryngeal nerve, similar to the oropharynx, which allows patients to localize proximal FBs accurately (see **Fig. 2**).[18]

There are 3 areas of physiologic narrowing along the adult esophagus where blunt FBs most commonly become impacted (**Fig. 3**). The first area is located posterior to the cricoid cartilage, at the level of the C-6 vertebra, where the esophagus begins with the upper esophageal "sphincter" (UES) or cricopharyngeus muscle. The UES is the most common site of impaction in pediatric patients (**Fig. 4**).[3,4,32] The second is at the level of T-4 where the distal aortic arch descends posterior to the mid-esophagus. Distally there is also an area of narrowing at the lower esophageal sphincter (LES). The LES is the narrowest point of the entire gastrointestinal tract in adults, and it is the location where most FBs become impacted (**Fig. 5**).[4,32] Patients with an anatomic abnormality or motor disturbance of the esophagus are more prone to entrapment of food or other objects, and will usually present with a history of chronic swallowing problems. Anatomic abnormalities include strictures, webs, rings, diverticula, and malignancies.[6,7] Motor disturbances are much rarer and include achalasia, scleroderma, diffuse esophageal spasm, or nutcracker esophagus.[6,7]

Epidemiology

Patients with retained esophageal FBs usually fall into 1 of 4 groups: pediatric, intentional adult ingestions, denture users, and adults with underlying esophageal

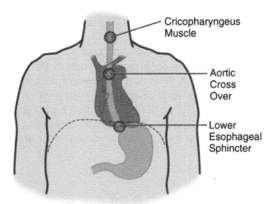

Fig. 3. The 3 anatomic areas of narrowing where esophageal FBs most commonly become impacted: the cricopharyngeus muscle, the aortic crossover, and the lower esophageal sphincter. (*From* Munter DW. Esophageal foreign bodies. In: Roberts JR, Hedges JR, eds. Clinical Procedures in Emergency Medicine, 5th ed. Philadelphia: Elsevier, 2010; with permission.)

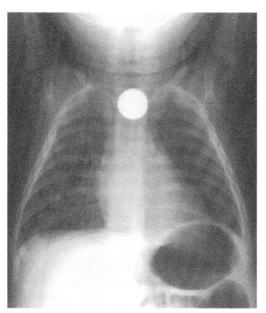

Fig. 4. Posteroanterior radiograph of an impacted esophageal coin at the level of the crico-pharyngeus muscle. This is the most common area of esophageal FB impaction in children. (*From* Munter DW. Esophageal foreign bodies. In: Roberts JR, Hedges JR, eds. Clinical Procedures in Emergency Medicine, 5th ed. Philadelphia: Elsevier, 2010; with permission.)

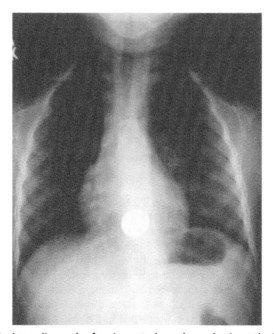

Fig. 5. Posteroanterior radiograph of an impacted esophageal coin at the level of the lower esophageal sphincter. This is the most common area of esophageal FB impaction in adults. (*From* Munter DW. Esophageal foreign bodies. In: Roberts JR, Hedges JR, eds. Clinical Procedures in Emergency Medicine, 5th ed. Philadelphia: Elsevier, 2010; with permission.)

pathology. Pediatric patients account for approximately 80% of retained esophageal FBs, with the peak incidence at 18 to 48 months.[11,22,23,33–39] These small children habitually place objects in their mouths and can inadvertently swallow or aspirate them. The most commonly ingested objects in this age group are coins,[5,6,36,40,41] but other small objects such as buttons and marbles are also commonly ingested.[5,11,33,36,42] Unusual or multiple FBs should alert the examining clinician to possible child abuse.[43] Patients with esophageal dysmotility are prone to impaction from even relatively small pieces of swallowed food.[5–7,42]

Complications

Many complications may arise from esophageal FBs, ranging from superficial mucosal injury to vocal cord paralysis, perforation, and life-threatening conditions such as retropharyngeal abscess and vascular injuries such as aortoesophageal fistula.[44–50] Complications are more likely with FBs that have been impacted for more than 24 hours and with sharp objects.[5,33] Most mortality from ingested FBs occurs because of complications from esophageal perforation.[1,23]

Presentation

Patients with an impacted esophageal FB usually present shortly after ingesting the object, and most adults and older children are able to provide a clear history of ingestion. The object is easily localized by the patient when it is located at the UES and upper third of the esophagus; however, when the object is located lower in the esophagus the patient may only have vague symptoms such as dysphagia, odynophagia, or a dull FB sensation that is not easily localizable. FBs at the UES may also cause gagging or vomiting.[42] Drooling or the inability to handle secretions suggests complete esophageal obstruction.[6]

Patients in the 18- to 48-month-old age group, which has the highest incidence of FB ingestion, may present with carers who are unable to provide a history of FB ingestion. A high index of suspicion is required, and clinicians should inquire about an object that was in the patient's mouth that "disappeared" or a transient history of coughing or gagging. An estimated 40% of FB ingestions in children are unwitnessed, and up to 50% never develop symptoms.[51–56] Symptoms are nonspecific and include irritability, poor feeding, vomiting, coughing, wheezing, behavioral changes, and failure to thrive.[6,14,51,57–59] Children are more likely than adults to have respiratory symptoms from an impacted esophageal FB, as their airway is softer and more compressible. Additional respiratory symptoms may include stridor, airway obstruction, and cardiac arrest.

Evaluation

When evaluating for an esophageal FB, the physical examination is usually normal.[6,7] As noted, drooling suggests complete obstruction.[6] Subcutaneous emphysema in the cervical region suggests esophageal perforation. Airway symptoms should be sought in children due to their softer and more compliant trachea.[32]

Because many patients are asymptomatic, and physical examination is usually normal, there should be a low threshold for obtaining plain radiographs.[5] Plain films usually detect radiopaque FBs such as glass and metal, but most ingested objects (food bolus, toothpick, aluminum beverage pull-tab, and many fish and chicken bones) are missed by plain films.[20,21,25,26,30,60] Because FBs preferentially become lodged at the UES in children and at the LES in adults, they will appear posterior to the tracheal air column on lateral view in children and beyond it in adults. Flat FBs are typically found to be lying in the frontal plane (see **Figs. 4** and **5**).[61]

For most patients with a food bolus impaction a plain film prior to propulsive therapy is prudent, as it may identify identification of a sharp fragments or other unanticipated disease in the thorax. If the diagnosis is in doubt, a contrast esophagogram may be obtained, although this decision is likely to make esophagoscopy much more difficult if it is required and is not without risk of aspiration, especially with high-grade obstructions.[60,62,63] Esophagograms are also limited by high reported false-positive (19%–26%) and false-negative (40%–55%) rates.[21,64] Barium is preferred to gastrografin unless there is risk of esophageal perforation, because it is much less toxic if aspirated. Newer nonionic solutions have been shown to be safe in either situation, but they are costly and may not be widely available.[7,42] Consultation with an endoscopist, if available, is prudent before performing a contrast swallowing study.

An increasingly widely available alternative to both esophagograms and esophagoscopy is noncontrast CT of the neck and mediastinum (**Fig. 6**).[19,62,65] In one study, CT found all impacted bony FBs located by endoscopy. In this study there was one false positive caused by esophageal calcification, and no false negatives.[30] Another study also demonstrated 100% sensitivity of CT for localizing esophageal FBs as well as demonstrating that CT may provide the additional benefit of identifying complications, including an esophageal perforation that was not seen with barium swallow.[31] A different study demonstrated this same benefit by locating an aortoesophageal fistula 7 days after the ingestion of a bone splinter.[66]

Management

The management strategy for esophageal FBs depends on their nature, location, and duration of impaction. As a general rule esophageal FBs are either urgently removed or seen to have passed into the stomach prior to patient discharge.

Esophagoscopy

Esophagoscopy is the best available technique for retrieval of most esophageal FBs, and allows for evaluation of secondary injury.[23,39] In many EDs the availability of esophagoscopy is limited, in which case other techniques described in this article may be needed. Clinical indications for immediate esophagoscopy include airway

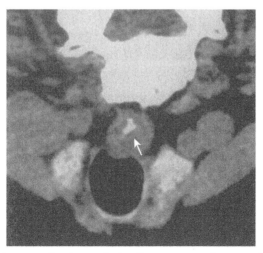

Fig. 6. Computed tomography demonstrates the presence of an esophageal FB (*arrow*). (*From* Munter DW. Esophageal foreign bodies. In: Roberts JR, Hedges JR, eds. Clinical Procedures in Emergency Medicine, 5th ed. Philadelphia: Elsevier, 2010; with permission.)

compromise (including stridor, coughing, or wheezing), evidence of obstruction or any FB that has been impacted for more than 24 hours, or if signs of perforation are present.[5,39,40,67] Sharp or elongated FBs should be removed endoscopically, as there is a high risk of perforation (**Fig. 7**). Button batteries that cannot be passed into the stomach with swallowed water require immediate endoscopic removal. Patients with signs of obstruction should be encouraged to sit in whatever position is most comfortable for them (upright in most cases) and should be allowed to suction their own secretions. For obtunded or gagging patients, placement of a nasogastric tube in the esophagus above the obstruction may succeed in draining pooled secretions.

If esophagoscopy is not immediately available, the patient should be transferred to a facility where an experienced endoscopist is on hand. The success rate for the endoscopic removal of a sharp object is between 94% and 100%.[23,39,68] Endoscopy should be performed under procedural sedation to prevent patient movements that may result in perforation or loss of the object into the patient's airway. Failed endoscopic removal will require removal in the operating room.

Button batteries

Button batteries contain an alkaline solution that can rapidly cause liquefaction necrosis of the esophageal mucosa (**Fig. 8**). Perforation may occur within 4 hours, with catastrophic complications such as esophagotracheal or esophagoaortic fistula.[49,69] If a child can cooperate, an attempt should be made to pass the battery into the stomach with swallowed water. Endoscopic removal of a button battery is challenging because of their smooth edges, and a collective review demonstrated that endoscopic removal failed 62.5% of the time.[70] When removal fails, the battery can be pushed distally to the stomach where it will likely pass through the gastrointestinal tract without difficulty.[70–73] Management of button batteries in the stomach is

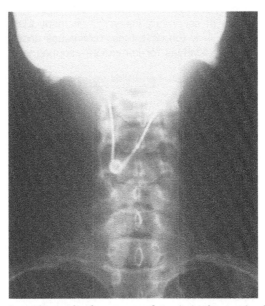

Fig. 7. Posteroanterior radiograph of on open safety pin in the proximal esophagus. Sharp FBs lodged in the esophagus should be removed endoscopically. (*From* Munter DW. Esophageal foreign bodies. In: Roberts JR, Hedges JR, eds. Clinical Procedures in Emergency Medicine, 5th ed. Philadelphia: Elsevier, 2010; with permission.)

described in the section "Stomach and duodenal foreign bodies." Follow-up with barium swallow studies to evaluate for a fistula or stricture is usually recommended at 24 to 36 hours and 10 to 14 days after the battery has been removed from the esophagus.[23] Antibiotics are recommended when significant mucosal damage is present.

Coins

As with other esophageal FBs, coins tend to lodge at the level of the cricopharyngeus in children and the LES in adults (see **Figs. 4** and **5**).[23] In young adults, accidental coin ingestion has become more common, due to a popular college drinking game called "Quarters."[5] Because coins in either the GI tract or the airway may cause similar symptoms, plain radiographs should be taken to determine the location of the coin.[74–77] Mouth to anus films are indicated in the pediatric population to determine if more than one FB is present.[5]

Coins lodged in the proximal or mid esophagus should undergo prompt extraction to avoid complications that are correlated with impaction times of longer than 24 hours.[33,78–80] Although some authorities state that an asymptomatic patient with a coin in the distal esophagus may be given 12 to 24 hours to allow the coin to pass into the stomach, this approach may not be practical in settings with limited and unreliable follow-up.[34–36,81,82] In most cases, impacted esophageal coins should be removed expeditiously, usually by endoscopy or, in children, by bougienage.[5,68,81] The catheter technique for removal of esophageal coins and other foreign objects was widely practiced in the era prior to the wide availability of endoscopy (**Fig. 9**). Many complications can ensue, including esophageal perforation, laceration, regurgitation with or without aspiration, and airway obstruction. These risks are compounded by most emergency physicians' lack of experience or familiarity with this techniques and the fact that more than 24 hours' impaction, one of the indications for intervention, is itself a contraindication to Foley extraction. The technique may still be useful in remote or austere settings where endoscopy is not available. If it is undertaken, all precautions should be taken to protect the airway. The Foley catheter should be placed orally rather than nasally to ensure that the coin is not pulled into the nasopharynx, and the patient should be placed in deep Trendelenburg to minimize the risk of aspiration. Fluoroscopy may make this procedure safer.[83,84]

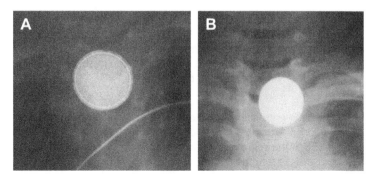

Fig. 8. (*A, B*) Two examples of button batteries lodged in the proximal esophagus. The appearance of button batteries on plain radiographs may mimic that of coins. Button batteries may cause liquefaction necrosis and perforation of the esophageal wall within 4 hours, and expedited removal should be arranged. (*From* Munter DW. Esophageal foreign bodies. In: Roberts JR, Hedges JR, eds. Clinical Procedures in Emergency Medicine, 5th ed. Philadelphia: Elsevier, 2010; with permission.)

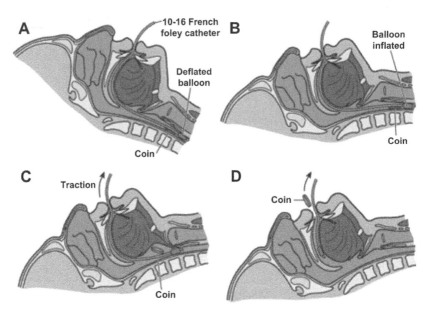

Fig. 9. (*A–D*) Technique for Foley catheter extraction of esophageal FBs. (*A*) The catheter is inserted orally into the esophagus distal to the coin. (*B*) The balloon is inflated. Gentle traction moves the coin proximally. (*C*) The coin is moved past the glottis. (*D*) The coin is brought into the mouth and grasped by the operator. This procedure has many complications and should only be performed where endoscopy is not available. Fluoroscopy may make the procedure safer. (*From* Munter DW. Esophageal foreign bodies. In: Roberts JR, Hedges JR, eds. Clinical Procedures in Emergency Medicine, 5th ed. Philadelphia: Elsevier, 2010; with permission.)

Bougienage, which has been successfully used to dislodge impacted esophageal coins in children, attempts to blindly advance the coin into the stomach. This technique has been used effectively by emergency physicians in pediatric patients, with a greater than 95% success rate and few reported complications, and results in significant reductions in ED length of stay and costs.[38,85–88] However, the technique requires equipment that is not available in many EDs (a Hurst-type bougie in a variety of sizes), and has been reported in settings where the emergency physicians have received special training in centers that have developed extensive experience in the technique. Postprocedure films should be obtained to document coin location. Patients may be discharged home with instructions to obtain follow-up radiographs if the coin is not noted in the stool within a week. All adults should obtain follow-up to evaluate for an underlying esophageal disorder.[5]

Pharmacologic therapies

FBs that pass the LES are usually able to pass along the remainder of the GI tract without complication. Several pharmacologic therapies have been developed to aid a blunt or smooth FB at the LES to pass into the stomach. Some of these such as atropine, meperidine, and diazepam have been shown to have success rates lower than observation alone.[33,42] Papain was used in the past to dissolve impacted meat,[89] but this practice has been abandoned because it can also dissolve the esophageal mucosa, resulting in esophageal rupture.[90,91] Glucagon, nitroglycerin, nifedipine, and gas-forming agents have proved to be the most effective pharmacologic agents in the management of distal blunt esophageal FB impactions, and are discussed individually here. Anxiolysis and pain control are also an important aspect of FB management, and may account for some of the success of the other pharmacologic agents discussed.[92]

Glucagon

The action of glucagon is thought to result from relaxation of the smooth muscle found in the distal esophagus and a decrease in the LES resting pressure.[93] Glucagon has no effect on the striated muscle of the proximal esophagus, where children often have impacted FBs. The therapeutic dose is 0.25 to 2.0 mg administered intravenously.

A common side effect of glucagon, if administered too rapidly, is nausea and vomiting. This effect may be responsible for some of the drug's success in clearing obstruction[94]; however, there is a theoretical risk of rupture of an obstructed esophagus with vomiting, so slow injection over 1 to 2 minutes is recommended. Mild elevation of blood glucose may also occur, but blood glucose does not need to be monitored.

The onset of action is less than a minute and the effects last about 25 minutes. After administration, the patient should be sitting upright and should be encouraged to take a sip of water approximately 1 minute after injection to induce esophageal peristalsis. A second dose may be used if the first is not successful. Glucagon is often thought of as a first-line agent. Its success rate of less than 38% can be improved when combined with gas-forming agents or carbonated beverages.[95-97]

Nitroglycerin and nifedipine

Sublingual nitroglycerin and nifedipine have been used in a manner analogous to that of glucagon for the disimpaction of distal blunt esophageal FBs.[98-100] Nitroglycerin reduces distal esophageal spasm and contraction, and nifedipine relaxes the LES in a manner similar to glucagon. Either may be used in combination with glucagon, but nitroglycerin and nifedipine should not be used simultaneously. The therapeutic dose is 1 to 2 (0.4 μg) sublingual nitroglycerin tablets or 5 to 10 mg of nifedipine. Patients with impacted esophageal FBs may be dehydrated because of an inability to swallow, and may be extremely sensitive to these agents, placing them at risk of iatrogenic hypotension. Intravenous access with a widely patent line sufficient for volume resuscitation should be placed, and the patient adequately hydrated before administration of these medications.

Gas-forming agents

Gas-forming agents and carbonated beverages have been used successfully for the treatment of distal esophageal food impactions. These solutions produce carbon dioxide, which is thought to distend the esophagus, relaxing the LES, and pushing the FB distally into the stomach.[96,101,102] Their use may increase the success of other spasmolytic agents.[101,103] Solutions described in the literature include a combination of 15 mL tartaric acid (solution of 18.7 g/100 mL water) followed immediately by 15 mL of sodium bicarbonate (10 g/100 mL water) or 1.5 to 3 g of tartaric acid dissolved in 15 mL of water followed by 2 to 3 g of sodium bicarbonate in 15 mL of water.[96,101] Commercially available gas-forming granules have also been used successfully.[104] Carbonated beverages (100 mL) may also work, and are more likely to be readily available in the ED.[97,102] Gas-forming agents should not be used if the FB has been impacted for more than 6 hours; if the patient is complaining of chest pain suggestive of esophageal injury; or if there is concern for obstruction, as there have been rare reports of esophageal perforation.[96,101,105]

If the patient has improvement of symptoms after pharmacologic intervention, a postprocedure radiograph or contrast study may be obtained to confirm passage into the stomach. Adult patients may be discharged home after successful disimpaction of an esophageal FB, but they should have close follow-up, as the majority will have an underlying esophageal disorder.[23] Patients who have had an esophageal FB dislodged by any method should be instructed to return to the ED with any chest or abdominal pain, persistent vomiting, hematemesis, difficulty swallowing, or shortness of breath.[96]

STOMACH AND DUODENAL FOREIGN BODIES

The vast majority of FBs that enter the stomach pass through the entire GI tract uneventfully. Objects longer than 5 cm may have difficulty negotiating the tight curve of the duodenum, and objects larger than 2 cm in diameter may have difficulty passing the pylorus or ileocecal valve.[106,107] Less than 1% of FBs that enter the stomach cause perforation of the bowel[108]; however, some investigators describe an intestinal perforation rate of 35% with sharp objects (usually at the ileocecal valve) whereas others, especially in the pre-endoscopic era, reported much lower rates.[78,109]

Most patients with an FB in the stomach are asymptomatic on presentation. Symptoms from an FB in the stomach may include pain, nausea, vomiting, hematemesis, or fever, and usually are secondary to a complication such as bleeding, obstruction, or perforation. Infants may present with failure to thrive. In young children, the symptoms that the patient is experiencing may be the first suggestion that an FB was ingested if the parents did not witness the event. Because the most common management of blunt FBs in the stomach is serial plain films over a period of weeks, a patient with a known FB may return to the ED with new symptoms or with asymptomatic failure of the object to pass.

Management of the patient with an FB in the stomach or duodenum varies depending on the nature of the FB and the patient's symptoms. Emergent endoscopy is a high priority if objects are long (>5 cm), of large diameter (>2 cm), or sharp, especially needles or toothpicks.[5,40,67,110] Small blunt objects can be observed and followed with serial radiographs.[6] If an object remains in the stomach for more than 7 days, the patient should be referred to a gastroenterologist for removal. If a patient becomes symptomatic, the object should be removed. Button batteries and drug packets require special attention and are discussed further.

Button Batteries in the Stomach

Button batteries should be followed with daily radiographs. Up to 85% will pass through the entire GI tract within 72 hours.[69,81] A button battery should be removed endoscopically if it remains in the stomach for more than 36 to 48 hours or if the patient becomes symptomatic. H2 blockers have been suggested to decrease the stomach acid reaction with the battery, but no benefit from this therapy has been confirmed.[69] Once past the duodenum, FB are no longer endoscopically accessible. Radiographs are needed only every 3 to 4 days to document progression if the FB has not been identified in the stool. A button battery that fails to pass or becomes symptomatic must be removed surgically. Although extremely rare, toxic serum concentrations of mercury have been reported, especially if the integrity of the battery (as determined by history or radiograph) has been disrupted, and may require chelation therapy.[69,111–113]

Illicit Drug Ingestion

Drug packets are ingested intentionally by "drug packers" and "drug stuffers." The preparation and quantity of drug ingested by these 2 groups typically have characteristic differences.[114,115] Drug packers are usually smugglers who ingest large quantities of drugs that have been carefully packaged to withstand transit through the GI tract.[116] Condoms and toy balloons wrapped in multiple layers have been the packaging material used most frequently; however, more precisely crafted wrappers have been reported in recent years.[111,116–118] Cocaine and heroin are the most commonly packed drugs, although other drugs are smuggled using this method as well.[119] Body packers may carry up to 1 kg of drug divided into 50 to 100 individual packets, although more than 200 packets have been reported.[119–121] Each packet contains a lethal dose of drug.[116,119,122,123] Drug stuffers are typically drug dealers or users who quickly ingest drug that has been loosely wrapped in plastic, foil, or poorly sealed containers while being pursued by law enforcement officials. Although the quantity of drug ingested by drug stuffers is typically much less than that of drug packers, the packaging is more likely to leak and cause symptoms. On rare occasion, the amount of drug ingested by a drug stuffer may be a lethal dose.

Both body packers and stuffers may present to the ED with a toxicologic emergency or under the custody of law enforcement officials wanting medical assessment of the patient and possible drug retrieval for evidence. Body packers may also present with bowel obstruction. "Body packer syndrome" should be considered in any recent international traveler who presents to the ED with seizures or a toxidrome consistent with illicit drug overdose.[123] Patient history is often unreliable, but should focus on the type and quantity of drug ingested as well as the nature of the packaging. History and physical examination findings to suggest a toxidrome should be sought. Evaluation should include plain radiography, which will demonstrate 85% to 90% of ingested drug packets but is less likely to identify small numbers of drug packets.[111,116,119] CT or barium-enhanced radiography may be used when plain films are not diagnostic.[124,125] A drug toxicology screen may be helpful in identifying the substance ingested if the patient is symptomatic. In asymptomatic patients, testing has low sensitivity, and positive tests may be unrelated to the packed substance.[126]

Body packers and stuffers who present with a toxicologic emergency should be treated accordingly. All drug stuffers should immediately be placed on continuous cardiac monitoring with large-bore intravenous access. Any sign of cocaine toxicity requires emergent transport of the patient to the operating room.[119] Intravenous benzodiazepines should be used liberally to control sympathomimetic symptoms, hypertension, or seizures. Hypertonic sodium bicarbonate and lidocaine may be used for ventricular dysrhythmias, and phentolamine or sodium nitroprusside may be used for hypertension. A more detailed discussion of the management of cocaine toxicity can be found elsewhere, and consultation with a medical toxicologist may be helpful.[119,127] Heroin leakage in body packers is less commonly fatal with naloxone, airway protection, and respiratory support as needed. In the asymptomatic body packer, it is reasonable to administer activated charcoal (1 g/kg) and perform continuous whole bowel irrigation with polyethylene glycol. Irrigation should continue in the intensive care unit until there is passage of clear polyethylene glycol solution. CT may be performed to verify passage of all packets.[119] Asymptomatic body stuffers may be treated with activated charcoal and observation. Whole bowel irrigation is warranted with drug intoxication in body stuffers as well.[128]

FOREIGN BODIES OF THE SMALL AND LARGE INTESTINE

Once in the small intestine, the most common impaction point is the ileocecal valve, followed by the hepatic and splenic flexures. Sharp objects tend to turn so that the blunt end leads and the sharp end trails.[5] Management of sharp FBs in the intestine includes daily radiographs to document progression of the FB. If there is no distal progression over a 3-day period or if the patient becomes symptomatic, emergent surgical consultation should be obtained.[5]

RECTAL FOREIGN BODIES

A wide variety of rectal FBs as well as complications from retained FBs have been reported. Anorectal FBs may infrequently be the result of an orally ingested sharp object that becomes impacted; however, the majority are the result of objects that are inserted through the anal canal.[6,129] Sharp ingested FBs usually present with symptoms of impaction such as bleeding, perforation, or abscess. The patient does not usually remember the ingestion and the object is identified during surgery.

Most rectal FBs have been inserted deliberately by the patient or a sexual partner. Objects inserted for sexual stimulation are typically blunt, and often resemble a penis in size and shape.[130–135] Repeated insertion of rectal FBs results in increasingly lax rectal tone, which allows patients to insert progressively larger objects that may be more difficult to remove. There are reports of psychiatric patients inserting sharp FBs to injure the clinician performing a digital rectal examination.[32] Assault victims may present with retained objects or fragments that may be blunt or sharp. Drug users may hide drugs or drug paraphernalia in their rectum, and prisoners have been found to conceal weapons in their rectum. Similar to ingested objects, inserted FBs may cause complications, but they are more frequently brought to the clinician's attention because of an inability to remove the object.

An accurate history may be impeded by the patient's embarrassment, which is also responsible for delays in presentation.[136] Fabricated histories are not uncommon, but gastrointestinal symptoms such as rectal or abdominal pain, decreased bowel movements, or bloody stools may signal real complications. The physician should seek an accurate history in a nonjudgmental and supportive manner, obtaining information about the substance, size, and shape of the object, duration of impaction, attempts at removal, and any symptoms that have occurred since insertion. The patient should be questioned regarding the possibility of assault.[132]

Abnormalities in vital signs and abdominal findings suggesting perforation or obstruction should be sought.[136] An examination of the anus followed by a digital rectal examination or anoscopy may reveal the FB location or signs of trauma. If there is the possibility of a sharp object, digital rectal examination should be replaced with anoscopy or may be delayed pending radiography. Plain radiographs are indicated in almost all cases except those that have clinical indications for CT, obviating the need for plain films. Air-filled objects such as plastic bottles may appear as a gas pattern in the shape of the FB. Rectal contrast can be given to outline radiolucent FBs. Free air and signs of obstruction should be sought.

Management of a rectal FB depends on the location and nature of the object. Rectal FBs are classified by location into 2 categories: low-lying and high-lying. Low-lying FBs are located within the rectal ampulla, are usually palpable on a digital rectal examination, and can often be removed by an emergency physician. High-lying FBs are located proximal to the rectosigmoid junction and require sigmoidoscopy for removal, often under general anesthesia.[6,137] These FBs are often long straight objects that are unable to navigate the curvature of the anorectal angle.[138] Removal of the FB by an emergency physician is contraindicated when there are signs of perforation, if sharp objects such as broken glass are present, or when the FB is high-lying. In these circumstances, or if attempts at removal by the emergency physician have failed, a surgical consultation is needed.

Before attempting to remove a rectal FB, premedication with a benzodiazepine calms the patient and relaxes the anal sphincter. However, procedural sedation may impede the patient's ability to assist with expulsion of the FB by performing the Valsalva maneuver.[132] A perianal block using local infiltration of 1% lidocaine and 0.5% bupivacaine will allow greater dilation of the anal sphincter.[136,139] The patient may be placed in the Sims, knee-chest, or lithotomy position during the extraction. The most appropriate position is determined by the character of the particular FB being removed. If the lithotomy position is used, the clinician may use suprapubic pressure to assist in expulsion of the FB.

Several methods for removal have been described. The simplest is to use suprapubic pressure from above the object while the examiner grasps the object with a finger from below.[139] If the FB has an accessible edge, an instrument such as a forceps may be used to grasp and remove the object under direct visualization with an anoscope or Parks retractor.[139] Most FBs in the rectum do not have a convenient edge to grasp, and attempts to withdraw them may be made using a Foley catheter or endotracheal tube with the balloon inflated beyond the object. The stiffness of an endotracheal tube allows passage past the object, but might increase the risk of perforation. If a Foley is employed, the stiffness of a fairly large (20–26 French) 3-way catheter with a 30-cc balloon is required. Hollow objects such as jars or bottles create a vacuum as they are pulled distally in the rectum, making removal difficult. In these cases, the Foley or endotracheal tube with its tip beyond the object can relieve the vacuum, if necessary with the assistance of gently insufflated air (**Fig. 10**). Many other techniques for

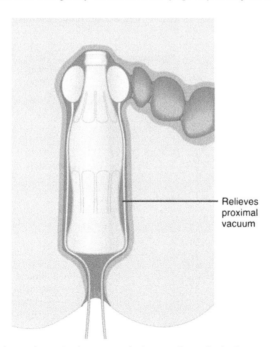

Relieves proximal vacuum

Fig. 10. Using a Foley catheter in the removal of a rectal FB. The balloon is placed proximally to the foreign object and inflated. More than one catheter may be used. The use of a Foley catheter or an endotracheal tube may be especially useful in the removal of hollow objects such as jars or bottles, so that the vacuum created by pulling on these objects is relieved. (*From* Coates WC. Anorectal Procedures. In: Roberts JR, Hedges JR, eds. Clinical Procedures in Emergency Medicine, 5th ed. Philadelphia: Elsevier, 2010; with permission.)

removing FBs from the rectum have been described, but are beyond the scope of this article, and should be reviewed in standard texts of emergency medicine procedures.

Serious complications from FB removal include deep mucosal tears, hemorrhage, and perforation. Even after an easy extraction, flexible sigmoidoscopy with or without plain radiography has been recommended for all patients. Observation with serial abdominal examinations may also be required.[136,137] Patients with symptoms or signs of perforation should be observed even after a normal sigmoidoscopic examination. Discharge instructions should include strict return precautions and education regarding symptoms of bleeding, perforation, or infection.

ANORECTAL EMERGENCIES

Anorectal disorders are commonly encountered in the ED setting. While the minority is life-threatening, there are many conditions that cause considerable discomfort. An understanding of anorectal anatomy is essential to understanding the disease processes that occur in this region. This section focuses on diseases that are commonly encountered or may require emergent management.

Anatomy

The anorectum is the terminal portion of the GI tract. The rectum is continuous prox-imally with the sigmoid colon and distally with the anal canal (**Fig. 11**). The flexure of the rectosigmoid junction lies anterior to the S3 vertebra. The rectum, about 15 cm in length, lies on the curved anterior surface of the sacrum and coccyx. The dilated terminal portion of the rectum is where the accumulating fecal mass is held until

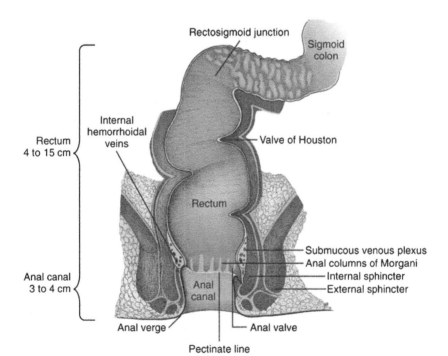

Fig. 11. Normal anatomy of the terminal gastrointestinal tract. (*From* Coates WC. Anorectal Procedures. In: Roberts JR, Hedges JR, eds. Clinical Procedures in Emergency Medicine, 5th ed. Philadelphia: Elsevier, 2010; with permission.)

defecation in the rectal ampulla. The rectal ampulla narrows and forms a 90° angle with the anal canal, which traverses the pelvic diaphragm consisting of the levator ani and coccygeus muscles.[140,141] The anus is 2.5 to 5 cm long. The anal canal is surrounded by the internal and external anal sphincters. The internal anal sphincter is a thickened extension of the circular smooth muscle layer of the rectum, and receives support from the levator ani muscles. It is innervated by parasympathetic fibers of the pelvic splanchnic nerves and, except during defecation, is tonically contracted. The external anal sphincter is a large broad circumferential band of voluntary muscle that is an extension of the levator ani and puborectalis muscles, and surrounds the entire length of the anal canal. It is innervated mainly by S4 fibers of the inferior rectal nerve. When feces or gas distends the rectal ampulla, the internal anal sphincter relaxes, requiring voluntary contraction of the external anal sphincter to prevent incontinence.[140]

The mucosa of the anal canal transitions from columnar epithelium at the dentate line to squamous epithelium at the orifice. Superior to the dentate line, folds of mucosa extend longitudinally to form the columns of Morgagni. Between these columns are anal crypts that contain mucus-forming glands responsible for lubricating the feces to facilitate evacuation. If these glands become obstructed, they can become infected and form abscesses or fistulae.[141]

The superior rectal artery supplies the rectum superior to the pectinate line, and the two inferior rectal arteries supply the anal canal. Superior to the pectinate line, blood drains from the internal rectal plexus through the superior rectal vein to the portal system. Distally the inferior rectal plexus drains through the inferior rectal veins to the caval system.[140]

The nerve supply superior to the pectinate line contains visceral fibers from the inferior hypogastric plexus and sympathetic trunk. Inferior to the pectinate line, somatic fibers from branches of the pudendal nerve are the reason thrombosed external hemorrhoids and anal fissures cause sharp localized pain.[140]

Hemorrhoids

The hemorrhoidal venous plexus is a series of vascular cushions composed of small blood vessels and smooth muscle fibers, which are thought to contribute to anal continence.[142] Symptoms occur when they become (for reasons that are disputed) engorged, inflamed, thrombosed, or prolapsed. As early as the third decade of life the connective tissue supporting the cushions begins to deteriorate, and venous distention may occur when there is interference with venous drainage. There is controversy as to whether the increased intra-abdominal pressure from constipation and/or straining at stool is sufficient to cause hemorrhoidal distension.[143–147] Pregnancy predisposes women to symptomatic hemorrhoids; however, most symptoms resolve after pregnancy.[142] Portal hypertension was long thought to be associated with symptomatic hemorrhoids; however, adult patients with portal hypertension have the same incidence of symptomatic hemorrhoids as normal controls.[148–150]

Patients may attribute any perianal condition to hemorrhoids, so a careful history and physical examination are important. Symptoms attributable to hemorrhoids can be divided into conditions associated with internal hemorrhoids and those associated with external hemorrhoids. Internal hemorrhoids are located in 3 major cushions (left lateral, right posterior, right anterior) above the pectinate line where there are no somatic sensory nerves, so they do not cause localized somatic pain. Patients often present with painless bleeding or prolapse. Internal hemorrhoids are classified into 4 degrees according to severity of prolapse. First-degree internal hemorrhoids protrude into the anal canal and may cause a sensation of fullness. Second-degree internal hemorrhoids prolapse externally during defecation, but spontaneously reduce after the bowel movement. Third-degree internal hemorrhoids may prolapse spontaneously or during a bowel movement and remain outside the anal canal until manually reduced. Spasm of the sphincter complex about the hemorrhoid may cause pain, which is relieved with reduction. Fourth-degree hemorrhoids are permanently prolapsed. Pain may induce sphincter spasm that can cause thrombosis, which may subsequently progress to gangrene. External hemorrhoids are located anywhere circumferentially along the anoderm and are innervated by cutaneous branches of the pudendal nerve and the sacral plexus. Symptoms of external hemorrhoids are usually related to acute pain with thrombosis or to pruritus.

Treatment of hemorrhoids should be pursued only if the patient is experiencing symptoms. Patients with discomfort from nonthrombosed external hemorrhoids or first-degree internal hemorrhoids may be treated conservatively with the W.A.S.H. regimen[151] (**Box 1**) and oral analgesics. Bathing in a tub of warm water is thought to relieve anal discomfort by relaxing the anal sphincter.[152] Application of ice cubes may also provide relief by reducing inflammation and causing vasoconstriction in the area. The average American diet consists of 8 to 15 g of fiber per day. A high-fiber diet consisting of 25 to 30 g of dietary fiber daily allows easier passage of stool, and with water intake should be prescribed to avoid constipation and promote regular well-formed stools that can be passed without straining. Stool softeners may be used acutely for patients with hard stools. Topical hydrocortisone may relieve bleeding from internal hemorrhoids or itching from external hemorrhoids; however, it should be used for limited periods to avoid atrophic changes in the skin.[143] Dibucaine ointment is available over the counter, and can be applied to relieve pain or itching. Topical nifedipine and nitrates have also been used successfully.[153,154]

Patients with second-degree or third-degree internal hemorrhoids may also benefit from the W.A.S.H. regimen; however, they should be referred to a surgeon for definitive management. Banding, sclerotherapy, photocoagulation, and laser ablation are definitive therapeutic options. If a fourth-degree hemorrhoid is thrombosed or gangrenous, the patient should undergo emergent hemorrhoidectomy.[143]

Acutely thrombosed external hemorrhoids may be excised in the ED. If not excised, the thrombus will begin to spontaneously resolve within 72 hours and will completely resolve in 10 to 14 days, so patients who present late or with diminishing pain should be managed conservatively.[142,155] Conversely, patients who present within 48 hours of symptom onset are most likely to benefit from excision.[155–157] When excising a thrombosed external hemorrhoid, a local anesthetic agent is applied either just under the skin surface of the hemorrhoid or in a field block under its base. After anesthesia, an elliptical piece of skin is excised and the underlying thrombus is removed (**Fig. 12**). If an area of skin is not excised, recurrence and/or skin tag formation are

---

Box 1
The W.A.S.H. Regimen

Warm water

Analgesic agents

Stool softeners

High-fiber diet

From Coates WC. Disorders of the anorectum. In: Marx JA, Hockberger RS, Walls RM. Rosen's Emergency Medicine: Concepts and Clinical Practice, 7th ed. Philadelphia: Elsevier, 2010; with permission.

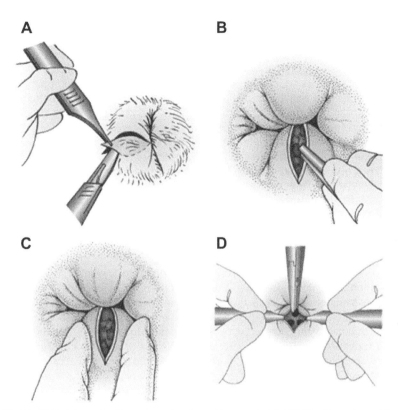

Fig. 12. (*A–D*) Excision of a thrombosed external hemorrhoid. (*A*) The thrombosed hemorrhoid is unroofed using an elliptical or triangular incision. The overlying skin is removed to prevent recurrence or skin tag formation. (*B*) Blood clots are removed with forceps or a small hemostat. (*C*) Multiple clots may be present. All clots should be removed. (*D*) Once the initial clot is removed, an assistant spreads the edges of the incision so that other clots that may be present can be identified and removed. (*From* Coates WC. Anorectal Procedures. In: Roberts JR, Hedges JR, eds. Clinical Procedures in Emergency Medicine, 5th ed. Philadelphia: Elsevier, 2010; with permission.)

more likely.[158,159] The skin margins are left open and dressed when bleeding is controlled, occasionally requiring the application of a hemostatic agent such as gelfoam. The patient should be instructed to avoid the use of toilet paper, and to wash with mild soap and water in the shower after bowel movements. Topical creams such as Preparation H or Anusol HC may provide some relief of anal discomfort. Antibiotics are not indicated.

Anal Fissures

Anal fissures are the most common cause of painful rectal bleeding and may extend from the anal verge as far as the pectinate line. Fissures are usually caused by the forceful passing of a large hard stool, but may be related to prolonged diarrhea.[142] Anal fissures can be exquisitely painful and may last for months if not treated promptly, and are most common among infants and patients between 30 and 50 years of age.[160,161] Most fissures occur along the posterior midline. Ten to fifteen percent of fissures occur at the anterior midline, and are more common among women.[142,161] Multiple fissures or fissures in other locations should raise the suspicion of systemic diseases such as Crohn disease, human immunodeficiency virus (HIV), tuberculosis, syphilis, or leukemia.[162] If fissures are not treated early they result in a vicious cycle of anal spasm, incomplete evacuation, constipation, and further injury during the next stool passage. Chronic fissures may display the classic "fissure triad" of a deep ulcerated crater with raised edges, sentinel pile, and enlarged anal papillae. The sentinel pile is a prominent posterior skin tag that may be large enough to be confused with an external hemorrhoid or to mask the presence of the fissure. This chronically inflamed tissue resists healing.

The initial symptom of an anal fissure is sudden sharp pain that may be accompanied by a small amount of bright red blood on the stool or toilet paper. This initial pain is followed by a dull ache that may last for hours, due to sphincter spasm. Subsequent bowel movements cause similar symptoms. Because most internal hemorrhoids cause painless bleeding, and external hemorrhoids are not painful unless thrombosed, these conditions should not be confused with a fissure. The fissure is usually visible with manual retraction of the buttocks with the patient in the knee-chest position. Reflex spasm and edema may also be noted. White connective tissue bands of the internal anal sphincter may be visible at the base of the deep chronic fissures.[142]

Management of anal fissures focuses on early healing to prevent chronic or permanent alteration of the inflamed tissue. This aspect is important because acute fissures almost always respond to medical therapy whereas chronic fissures have much higher failure rates with medical therapy, and surgical therapy, while successful most of the time, is frequently complicated by incontinence. Management begins with the W.A.S.H. regimen (see **Box 1**).[151] Further relaxation of sphincter spasm may be achieved with a variety of oral, transdermal, and topical formulations of nitrates and/or calcium channel blockers.[161,163–165] Local injection of botulinum toxin may also obviate the need for surgical intervention, though it can cause temporary incontinence.[166–169] Most patients experience some relief with conservative management within 2 to 3 days, and acute fissures may completely resolve within a month if treated adequately. Acute care of patients with chronic fissures also focuses on analgesia and reduction of sphincter tone, but may ultimately require sphincterotomy.[142]

Anorectal Abscesses

Anorectal abscesses result when drainage of the mucus-producing glands is prohibited by obstruction of the anal crypts, stasis, suppuration, and abscess formation. Bacterial cultures are usually polymicrobial and often include *Staphylococcus aureus*, *Escherichia coli*, *Streptococcus*, *Proteus*, and *Bacteroides* species. A smaller number of abscesses result from inflammatory bowel disease, trauma, or an atypical infection such as tuberculosis, actinomycosis, or lymphogranuloma venereum.[170–172] For clinical purposes, there are two categories of anorectal abscesses. Perianal abscesses, which do not involve the deep tissue spaces of the pelvis, can often be managed in ED with caution. Perirectal abscesses should be managed operatively.

Perianal abscesses present with severe pain and swelling in the region of the external anal orifice, which makes sitting or defecating painful. These abscesses occur at the anal verge and the lowest portion of the anal canal. This region is separated from the ischiorectal space by a horizontal fascial septum and is continuous with the fat of the gluteal region; nevertheless these abscesses, like perirectal abscesses, originate from the anal crypts, and therefore extend between the layers of the internal sphincter and those of the superficial and subcutaneous bands of the external sphincter (the intersphincteric space). Physical examination reveals an area of tenderness and induration with or without central fluctuance. The abscesses may extend laterally into the gluteal region, with associated cellulitis.[173] A sinus tract leading from the obstructed crypt may be palpated as a cord within the anal canal (if the patient can tolerate a rectal examination). The diagnosis of superficial perianal abscess cannot be made with certainty until a thorough digital rectal examination has evaluated the rectal walls above the anal sphincter for fullness, induration, or tenderness. If the diagnosis is in doubt, there should be a low threshold for pelvic CT (preferably with intravenous contrast).

Superficial well-localized perianal abscesses may be managed with incision and drainage in the ED. A single linear incision may be made over the area of maximal fluctuance, with subsequent packing as is performed with other cutaneous abscesses. If a cruciate incision is made, the resulting flaps should be excised to avoid premature closure and recurrence of the abscess.[174] Probing and breaking up loculations to adequately drain a perianal abscess can be extremely painful, so liberal analgesia is advised. Procedural sedation may be necessary. Procedural sedation before making the incision often allows the clinician the opportunity to perform a more thorough rectal examination to confirm that the abscess does not extend into any of the perirectal spaces. If it does, the procedure should be aborted and surgical consultation obtained. Inadequate analgesia resulting in inadequate drainage is likely the reason why up to 40% of drained perianal abscesses recur and/or form fistulae.[170,175,176]

Perirectal abscesses also arise from obstructed anal crypts but, because of suppurative extension in directions other than the anal orifice, result in abscess formation in one or more of the deep spaces of the pelvis. These abscesses cannot be adequately drained without operative intervention under general anesthesia.[142,174] These potential spaces are large and are filled with relatively hypovascular areolar adipose tissue that has limited resistance to a spreading infection. The spaces include the ischiorectal space, the postanal space (connecting the ischiorectal spaces on either side), the intersphincteric space between the internal and external anal sphincters, and the supralevator space.[177,178] Supralevator abscesses are more frequently associated with diabetes, neoplasia, and Crohn disease. Patients with deep abscesses present with poorly localized pelvic and rectal pain exacerbated prior to defecation (due to the previously described relaxation and contraction of the anal sphincters, all of which are directly affected by the inflammatory process) or during defecation. Patients may also describe deep pelvic pain with micturition (due to alterations in the shape of the bladder) and, in women, the vagina, especially with intercourse.

On examination, these patients may have fever or other systemic signs of toxicity. Digital rectal examination, if it can be tolerated by the patient, may reveal exquisite tenderness, fullness, and induration adjacent to the anus or rectum. Even in patients who are unable to tolerate rectal examination, the diagnosis of perirectal abscess is almost certain if there is a history suggesting anorectal infection and if a simple perianal abscess cannot be identified by gentle palpation around the anal orifice. Such patients should be sent for CT of the pelvis to determine the location of the abscess before surgery.[179,180] Conversely, as previously noted, the presence of a tender mass at the anal verge does not definitively rule in a superficial perianal process, because deep abscesses can finally point beyond the anal margin after suppuration along a long and serpinginous tract through the deep perirectal spaces. Perirectal abscesses should be treated operatively.

Pilonidal Disease

Pilonidal disease describes a spectrum of clinical presentations, beginning with asymptomatic hair-containing cysts and sinuses, which may result in sacrococcygeal abscesses that have a tendency to recur.[181] The etiology of these infections, though still debated, probably involves acute inflammation of ingrowing hair follicles, often precipitated by pressure or trauma to the region.[182–185] Some patients simply present with an asymptomatic sinus tract in the region of the gluteal cleft, but in the ED patients are more likely to complain of a swollen painful area consistent with an abscess. Acute management involves incision, drainage, and packing of the abscess. The patient should be rechecked in the ED or by a primary physician in 2 days for resolution of symptoms and removal of packing. For large abscesses it may not be possible to remove all the packing after 2 days, mandating a further recheck in 2 days. The patient should be advised to seek evaluation by a surgeon in 1 to 2 weeks so that definitive management can be arranged. Follicle removal and unroofing or excision of the sinus tract may be performed; however, there is evidence that conservative management with local hygiene and shaving the region every 1 to 3 weeks may be as effective as surgery.[181]

Pruritus Ani

Severe perianal itch is a symptom most frequently seen in aging men. The itch is typically worse during the summer months and at night. There are many causes, but the most common is poor perianal hygiene. Changes in anal anatomy including hemorrhoids, skin tags, fissures, fistulae, obesity, or prolapse make cleaning the perianal region more difficult. Conversely, overzealous anal hygiene may itself be the cause of pruritus, due to the removal of essential oils that maintain the homeostasis of the anal epithelium. Spicy foods, caffeine, milk, tomatoes, and alcohol may alter the pH of feces, exacerbating its irritating effect. Poorly formed or liquid stools also impede anal hygiene. Medications that cause GI irritation or certain antibiotics such as tetracyclines also cause perianal itching.[142,186] Other causes of anal itching include contact dermatitis, psoriasis, and systemic diseases such as diabetes, renal failure, and iron deficiency. Chronic low-grade trauma from anal sexual practices, sexually transmitted infections, and local infections such as pinworm, scabies, or fungal infections may also cause pruritus. Regardless of the original cause, many cases of pruritus ani become self-perpetuating as a result of the trauma inflicted to the delicate anal skin by scratching and an ensuing itch-scratch cycle. Treatment is based on etiology that can often be identified by history, which should focus on anal hygiene, systemic illnesses, sexual history, and diet. Examination of the patient's skin often reveals the erythematous thickened skin resulting from prolonged scratching. Other findings may include external hemorrhoids, prolapse, or skin tags. Specimens should be obtained for microscopic testing for *Candida* or for pinworm eggs as mandated by clinical findings. A rectal examination should be performed to exclude the presence of a fistula, malignancy, or other lesions.

When poor hygiene is the cause or pruritus ani, the patient should be educated on proper anal hygiene. These patients benefit from washing the perianal region with warm water after bowel movements. As noted, patients should be warned regarding overzealous washing or the use of soaps, scents, or detergents in the region. The area should be patted dry rather than wiped, which may cause further skin trauma. Loose-fitting cotton underwear to promote air circulation and decrease perspiration is helpful. Tepid sitz baths and/or application of ice may provide temporary relief, especially in the evening when symptoms are worse. Patients should receive dietary fiber supplements, and be advised about ways to maintain a high-fiber diet and good oral hydration to promote regular bowel movements with well-formed stools. Specific causes of pruritus should be managed accordingly.[186]

Rectal Prolapse

Rectal prolapse may include all layers of the rectum (procidentia) or the mucosal layer alone (**Fig. 13**).[187–189] Internal prolapse (internal intussusception) may also occur,

A

B

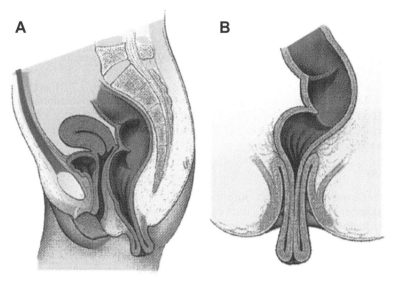

Fig. 13. Rectal prolapse. (*A*) Complete procidentia or rectal prolapse involving all layers of the rectum. (*B*) Intussusception of the sigmoid colon beyond the anus. (*From* Kratzer GL, Demarest RJ. Office Management of Colon and Rectal Disease. Philadelphia: WB Saunders, 1985; with permission.)

usually in elderly women, but is not discussed here. Procidentia is more common in elderly women with chronic constipation, and may be accompanied by uterine prolapse and/or cystocele. Patients often present with the sensation of an anal mass at defecation that usually retracts when the patient stands up.[187] As the disease progresses the mass no longer retracts spontaneously, and will eventually prolapse spontaneously during daily activities (**Fig. 14**). Mucosal prolapse may also be seen in children younger than 3 years, and is most often associated with cystic fibrosis or malnutrition.[190] The parent may report protrusion during defecation, and there may be small amounts of blood or mucous in the stools.

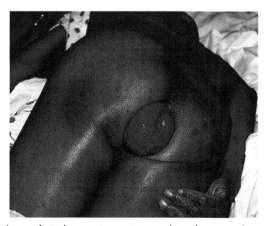

Fig. 14. Rectal prolapse that does not spontaneously reduce requires manual reduction. (*From* Coates WC. Anorectal Procedures. In: Roberts JR, Hedges JR, eds. Clinical Procedures in Emergency Medicine, 5th ed. Philadelphia: Elsevier, 2010; with permission.)

Manual reduction of procidentia or mucosal prolapse is performed by gentle constant pressure on the mass over several minutes. Sedation or a field block with local anesthesia may be necessary for successful reduction. Granulated sugar applied to the prolapsed rectum may aid in reduction by desiccation of the mucosa, thus reducing edema.[191] After successful reduction, both adults and children should be referred for outpatient evaluation for an underlying etiology.[181,192–196] Parents should be instructed on the use of increased dietary fiber and oral hydration to prevent constipation.[189] If reduction is unsuccessful or if the procidentia is incarcerated, ischemic, extensively ulcerated, or severely traumatized, immediate surgical consultation should be obtained.[189]

SUMMARY

Ingested FBs are usually benign, but impacted FBs are potentially life-threatening. The ED management of FBs in the GI tract varies depending on the nature of the object, its anatomic location, and the symptoms experienced by the patient.

Anorectal disorders are frequently encountered in the ED. An understanding of anorectal anatomy and common disorders allows the emergency physician to provide relief and resolution in the majority of cases.

REFERENCES

1. Schwartz GF, Polsky HS. Ingested foreign bodies of the gastrointestinal tract. Am Surg 1976;42(4):236–8.
2. Erbes J, Babbitt DP. Foreign bodies in the alimentary tract of infants and children. Appl Ther 1965;7(12):1103–9.
3. Cheng W, Tam PK. Foreign-body ingestion in children: experience with 1,265 cases. J Pediatr Surg 1999;34(10):1472–6.
4. Conway WC, Sugawa C, Ono H, et al. Upper GI foreign body: an adult urban emergency hospital experience. Surg Endosc 2007;21(3):455–60.
5. Webb WA. Management of foreign bodies of the upper gastrointestinal tract: update. Gastrointest Endosc 1995;41(1):39–51.
6. Lyons MF, Tsuchida AM. Foreign bodies of the gastrointestinal tract. Med Clin North Am 1993;77(5):1101–14.
7. Brady PG. Esophageal foreign bodies. Gastroenterol Clin North Am 1991;20(4): 691–701.
8. Rosenow EC. Foreign bodies of the esophagus. In: Payne WS, Olsen AM, editors. The esophagus. Philadelphia: Lea & Febiger; 1974. p. 159–70.
9. Gunn A. Intestinal perforation due to swallowed fish or meat bone. Lancet 1966; 1(7429):125–8.
10. Bunker PG. The role of dentistry in problems of foreign body in the air and food passage. J Am Dent Assoc 1962;64:782–7.
11. Binder L, Anderson WA. Pediatric gastrointestinal foreign body ingestions. Ann Emerg Med 1984;13(2):112–7.
12. Velitchkov NG, Grigorov GI, Losanoff JE, et al. Ingested foreign bodies of the gastrointestinal tract: retrospective analysis of 542 cases. World J Surg 1996; 20(8):1001–5.
13. Wu I, Ho T, Chang C, et al. Value of lateral neck radiography for ingested foreign bodies using the likelihood ratio. J Otolaryngol Head Neck Surg 2008;37(2):292–6.
14. Nandi P, Ong GB. Foreign body in the oesophagus: review of 2394 cases. Br J Surg 1978;65(1):5–9.
15. Phillipps JJ, Patel P. Swallowed foreign bodies. J Laryngol Otol 1988;102:235–41.

16. Jones NS, Lannigan FJ, Salama NY. Foreign bodies in the throat: a prospective study of 388 cases. J Laryngol Otol 1991;105(2):104–8.

17. Bizakis JG, Segas J, Haralambos S, et al. Retropharyngeal abscess associated with a swallowed bone. Am J Otolaryngol 1993;14(5):354–7.

18. Connolly AA, Birchall M, Walsh-Waring GP, et al. Ingested foreign bodies: patient-guided localization is a useful clinical tool. Clin Otolaryngol 1992;17:520.

19. Braverman I, Gomori JM, Polv O, et al. The role of CT imaging in the evaluation of cervical esophageal foreign bodies. J Otolaryngol 1993;22(4):311–4.

20. Sundgren PC, Burnett A, Maly PV. Value of radiography in the management of possible fishbone ingestion. Ann Otol Rhinol Laryngol 1994;103(8):628–31.

21. Derowe A, Ophir D. Negative findings of esophagoscopy for suspected foreign bodies. Am J Otolaryngol 1994;15(1):41–5.

22. Hess GP. An approach to throat complaints: foreign body sensation, difficulty swallowing and hoarseness. Emerg Med Clin North Am 1987;5(2):313–34.

23. Webb WA. Management of foreign bodies of the upper gastrointestinal tract. Gastroenterology 1988;94(1):204–16.

24. Ngan JH, Fok PJ, Lai EC, et al. A prospective study on fish bone ingestion: experience of 358 patients. Ann Surg 1990;211(4):459–62.

25. Evans RM, Ahuja A, Rhys Williams S, et al. The lateral neck radiograph in suspected impacted fishbones—does it have a role? Clin Radiol 1992;46(2):121–3.

26. Marais J, Mitchell R, Wightman AJA. The value of radiographic assessment of oropharyngeal foreign bodies. J Laryngol Otol 1995;109(5):452–4.

27. Lue AJ, Fang WD, Manolidis S. Use of plain radiography and computed tomography to identify fish bone foreign bodies. Otolaryngol Head Neck Surg 2000;123(4):435–8.

28. Nehme Kingsley A, Abcarian H. Colorectal foreign bodies: management update. Dis Colon Rectum 1985;28(12):941–4.

29. Flom LL, Ellis GL. Radiologic evaluation of foreign bodies. Emerg Med Clin North Am 1992;10(1):163–77.

30. Eliashar R, Dano I, Dangoor E, et al. Computed tomography diagnosis of esophageal bone impaction: a prospective study. Ann Otol Rhinol Laryngol 1999;108(7):708–10.

31. Marco de Lucas E, Sadaba P, Lastra Garcia-Baron P, et al. Value of helical computed tomography in the management of upper esophageal foreign bodies. Acta Radiol 2004;45(4):369–74.

32. Stack LB, Munter DW. Foreign bodies in the gastrointestinal tract. Emerg Med Clin North Am 1996;14(3):493–521.

33. Chaikhouni A, Kratz JM, Crawford FA. Foreign bodies of the esophagus. Am Surg 1985;51(4):173–9.

34. Myer C. Potential hazards of esophageal foreign body extraction. Pediatr Radiol 1991;21(2):97–8.

35. Conners GP, Cobaugh DJ, Feinberg R, et al. Home observation for asymptomatic coin ingestion: acceptance and outcomes. The New York State Poison Control Center Coin Ingestion Study Group. Acad Emerg Med 1999;6(3):213–7.

36. Gracia C, Frey CF, Bodai BI. Diagnosis and management of ingested foreign bodies: a ten-year experience. Ann Emerg Med 1984;13(1):30–4.

37. Giordano A, Adams G, Boies L, et al. Current management of esophageal foreign bodies. Arch Otolaryngol 1981;107(4):249–51.

38. Kelley JE, Leech MH, Carr MG. A safe and cost-effective protocol for the management of esophageal coins in children. J Pediatr Surg 1993;28(7):898.

39. Ricote GC, Torre LR, De Ayala VP, et al. Fiberendoscopic removal of foreign bodies of the upper part of the gastrointestinal tract. Surg Gynecol Obstet 1985;160(6):499–504.
40. Rosch W, Classen M. Fiberendoscopic foreign body removal from the upper gastrointestinal tract. Endoscopy 1972;4:193–7.
41. Vizcarrondo FJ, Brady PG, Nord HJ. Foreign bodies of the upper gastrointestinal tract. Gastrointest Endosc 1983;29(3):208–10.
42. Taylor R. Esophageal foreign bodies. Emerg Med Clin North Am 1987;5(2):301.
43. Nolte KB. Esophageal foreign bodies as child abuse: potential fatal mechanisms. Am J Forensic Med Pathol 1993;14(4):323–6.
44. Weissberg D, Refaely Y. Foreign bodies in the esophagus. Ann Thorac Surg 2007;84(6):1854–7.
45. Samarasam I, Chandran S, Shukla V, et al. A missing denture's misadventure! Dis Esophagus 2006;19(1):53–5.
46. Kay M, Wyllie R. Pediatric foreign bodies and their management. Curr Gastroenterol Rep 2005;7(3):212–8.
47. Bhasin A, Elitsur Y. Esophageal stenosis, a rare complication of coin ingestion: case report. Gastrointest Endosc 2004;59(1):152–4.
48. Kinzer S, Pfeiffer J, Becker S, et al. Severe deep neck space infections and mediastinitis of odontogenic origin: clinical relevance and implications for diagnosis and treatment. Acta Otolaryngol 2009;129(1):62–70.
49. Blatnik BS, Toohill RJ, Lehman RH. Fatal complications from an alkaline battery foreign body in the esophagus. Ann Otol Rhinol Laryngol 1977;86(5):611–5.
50. Kelly SL, Peters P, Ogg MJ, et al. Successful management of an aortoesophageal fistula caused by a fish bone–case report and review of literature. J Cardiothorac Surg 2009;8(4):21.
51. Dahshan A. Management of ingested foreign bodies in children. J Okla State Med Assoc 2001;94(6):183–6.
52. Arana A, Hauser B, Hachimi-Idrissi S, et al. Management of ingested foreign bodies in childhood and review of the literature. Eur J Pediatr 2001;160(8): 468–72.
53. Macpherson RI, Hill JG, Othersen HB, et al. Esophageal foreign bodies in children: diagnosis, treatment, and complicatins. Am J Roentgenol 1996; 166(4):919.
54. Caravati EM, Bennett DL, McElwee NE. Pediatric coin ingestion: a prospective study on the utility of routine roentgenograms. Am J Dis Child 1989;143(5): 549–51.
55. Conners GP, Chamberlain JM, Ochsenschlager DW. Symptoms and spontaneous passage of esophageal coins. Arch Pediatr Adolesc Med 1995;149(1): 36.
56. Hodge D, Tecklenberg F, Fleisher G. Coin ingestion: does every child need a radiograph? Ann Emerg Med 1985;14(5):443.
57. Chen MK, Beierle EA. Gastrointestinal foreign bodies. Pediatr Ann 2001;30(12): 736–42.
58. Eisen GM, Baron TH, Dominitz JA, et al. Guideline for the management of ingested foreign bodies. Gastrointest Endosc 2002;55(7):802–6.
59. Bailey P. Pediatric esophageal foreign body with minimal symptomatology. Ann Emerg Med 1983;12(7):452–4.
60. Watanabe K, Kikuchi T, Katori Y, et al. The usefulness of computed tomography in the diagnosis of impacted fish bones in the oesophagus. J Laryngol Otol 1998;112(4):360–4.

61. McGahren ED. Esophageal foreign bodies. Pediatr Rev 1999;20(4):129–33.
62. Ekberg O. Normal anatomy and techniques of examination of the esophagus: fluoroscopy, CT, MRI, and scintigraphy. In: Freeny PC, Stevenson GW, editors. Margulis and Burhennes's alimentary tract radiology. 5th edition. St Louis (MO): Mosby; 1994. p. 183.
63. Ginsberg GG. Management of ingested foreign objects and food bolus impactions. Gastrointest Endosc 1995;41(1):33–8.
64. Herranz-Gonzalez J, Martinesz-Vidal J, Garcia-Sarandese A, et al. Oesophageal foreign bodies in adults. Otolaryngol Head Neck Surg 1991;105(5):649–54.
65. Akazawa Y, Watanabe S, Nobukiyo S, et al. The management of possible fishbone ingestion. Auris Nasus Larynx 2004;31(4):413–6.
66. Pons J, Demoux R, Campan P, et al. A fatal aorto-esophageal fistula due to a foreign body: a foreseeable accident? Presse Med 1999;28(4):781.
67. Carp L. Foreign bodies in the intestine. Ann Surg 1927;85(4):575–91.
68. Berggreen PJ, Harrison ME, Sanowski RA, et al. Techniques and complications of esophageal foreign body extraction in children and adults. Gastrointest Endosc 1993;39(5):626–30.
69. Litovitz TL, Schmitz BF. Ingestion of cylindrical and button batteries: an analysis of 2382 cases. Pediatrics 1992;89(4):747–57.
70. Litovitz TL. Button battery ingestions. JAMA 1983;249(18):2495–500.
71. Litovitz TL. Battery ingestions: product accessibility and clinical course. Pediatrics 1985;75(3):468–76.
72. Maves MD, Carithers JS, Birck HG. Esophageal burns secondary to disc battery ingestion. Ann Otol Rhinol Laryngol 1984;93(4):364–9.
73. Mofenson HC, Greensher J, Caraccio TR, et al. Ingestion of small flat disc batteries. Ann Emerg Med 1983;12(2):88–90.
74. Nahman BV, Mueller CF. Asymptomatic esophageal perforation by a coin in a child. Ann Emerg Med 1984;13(8):627–9.
75. Morioka WT, Smith TW, Maisel RH, et al. Unexpected radiographic findings related to foreign bodies. Ann Otol Rhinol Laryngol 1975;84(5):627–30.
76. Spitz L, Hirsig J. Prolonged foreign body impaction in the esophagus. Arch Dis Child 1982;57(7):551–3.
77. Handler SD, Beaugard ME, Canalis RF, et al. Unsuspected esophageal foreign bodies in adults with upper airway obstruction. Chest 1981;80:234–6.
78. Maleki M, Evans WE. Foreign body perforation of the intestinal tract: report of 12 cases and a review of the literature. Arch Surg 1970;101(4):475–7.
79. Spitz L. Management of ingested foreign bodies in childhood. BMJ 1971; 4(5785):469–72.
80. Wu MH, Lai WW. Aortoesophageal fistula induced by foreign bodies. Ann Thorac Surg 1992;54(1):155–6.
81. Waltzman ML. Management of esophageal coins. Curr Opin Pediatr 2006;18(5): 571–4.
82. Conners GP, Frey CF, Bodao BI, et al. Conservative management of pediatric distal esophageal coins. J Emerg Med 1996;14(6):723–6.
83. Campbell JB, Quattromani FL, Foley LC. Foley catheter removal of blunt esophageal foreign bodies. Experience with 100 consecutive children. Pediatr Radiol 1983;13(3):116–9.
84. Ginaldi S. Removal of esophageal foreign bodies using a Foley catheter in adults. Am J Emerg Med 1985;3(1):64–6.
85. Calkins CM, Christians KK, Sell LL. Cost analysis in the management of esophageal coins: endoscopy versus bougienage. J Pediatr Surg 1999;34(3):412–4.

86. Emslander HC, Bonadio W, Klatzo M. Efficiency of esophageal bougienage by emergency physicians in pediatric coin ingestion. Ann Emerg Med 1996;27(6): 726–9.

87. Bonadio WA, Jona JZ, Glicklich M, et al. Esophageal bougienage technique for coin ingestion in children. J Pediatr Surg 1988;23(10):917–8.

88. Arms JL, Mackernberg-Mohn MD, Bowen MV, et al. Safety and efficacy of a protocol using bougienage or endoscopy for the management of coins acutely lodged in the esophagus: a large case series. Ann Emerg Med 2008;51(4): 367–72.

89. Cavo JW, Koops HJ, Gryboski RA. Use of enzymes for meat impactions in the esophagus. Laryngoscope 1977;87(4):630–4.

90. Andersen HA, Bernatz PE, Grandlay JH. Perforation of the esophagus after use of a digestive agent: report of a case and experimental study. Ann Otol Rhinol Laryngol 1959;68:890–6.

91. Holsinger JW, Fuson RL, Sealy WC. Esophageal perforation following meat impaction and papain ingestion. JAMA 1968;204(2):188–9.

92. Tibbling L, Bjorkhoel A, Jansson E, et al. Effect of spasmolytic drugs on esophageal foreign bodies. Dysphagia 1995;10:126–7.

93. Colon V, Grad A, Pulliam G, et al. Effect of doses of glucagon used to treat food impaction on esophageal motor function of normal subjects. Dysphagia 1999; 14(1):27–30.

94. Maglinte DD. Pharmacoradiologic disimpaction of lower esophageal foreign bodies: should we abandon it? Dysphagia 1995;10(2):128–30.

95. Arora S, Galich P. Myth: glucagon is an effective first-line therapy for esophageal foreign body impaction. CJEM 2009;11(2):169–71.

96. Zimmers T, Chan SB, Kouchoukos PL, et al. Use of gas-forming agents in esophageal food impactions. Ann Emerg Med 1988;17(7):693–5.

97. Karanjia ND, Rees M. The use of Coca-Cola in the management of bolus obstruction in benign oesophageal stricture. Ann R Coll Surg Engl 1993;75(2):94–5.

98. Bell AF, Eibling DE. Nifedipine in the treatment of distal esophageal food impaction [letter]. Arch Otolaryngol Head Neck Surg 1988;114(6):682–3.

99. Gibson MS. Nitroglycerin use in esophageal disorders [letter]. Ann Emerg Med 1980;9(5):280.

100. Goldberg GJ. Emergency department treatment of esophageal obstruction [letter]. Ann Emerg Med 1980;9(5):280.

101. Rice B, Spiegel P, Dombrowski P. Acute esophageal food impaction treated by gas forming agents. Radiology 1983;146(2):299–301.

102. Mohammed S, Hegedus V. Dislodgment of impacted oesophageal foreign bodies with carbonated beverages. Clin Radiol 1986;37(6):589–92.

103. Kaszar-Seibert DJ, Korn WT, Bindman DJ, et al. Treatment of acute esophageal food impaction with a combination of glucagon, effervescent agent, and water. AJR Am J Roentgenol 1990;154(3):533–4.

104. Smith JC, Janower ML, Geiger AH. Use of glucagon and gas-forming agents in acute esophageal food impaction. Radiology 1986;159(2):567–8.

105. Rohrmann CA Jr, Acheson MB. Esophageal perforation during double-contrast esophagram. AJR Am J Roentgenol 1985;145(2):283–4.

106. Knight LC, Lesser TH. Fish bones in the throat. Arch Emerg Med 1989;6(1): 13–6.

107. Koch H. Operative endoscopy. Gastrointest Endosc 1977;24(2):65–8.

108. Johnson WE. On ingestion of razor blades. JAMA 1969;208(11):2163.

109. Henderson FF, Gaston EA. Ingested foreign bodies in the gastrointestinal tract. Arch Surg 1938;36:66–95.
110. Paul RI, Jaffe DM. Sharp object ingestions in children: illustrative cases and literature review. Pediatr Emerg Care 1988;4(4):245–8.
111. Caruana DS, Weinbach B, Goerg D, et al. Cocaine packet ingestion. Diagnosis, management, and natural history. Ann Intern Med 1984;100(1):73–4.
112. Kulig K, Rumack CM, Rumack BH, et al. Disk battery ingestion. Elevated urine mercury levels and enema removal of battery fragments. JAMA 1983;249(18): 2502–4.
113. Mant TGK, Lewis JL, Mattoo TK, et al. Mercury poisoning after disc-battery ingestion. Hum Toxicol 1987;6(2):179–81.
114. Booker RJ, Smith JE, Rodger MP. Packers pushers and stuffers—Managing patients with concealed drugs in UK emergency departments: a clinical and medicolegal review. Emerg Med J 2009;26(5):316–20.
115. Pollack CV, Biggers DW, Carlton FB, et al. Two crack cocaine body stuffers. Ann Emerg Med 1992;21(11):1370–80.
116. McCarron MM, Wood JD. The cocaine "body packer" syndrome: diagnosis and treatment. JAMA 1983;250(11):1417–20.
117. Suarez CA, Arango A, Lester JL. Cocaine-condom ingestion: surgical treatment. JAMA 1977;238(13):1391–2.
118. Pidoto RR, Agliata AM, Bertoline R, et al. A new method of packaging cocaine for international traffic and implications for the management of cocaine body-packers. J Emerg Med 2002;23(2):149–53.
119. Traub SJ, Hoffman RS, Nelson LS. Current concepts: body packing-the internal concealment of illicit drugs. N Engl J Med 2003;349(26):2519–26.
120. Gherardi RK, Baud FJ, Leporc P, et al. Detection of drugs in the urine of body-packers. Lancet 1988;1(8594):1076–8.
121. Bulstrode N, Banks F, Shrotria S. The outcome of drug smuggling by 'body-packers'—the British experience. Ann R Coll Surg Engl 2002;84(1):35–8.
122. Price KR. Fatal cocaine poisoning. J Forensic Sci Soc 1974;14(4):329–33.
123. Wetli CV, Wright RK. Death caused by recreational cocaine use. JAMA 1979; 241(23):2519–22.
124. Marc B, Baud FJ, Aelion MJ, et al. The cocaine body-packer syndrome: evaluation of a method of contrast study of the bowel. J Forensic Sci 1990;35(2): 345–55.
125. Hartoko TJ, Demey HE, De Schepper AMA, et al. The body packer syndrome— cocaine smuggling in the gastrointestinal tract. Klin Wochenschr 1988;66(22): 1116–20.
126. Bogusz MJ, Althoff H, Erkens M, et al. Internally concealed cocaine: analytical and diagnostic aspects. J Forensic Sci 1995;40(5):811–5.
127. Hollander JE, Hoffman RS. Cocaine. In: Goldfrank LR, Flomenbaum NE, Lewin NA, et al, editors. Goldfrank's toxicologic emergencies. 7th edition. New York: McGraw-Hill; 2002. p. 1004–19.
128. June R, Aks SE, Keys N, et al. Medical outcome of cocaine body stuffers. J Emerg Med 2000;18(2):221–4.
129. Moreira CA, Wongpakdee S, Gennaro AR. A foreign body (chicken bone) in the rectum causing extensive perirectal and scrota1 abscess: report of a case. Dis Colon Rectum 1975;18(5):407–9.
130. Thomson SR, Fraser M, Stupp C, et al. Iatrogenic and accidental colon injuries-What to do? Dis Colon Rectum 1994;37(5):496–502.

131. Fry RD. Anorectal trauma and foreign bodies. Surg Clin North Am 1994;74(6): 1491–505.
132. Johnson SO, Hartranft TH. Nonsurgical removal of a rectal foreign body using a vacuum extractor. Report of a case. Dis Colon Rectum 1996;39(8): 935–7.
133. Ooi BS, Ho YH, Eu KW, et al. Management of anorectal foreign bodies: a cause for obscure anal pain. Aust NZ J Surg 1998;68(12):852–5.
134. Losanoff JE, Kjossev KT. Rectal "oven mitt": the importance of considering a serious underlying injury. J Emerg Med 1999;17(1):31–3.
135. Clarke DL, Buccimazza I, Anderson FA, et al. Colorectal foreign bodies. Colorectal Dis 2005;7(1):98–103.
136. Goldberg JE, Steele SR. Rectal foreign bodies. Surg Clin North Am 2010;91(1): 173–84.
137. Eftaiha M, Hambrick E, Abcarian H. Principles of management of colorectal foreign bodies. Arch Surg 1977;112(6):691–5.
138. Barone JE, Sohn N, Nealton TF. Perforations and foreign bodies of the rectum: report of 28 cases. Ann Surg 1976;184(5):601–4.
139. Wigle RL. Emergency department management of retained rectal foreign bodies. Am J Emerg Med 1988;6(4):385–9.
140. Moore KL. Pelvis and perineum. In: Moore KL, Dalley DK, editors. Clinically oriented anatomy. 4th edition. Baltimore (MD): Williams and Wilkins; 1999. p. 395–400.
141. Barleben A, Mills S. Anorectal anatomy and physiology. Surg Clin North Am 2010;90(1):1–15.
142. Bullard Dunn KM, Rothenberger DA. Colon, rectum, and anus. In: Brunicardi FC, Andersen DK, Billiar TR, et al, editors. Schwartz's principles of surgery. 9th edition. McGraw-Hill Professional; 2009. Chapter 29. Available at: http://www.accessmedicine.com/content.aspx?aID=5014922. Accessed March 3, 2011.
143. Corman ML. Colon and rectal surgery. 4th edition. Philadelphia: JB Lippincott; 1998. p. 154–6.
144. Thomson WHF. The nature of haemorrhoids. Br J Surg 1975;62(5):542–52.
145. Gibbons CP, Bannister JJ, Read NW. Role of constipation and anal hypertonia in the pathogenesis of haemorrhoids. Br J Surg 1988;75(7):656–60.
146. Johanson JF, Sonnenberg A. The prevalence of hemorrhoids and chronic constipation. An epidemiologic study. Gastroenterology 1990;98(2):380–6.
147. Johanson JF, Sonnenberg A. Constipation is not a risk factor for hemorrhoids: a case-control study of potential etiological agents. Am J Gastroenterol 1994; 89(11):1981–6.
148. Bernstein WC. What are hemorrhoids and what is their relationship to the portal venous system? Dis Colon Rectum 1983;26(12):829–34.
149. Hosking SW, Smart HL, Johnson AG, et al. Anorectal varices, haemorrhoids, and portal hypertension. Lancet 1989;1(8634):349–52.
150. Johansen K, Bardin J, Orloff MJ. Massive bleeding from hemorrhoidal varices in portal hypertension. JAMA 1980;244(18):2084–5.
151. Coates A. Anorectum. In: Marx JA, Hockberger RS, Walls RM, editors. Rosen's emergency medicine, concepts and clinical practice. 6th edition. St Louis (MO): Mosby; 2006. p. 1511.
152. Dodi G, Bogoni F, Infantino A, et al. Hot or cold in anal pain? A study in the changes in internal sphincter pressure profiles. Dis Colon Rectum 1986; 299(4):248–51.

153. Gorfine SR. Treatment of benign anal disease with topical nitroglycerin. Dis Colon Rectum 1995;38(5):453–7.
154. Perrotti P, Antropoli C, Molino D, et al. Conservative treatment of acute thrombosed external hemorrhoids with topical nifedipine. Dis Colon Rectum 2001; 44(3):405–9.
155. Grosz CR. A surgical treatment of thrombosed external hemorrhoids. Dis Colon Rectum 1990;33(3):249.
156. Janicke DM, Pundt MR. Anorectal disorders. Emerg Med Clin North Am 1996; 14(4):757–88.
157. Greenspon J, Williams SB, Young HA, et al. Thrombosed external hemorrhoids: outcome after conservative or surgical management. Dis Colon Rectum 2004; 47(9):1493–8.
158. Orkin BA, Schwartz AM, Orkin M. Hemorrhoids: what the dermatologist should know. J Am Acad Dermatol 1999;41(3):449–56.
159. Sakulsky SB, Blumenthal JA, Lynch RH. Treatment of thrombosed hemorrhoids by excision. Am J Surg 1970;120(4):537–8.
160. Matt JG. Proctologic problems in infants and children: an analysis of 308 cases. Dis Colon Rectum 1960;3:511–22.
161. Metcalf AM. Anal fissure. Surg Clin North Am 2002;82(6):1291–7.
162. Rosen L, Abel ME, Gordon PH. Practice parameters for the management of anal fissure. Dis Colon Rectum 1992;35(2):206–8.
163. Nelson R. Non surgical therapy for anal fissure. Cochrane Database Syst Rev 2006;18(4):CDC003431.
164. Lund JN, Nystrom PO, Coremans G, et al. An evidence-based treatment algorithm for anal fissure. Tech Coloproctol 2006;10(3):177–80.
165. Kennedy ML, Sowter S, Nguyen H, et al. Glyceryl trinitrate ointment for the treatment of chronic anal fissure: results of a placebo-controlled trial and long-term follow-up. Dis Colon Rectum 1999;42(8):1000–6.
166. Brisinda G, Cadeddu F, Mazzeo P, et al. Botulinum toxin A for the treatment of chronic anal fissure. Expert Rev Gastroenterol Hepatol 2007;1(2): 219–28.
167. Mitka M. Colon and rectal surgeons are trying Botox treatment, too. JAMA 2002; 288(4):439–40.
168. Maria G, Cassetta E, Gui D, et al. A comparison of botulinum toxin and saline for the treatment of chronic anal fissure. N Engl J Med 1998;338:217.
169. Jost WH, Schrank B. Repeat botulin toxin injections in anal fissure: in patients with relapse and after insufficient effect of first treatment. Dig Dis Sci 1999; 44(8):1588–9.
170. Nelson R. Anorectal abscess fistula: what do we know? Surg Clin North Am 2002;82(6):1139–51.
171. Macdonald A, Wilson-Storey D, Munro F. Treatment of perianal abscess and fistula-in-ano in children. Br J Surg 2003;90(2):220–1.
172. Patient Care Committee of The Society for Surgery of the Alimentary Tract. Treatment of perineal suppurative processes. J Gastrointest Surg 2005;9:457.
173. Moreillon P, Que Y-A, Glauser MP. *Staphylococcus aureus* (including staphylococcal type shock). In: Mandell GL, Bennett JE, Dolin R, editors. Mandell, Douglas, and Bennett's principles and practice of infectious diseases. 6th edition. Philadelphia: Elsevier Churchill Livingstone; 2005. p. 2321.
174. Hyman N. Anorectal abscess and fistula. Prim Care 1999;26(1):69–80.
175. Hancock BD. ABC of colorectal diseases. Anal fissures and fistulas. BMJ 1992; 304(6831):904–7.

176. Hamalainen KP, Sainio AP. Incidence of fistulas after drainage of acute anorectal abscesses. Dis Colon Rectum 1998;41(11):1357–61.
177. Arko FR. Anorectal disorders. Am Fam Physician 1980;22(4):121–6.
178. Kodner IJ, Fry RD, Fleshman JW, et al. Colon, rectum, and anus. In: Schwartz SI, Shires GT, Spencer FC, et al, editors. Principles of surgery. 7th edition. New York: McGraw-Hill; 1999. p. 1265.
179. Chandwani D, Shih R, Cochrane D. Bedside emergency ultrasonography in the evaluation of a perirectal abscess. Am J Emerg Med 2004;22(4):315.
180. Tio TL, Mulder CJ, Wijers OB, et al. Endosonography of peri-anal and peri-colorectal fistula and/or abscess in Crohn's disease. Gastrointest Endosc 1990;36(4):331–6.
181. Hull TL, Wu J. Pilonidal disease. Surg Clin North Am 2002;82(6):1169–85.
182. da Silva JH. Pilonidal cyst: cause and treatment. Dis Colon Rectum 2000;43(8): 1146–56.
183. Humphries AE, Duncan JE. Evaluation and management of pilonidal disease. Surg Clin North Am 2010;90(1):113–24.
184. Haworth JC, Zachary RB. Congenital dermal sinuses in children—their relation to pilonidal sinus. Lancet 1955;2(6879):10.
185. Billingham RP. Anorectal miscellany: pilonidal disease, anal cancer, Bowen's and Paget's diseases, foreign bodies, and hidradenitis suppurativa. Prim Care 1999;26(1):171–7.
186. Bender JS, Duncan MD. Benign conditions of the anus and rectum. In: Barker LR, Burton JR, Zieve PD, editors. Principles of ambulatory medicine. 6th edition. Philadelphia: Lippincott Williams & Wilkins; 2003. p. 1542–54.
187. Toglia MR. Pathophysiology of anorectal dysfunction. Obstet Gynecol Clin North Am 1998;25(4):771–81.
188. Felt-Bersma RJ, Cuesta MA. Rectal prolapse, rectal intussusceptions, rectocele, and solitary rectal ulcer syndrome. Gastroenterol Clin North Am 2001;30(1): 199–222.
189. Harrison BP, Cespedes RD. Pelvic organ prolapse. Emerg Med Clin North Am 2001;19(3):781–97.
190. Corman ML. Rectal prolapse in children. Dis Colon Rectum 1985;28(7):535–9.
191. Coburn WM 3rd, Russell MA, Hofstetter WL. Sucrose as an aid to manual reduction of incarcerated rectal prolapse. Ann Emerg Med 1997;30(3):347–9.
192. de Hoog DE, Heemskerk J, Nieman FH, et al. Recurrence and functional results after open versus conventional laparoscopic versus robot-assisted laparoscopic rectopexy for rectal prolapse: a case-control study. Int J Colorectal Dis 2009;24(10):1201–6.
193. Sajid M, Siddiqui M, Baig M. Open versus laparoscopic repair of full thickness rectal prolapse: a re-meta-analysis. Colorectal Dis 2010;12(6):515–25.
194. Altomare DF, Binda G, Ganio E, et al. Long-term outcome of Altemeier's procedure for rectal prolapse. Dis Colon Rectum 2009;52(4):698–703.
195. Nigro ND. Procidentia of the rectum. Surg Clin North Am 1978;58(3):539–54.
196. Henry MM. Rectal prolapse. Br J Hosp Med 1980;24(4):302–7.

Abdominal Pain in Children

Jennifer R. Marin, MD, MSc[a],*, Elizabeth R. Alpern, MD, MSCE[b]

KEYWORDS

• Abdominal pain • Pediatric • Children

Abdominal pain is one of the most common reasons pediatric patients seek emergency medical care.[1–3] In the emergency department (ED), physicians must distinguish between emergent diagnoses that require immediate intervention, such as appendicitis, intussusception, and ovarian torsion, and self-limiting processes that are amenable to outpatient management and parental/guardian education, such as viral gastroenteritis and constipation. Abdominal pain also may be a presentation of extraabdominal processes, such as pneumonia and asthma.

HISTORY

The diagnosis of a child with abdominal pain can often be determined, or the differential diagnosis can at least be honed, with the aid of a good history and physical examination. Before even entering the room, the clinician can gain a wealth of information simply by observing the child from the doorway. For example, it can be reassuring to see a young child running around the room or sitting playing with toys on the bed, versus the child lying flat on the stretcher crying from pain. For many young children, being in the hospital or in the presence of health care workers can be intimidating and frightening. Therefore, the physician should minimize the child's anxiety. Some children fear even the sight of a white coat, and therefore its removal may provide some comfort. The physician should kneel or sit near the child as opposed to standing over the child, because being located near the child's eye level can be less daunting for them.

It may be difficult to elicit a detailed or even accurate history from the parent/guardian secondary to the age of the child. For instance, a child may present with inconsolable crying and it may not be apparent to the caregiver that the source of the pain is abdominal. However, as long as the physician maintains a high index of

The authors have no financial conflicts to report.

[a] Division of Emergency Medicine, Department of Pediatrics, Children's Hospital of Pittsburgh, 4401 Penn Avenue, AOB 2nd floor, Suite 2400, Pittsburgh, PA 15224, USA

[b] Division of Emergency Medicine, Department of Pediatrics, The Children's Hospital of Philadelphia, 34th Street and Civic Center Boulevard, Philadelphia, PA 19104, USA

* Corresponding author.

E-mail address: jennifer.marin@chp.edu

suspicion for an abdominal condition in these patients, the diagnosis is unlikely to be missed.

The history should be tailored to the age of the child. For example, it is important to obtain the sexual past and present history of an adolescent patient presenting with abdominal pain. Furthermore, this history should be gathered with family members out of the room in order to respect confidentiality and evoke a more accurate history. Birth and neonatal history become more relevant to the infant presenting with possible abdominal pain, versus the older adolescent patient. The history should be elicited from both the patient and the caregiver in the verbal child, whereas in the preverbal child, the history is obtained from the parent/guardian exclusively.

PHYSICAL EXAMINATION

The physical examination should begin with review of the vital signs. It is important to have knowledge of pediatric normal values for heart rate, respiratory rate, and blood pressure. Rather than memorizing ranges for each age group, it may be helpful to have a reference to which the clinician can refer when caring for a pediatric patient (Table 1).

It is important to focus not only on the abdominal portion of the physical examination of the child with abdominal pain, because extraabdominal causes may also present with abdominal pain. For example, the physician should perform a complete oropharyngeal, lung, back, skin, external genital, and possibly internal genital examination as part of the evaluation as well. When the physician is ready to examine the abdomen, the accuracy of the examination may be improved by using a toy as a distraction tool before auscultation or palpation.[2] If the child is already sitting in the lap of their caregiver, it may be useful to perform as much of the examination as possible with the child remaining there. The physician may initially palpate the caregiver's or a stuffed animal's abdomen in an effort to show the benign nature of the examination to the child. A school-age child may feel more comfortable if they are allowed to place their hand over or under the physician's hand as the abdomen is being palpated. Asking the older child questions about school, friends, and activities that they enjoy may serve as a distraction tool and facilitate examination.

The abdominal examination should begin with visualization of obvious abnormalities, such as distension, bruising, or masses. If palpation is hindered by voluntary guarding from the child, it is useful to bend the child's knees and attempt the distraction techniques mentioned earlier. When eliciting peritoneal signs, the child can be

Table 1 Pediatric normal vital signs							
	0–3 mo	3–6 mo	6–12 mo	1–3 y	3–6 y	6–12 y	>12 y
Heart rate (beats/min)	100–150	90–120	80–120	70–110	65–110	60–95	55–85
Respiratory rate (breaths/min)	35–55	30–45	25–40	20–30	20–25	14–22	12–18
Systolic blood pressure (mm Hg)	65–85	70–90	80–100	90–105	95–110	100–120	110–135
Diastolic blood pressure (mm Hg)	45–55	50–65	55–65	55–70	60–75	60–75	65–85

Data from Mathers LH, Frankel LR. Pediatric emergencies and resuscitation. In: Kliegman RM, Behrman RE, et al, editors. Nelson textbook of pediatrics, 18th edition. Maryland Heights (MO): WB Saunders, 2007.

asked to jump up and down if they are able to stand. Otherwise, with the child sitting on a caregiver's lap, the caregiver can be asked to bounce the child up and down and observe for signs of pain from the child. The rectal examination, evaluating for firm stool, blood, and a palpable mass, is not imperative in all children presenting with abdominal pain but may be useful in narrowing the differential diagnosis. In most children, it can be easily performed by partially introducing a small finger into the rectal vault.

DIFFERENTIAL DIAGNOSIS

It is helpful to consider the differential diagnosis of the child with abdominal pain in terms of the age of the child, because many diagnoses are seen more commonly in children of certain age groups (**Table 2**).

For purposes of this article, we consider select pediatric diagnoses in terms of surgical emergencies involving the abdomen and pelvis, nonsurgical gastrointestinal diseases, and extraabdominal diagnoses.

DIAGNOSES
Surgical

Appendicitis

Appendicitis is the most frequent surgical cause of abdominal pain in children presenting to EDs or outpatient clinics.[4,5] In one-third of children with appendicitis, the appendix ruptures before operative treatment.[6,7] This situation is particularly of concern in children less than 4 years of age. In this age group, despite not being a common diagnosis, the prevalence of perforation is high, with rates reported to be as high as 80% to 100%.[8-10] Moreover, because the omentum is less developed, perforations are less likely to be localized, leading to generalized peritonitis.[2]

The pathophysiology of appendicitis in children is different from that of adults because of the changing anatomic location and susceptibility of the appendix throughout childhood.[11] For example, neonatal appendicitis is infrequent because of their funnel-shaped appendix, soft diet, recumbent posture, and infrequent gastrointestinal and upper respiratory infections.[12,13] Around 1 to 2 years of age, the appendix becomes more susceptible to appendicitis as it assumes the adult shape. As the child ages, lymphoid follicle hyperplasia and size of the appendix gradually increase throughout childhood and peak in adolescence, which represents the highest incidence of appendicitis.[8,14]

The classic presentation of appendicitis (periumbilical abdominal pain migrating to the right lower quadrant associated with nausea, vomiting, and fever) is seen less often in pediatric patients compared with adults,[15] and its presence in children is not so strong a predictor for appendicitis as it is in adult patients.[11] Children often present earlier in the clinical process than adults, when only mild or nonspecific signs and symptoms are present. Furthermore, there are limited data indicating that signs such as rebound tenderness and Rovsing sign are accurate in children.[16] More common findings of appendicitis in children are right lower quadrant pain, vomiting, abdominal tenderness, and guarding.[16] In addition, the appendix may be located deep in the pelvis or rectocecally, which gives rise to back or pelvic pain, rather than the abdominal pain seen with the more common anterior appendix. Although difficult to elicit from caregivers, a history of abdominal pain preceding any emesis can be helpful to distinguish appendicitis from acute gastroenteritis (AGE).[2]

Laboratory testing can aid in the diagnosis of appendicitis; however, no test is 100% sensitive and specific for the diagnosis. The white blood cell count (WBC),[17-19]

Table 2
Pediatric diagnosis presenting with abdominal pain by age group[a]

Age Group	Infancy (<2 y)	Preschool Age (2–5 y)	School Age (>5 y)	Adolescent
Gastrointestinal	Colic Gastroesophageal reflux disease AGE Trauma (possible child abuse) Milk protein allergy	AGE Urinary tract infection Trauma Constipation Henoch-Schönlein purpura	AGE Trauma Urinary tract infection Functional abdominal pain Constipation Inflammatory bowel disease	AGE Gastritis Gastroesophageal reflux disease Inflammatory bowel disease Trauma Constipation Urinary tract infection Hepatitis Pancreatitis
Surgical abdominopelvic emergencies	Intussusception Incarcerated hernia Volvulus	Appendicitis Meckel's diverticulum Intussusception	Appendicitis Testicular torsion	Appendicitis Testicular torsion Ovarian torsion Ectopic pregnancy Cholecystitis
Extraabdominal		Pneumonia Asthma	Pneumonia Asthma Diabetes mellitus Group A streptococcal pharyngitis	Pneumonia Group A streptococcal pharyngitis Asthma Nephrolithiasis Pregnancy Pelvic inflammatory disease Dysmenorrhea Epididymitis

[a] Diagnoses are included in age groups in which they are most commonly seen. This strategy does not exclude the rare patient who may present with a diagnosis not commonly seen in that age group.

Data from Ruddy RM. Pain–abdomen. In: Fleisher G, Ludwig S, Henretig F, et al, editors. Textbook of pediatric emergency medicine, 5th edition. Philadelphia: Lippincott Williams & Wilkins; 2006.

C-reactive protein (CRP) test,[17,18,20–22] and urinalysis (UA) may be useful; however, the WBC count and CRP level may be increased in other conditions and normal in appendicitis. Furthermore, if the inflamed appendix is located adjacent to the ureter, the UA may reveal sterile pyuria or hematuria.[23]

Many scoring systems using a combination of signs, symptoms, and laboratory results to predict which patients have acute appendicitis have been developed and validated in children. These scoring systems have varying sensitivities (65%–98%) and specificities (32%–92%)[24–28] and are rarely used as definitive confirmation of the diagnosis.

Radiologic diagnosis of acute appendicitis before appendectomy has become increasingly more common as its availability in the ED has improved. Plain abdominal radiographs should not be routinely used in evaluating the patient with appendicitis, because only half of patients with surgically proved disease have abnormal findings, most of which are nonspecific.[29] Appendicoliths, which are believed to be the most specific finding of acute appendicitis, are visualized in only 5% to 15% of patients.[2,30,31] If a radiograph is obtained in the evaluation of the child with abdominal pain, **Box 1** lists findings that may be associated with acute appendicitis. Ultrasound has been increasingly used as the modality of choice in pediatric patients because of the lack of radiation exposure and need for contrast agents. As with ultrasound examinations for other indications, the test characteristics of ultrasound for diagnosing acute appendicitis depend on the experience and comfort level of the operator. In experienced hands, ultrasound can achieve sensitivities of 85% to 90% and specificities of 95% to 100%.[32–40] Using a graded compression technique, acute appendicitis is defined as an aperistaltic, noncompressible appendix larger than 6 mm in diameter. The presence of periappendiceal fluid may indicate inflammation or an early perforation. If present, an appendicolith may also be visualized by ultrasound. If ultrasound is unavailable, or is obtained and fails to visualize the appendix, a computed tomography (CT) scan becomes the test of choice. Sensitivity has been shown to be 88% to 97%, with specificities of 94% to 97% in pediatric studies,[41–43] and it also offers the advantage of identifying complications of appendicitis as well as alternative diagnoses. However, it is slower, may require oral or rectal contrast, which may be difficult to administer to a young child, and carries the risk of significant radiation exposure.

Children are at greater risk than adults from a given dose of radiation because they are inherently more radiosensitive and because they have more remaining years of life during which a radiation-induced cancer could develop.[44] Although no large-scale epidemiologic studies of the cancer risks associated with abdominal CT have been reported,[44] the cancer risks associated with the radiation exposure from CT scans have been estimated (**Fig. 1**). By adjusting for current CT usage, it can be estimated

---

Box 1
Abdominal radiograph findings in acute appendicitis

Sentinel loop

Air-fluid levels

Right-sided curvature of the spine

Fecolith

Mass in right lower quadrant

Loss of psoas sign

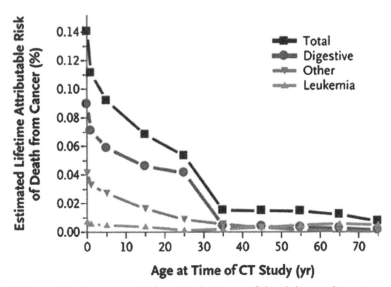

Fig. 1. Estimated lifetime cancer risk from single CT scan of the abdomen. (*From* Brenner DJ, Hall EJ. Computed tomography–an increasing source of radiation exposure. N Engl J Med 2007;357(22):2281; with permission.)

that about 1.5% to 2.0% of all cancers in the United States may be attributable to the radiation from CT studies.[44] If a CT is determined necessary, the question of which contrast agent or combination of agents to use (oral, intravenous, rectal) is a matter of debate in the radiology literature, is institutional-dependent, and should be decided on in concert with the radiologist or technician performing the study.

Despite the increased usage of radiologic modalities to confirm the diagnosis of acute appendicitis, when the clinician has a high suspicion for appendicitis, a surgeon should be consulted early in the patient course. While the diagnostic evaluation is being pursued, it is important to medically manage the patient until the diagnosis is confirmed and surgical management can occur. Children with appendicitis usually have decreased oral intake throughout the day, may have significant insensible losses if they are febrile, and also have third spacing secondary to intestinal inflammation, all leading to fluid losses, which should be replenished intravenously. Normal saline or lactated Ringer boluses should be given in order to establish euvolemia, followed by maintenance fluids until the child is taken to the operating room. Antibiotic coverage for gram-negative and anaerobic bacteria (such as ampicillin/sulbactam, piperacillin/tazobactam, or ampicillin/gentamicin/flagyl) should be started in the ED once the diagnosis is confirmed.

It is not uncommon for the diagnosis to remain unconfirmed, particularly in those children with a low or moderate suspicion for appendicitis. These patients should either be admitted to the hospital for serial abdominal examinations or if the suspicion for appendicitis is low, the patient seems well and has adequate oral intake, and there is reliable follow-up within 8 to 12 hours, the patient may be sent home with strict anticipatory guidance for when to return to the ED.

Intussusception

Intussusception is second to appendicitis as the most common cause of an acute abdominal emergency in children.[45] It is the most common cause of intestinal obstruction in children between 3 months and 6 years of age.[45] Although intussusception can occur at any age, the peak incidence occurs between 5 and 9 months of age,[46] and about half of patients are less than 1 year of age.[47]

Intussusception occurs when a segment of bowel (intussusceptum) invaginates into the distal bowel (intussuscipiens) (**Fig. 2**). This situation results in venous congestion and bowel wall edema initially; however, if unrecognized and untreated, this may lead to arterial obstruction with bowel necrosis and perforation.[48,49] Most intussusceptions in children (90%) are ileocolic and idiopathic in nature.[50] Presumably, idiopathic intussusception is caused by lymphoid hyperplasia, which has been suggested as the lead point.[51] Viral infections caused by adenovirus, rotavirus, and human herpesvirus 6 have been reported to be associated with intussusception.[52,53]

The clinician should have a high index of suspicion for intussusception in a young child with paroxysmal, colicky abdominal pain and vomiting. The classic triad of intermittent abdominal pain, red currant jelly stool (caused by venous congestion from obstruction), and a palpable mass occurs in a minority of patients (up to 40% of children with intussusception).[54,55] More common than grossly bloody stools is the presence of fecal occult blood, which is seen in approximately 50% of patients.[45]

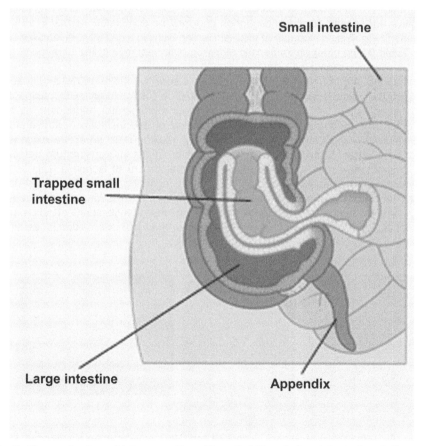

Fig. 2. The mechanism of intussusception. (*From* Del Mar, C. Royal Australian College of General Practitioners Complete Home Medical Guide, 2nd ed. Dorling Kindersley Australia; 2006; with permission.)

Therefore, the suspicion of intussusception should prompt the clinician to perform a rectal examination with testing for occult blood. Although it is an unusual presentation, some children with intussusception may present with lethargy or altered mental status, a feature that is postulated to be caused by the release of endogenous opioids secondary to the paroxysms of pain.[56,57] In addition, many children present with nonspecific signs and symptoms, which may lead to a delay or missed diagnosis in up to 60% of cases.[45] Specifically, infants younger than 4 months have a higher incidence of painless intussusception.[55] Also, up to 30% of patients with intussusception have diarrhea,[58] and therefore viral gastroenteritis is frequently entertained as the initial diagnosis. Intermittent intussusception is another entity that may prove challenging for the clinician, because these children may have resolution of their symptoms between episodes of obstruction.

When evaluating a child with suspected intussusception, the first step in diagnosis is obtaining 2 or 3 radiographic views of the abdomen. Left lateral decubitus radiographs are particularly helpful for this diagnosis, because the presence of air in the right lower quadrant makes the diagnosis of intussusception less likely. This situation is because most idiopathic intussusceptions occur at the level of the right upper quadrant, resulting in a paucity or absence of gas in the right lower quadrant, which can be confirmed in the decubitus position. However, plain abdominal films are neither sensitive nor specific for intussusception and may be completely normal in 25% of patients.[59] **Fig. 3** is an example of the plain radiographs in a patient with intussusception. **Table 3** lists other characteristic signs on plain radiograph and ultrasound that may be seen in patients with intussusception.

Ultrasound (**Fig. 4**) has recently emerged as a sensitive (98%–100%) and specific (88%–100%) diagnostic tool for the evaluation of children with suspected intussusception.[60–63] However, because ultrasound is operator dependent, its test characteristics for this indication vary depending on the institution. Ultrasound is a noninvasive, rapid, and nonionizing modality, making it an attractive diagnostic option in children. In addition, a lack of perfusion in the intussusceptum detected with color duplex imaging may indicate the development of ischemia. Ultrasound also has the advantage of providing information regarding a pathologic lead point mass, the presence of a small bowel intussusception, information regarding reducibility based on bowel wall findings, and in the identification of alternative diagnoses.[60,61,64,65] If ultrasound is unavailable or if an intussusception is identified

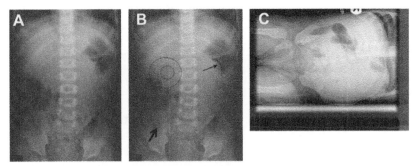

Fig. 3. (A–C) Upright (A unlabeled, B labeled) and left lateral decubitus (C) radiographs of a patient with intussusception. (B) Target sign (concentric circles), crescent sign (thin arrow with semicircle), paucity of gas in right lower quadrant (thick arrow). (C) Air-fluid levels and paucity of gas throughout abdomen.

Table 3
Radiologic findings of intussusception

Finding	Description	Radiograph or US
Soft-tissue mass in upper abdomen		Radiograph
Paucity/absence of air in right lower quadrant		Radiograph
Small bowel obstruction		Radiograph or US
Target sign	2 concentric, circular, radiolucent lines to the right of the spine superimposed on the kidney; caused by right upper quadrant mass with mesenteric fat of intussusceptum	Radiograph
Crescent/meniscus sign	Crescent of gas within the colonic lumen that outlines the apex of the intussusception	Radiograph
Pseudokidney sign	Hyperechoic tubular center with a hypoechoic rim on both sides, producing a kidneylike appearance in longitudinal plane	US
Donut sign	Hypoechoic outer rim of homogeneous thickness (intussuscipiens) with a central hyperechoic core (intussusceptum) representing layers of the intestine within the intestine in transverse plane	US

Abbreviation: US, ultrasound.
Data from Waseem M, Rosenberg HK. Intussusception. Pediatr Emerg Care 2008; 24(11):794.

by ultrasound, the patient should undergo a fluoroscopic barium or air enema, which is both diagnostic and therapeutic.

Although capable of showing intussusception, CT is usually not indicated because the diagnosis is reliably made either by ultrasound or radiographic barium or air enema. However, an abdominal CT scan may be useful in older children in excluding other diagnosis and in assessing for a lead point.

Treatment of confirmed intussusception begins with fluid resuscitation and maintenance of intravenous fluids, because most patients are dehydrated secondary to vomiting, poor oral intake, and third spacing.[45] Because intussusception may become a surgical condition, if radiographic barium or air enema reduction is unsuccessful, it is important that a pediatric surgeon be available before attempted reduction with enema. Nonoperative reduction of intussusception includes air, barium, or aqueous enema, typically under fluoroscopic guidance (**Fig. 5**). The decision about which agent to use is typically based on the comfort and preference of the radiologist performing the procedure. Success ranges up to 70% for barium[66] and 84% for air,[67,68] and is influenced by the duration of symptoms, with enema reduction being less successful the longer the delay in diagnosis.[69] Some pediatric radiologists have begun to incorporate the use of ultrasound-guided enema reduction as a treatment modality instead of traditional fluoroscopy-guided reduction, which carries the risk of ionizing radiation. This method has been used in other countries and has been shown to be safe and effective.[70–72]

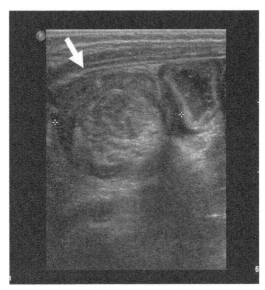

Fig. 4. Transverse ultrasonographic view of intussusception. Note the donut sign (*arrow*).

Operative reduction is required when radiographic enema reduction is either contraindicated, as in peritonitis, perforation, or profound shock,[73] or if reduction is unsuccessful.

The risk of recurrent intussusception after reduction is rare but more likely with nonoperative reduction. It has been reported in up to 15% of patients after undergoing hydrostatic reduction and up to 3% after operative reduction.[74] The risk is greatest in the first 24 hours after reduction, and therefore some institutions routinely admit these patients during this time for observation.

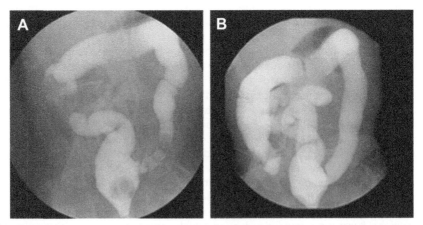

Fig. 5. (*A*) Fluoroscopic-guided enema showing contrast to the hepatic flexure at the level of the intussusception. (*B*) Successful enema reduction of intussusception. Note the presence of contrast filling the entire length of the large bowel.

Volvulus

Midgut volvulus is a surgical emergency in which a loop of bowel twists about its mesenteric attachment. It results from abnormal embryologic rotation of the midgut, known as malrotation. Malrotation occurs during the fifth to eighth week in embryonic life, when the intestine projects out of the abdominal cavity, rotates 270°, then returns into the abdomen. If the rotation does not occur correctly, the intestine does not develop a normal mesenteric attachment and is at risk for later twisting (**Fig. 6**). In addition, malrotated intestine is prone to obstruction by congenital bands of fibrous tissue (Ladd bands), which develop as a result of abnormal fixation of the colon to the right side of the retroperitoneum. Up to 75% of volvulus cases occur within the first month of life, and most (up to 90%) occur within the first year of life.[75,76]

Volvulus requires early detection in order to prevent irreversible loss of bowel. It should be suspected particularly in young infants with bilious emesis, and any infant with bilious vomiting should be considered to have a volvulus until proved otherwise. Volvulus may also present as failure to thrive, with severe feeding intolerance.[77] Pain and irritability are not prominent features in the neonate.[78] The abdomen is usually soft and nontender to palpation until strangulation of the bowel has developed, when it becomes distended and tender and the infant begins to have hematochezia.[79] In addition, an infant with already ischemic or necrotic bowel may present in shock and rapidly deteriorate clinically if the diagnosis is not recognized and surgically corrected.

The evaluation of a child with suspected volvulus should begin with abdominal plain films. These films may show a classic double-bubble sign (air bubbles located in the stomach and duodenum), other signs consistent with intestinal obstruction such as a paucity of gas, air-fluid levels, and dilated loops of bowel, or the radiograph most commonly may be entirely normal. Definitive diagnosis is made with an upper gastrointestinal (UGI) series to assess for the position of the ligament of Treitz. Normally the ligament of Treitz should be located at the level of the pylorus and just to the left of

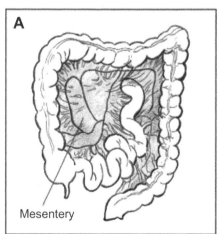
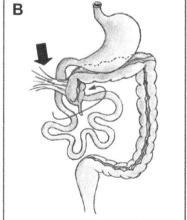

Fig. 6. (*A*) Normal bowel and mesentery position. (*B*) Positioning of the bowel and mesentery in malrotation. Note the cecum is not positioned correctly in the right lower quadrant, predisposing the bowel to twisting (*circular arrow*), and the tissue that normally holds it in place may cross over and block part of the small bowel (*thick arrow*). (*From* National Digestive Diseases Information Clearinghouse. Anatomic problems of the colon. NIH Publication No. 05–5120, February 2005. Available at: http://digestive.niddk.nih.gov/ddiseases/pubs/anatomiccolon/#Volvulus. Accessed January 3, 2009.)

midline, with the second portion of the duodenum coursing posteriorly on a lateral view.[80] The classic finding is that of the small intestine rotated to the right side of the abdomen (indicating malrotation), with contrast narrowing at the site of obstruction causing corkscrewing (indicating a volvulus) (**Fig. 7**). When the diagnosis is still in question, a contrast enema may provide additional information by showing an abnormal cecal position in association with malrotation.[81]

Ultrasound has also been used to make the diagnosis, but it is not as reliable as a UGI series. Ultrasound findings of volvulus include a distended, fluid-filled duodenum, increased peritoneal fluid, and dilated small bowel loops to the right of the spine.[82,83] Twisting of the small bowel around the superior mesenteric artery may also be seen.[84] The finding of inversion of the normal positions of the superior mesenteric artery and vein has been described as predictive of malrotation[83,85–89]; however, the true significance of this finding is controversial, and in addition, a normal relationship of the 2 vessels does not exclude malrotation.[84,90,91]

Treatment of volvulus should begin with aggressive fluid resuscitation with boluses of normal saline or lactated Ringer boluses and placement of a nasogastric tube. A pediatric surgeon should be immediately consulted once the diagnosis is suspected, because some surgeons explore the abdomen of such a child in the operating room without confirmatory diagnostic testing.[2]

Meckel's diverticulum

Meckel's diverticulum is the most common congenital malformation of the gastrointestinal tract.[92] Its presence is caused by the failure of the omphalomesenteric duct

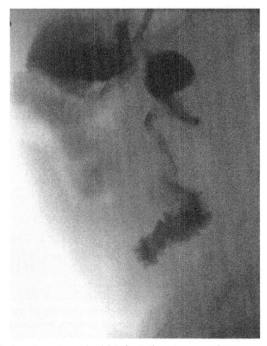

Fig. 7. UGI lateral view in a 1-week-old infant showing a corkscrew configuration of the distal duodenum and proximal jejunum in a patient with midgut volvulus. (*From* Williams H. Green for danger! Intestinal malrotation and volvulus. Arch Dis Child Educ Pract Ed 2007;92(3):90; with permission.)

to involute completely, resulting in patency of the ileal end of the duct.[93] It represents a true diverticulum because it is composed of all the layers of the intestinal wall.[94,95] The features of Meckel's diverticulum are commonly described by the rule of 2s[96]: present in 2% of the population, 2% of affected patients become symptomatic, the most common location is 2 feet from the ileocecal valve, nearly half of patients are less than 2 years of age, and the diverticulum is typically 2 inches (5 cm) long.

The classic presentation of Meckel's diverticulum is painless rectal bleeding caused by the heterotopic gastric mucosa when it is present. Other presentations may be seen depending on the complications that may arise from the presence of a Meckel's diverticulum, such as intussusception, obstruction, perforation, strangulation caused by a mesodiverticular band, diverticulitis, volvulus, hernia, and neoplasm.[97]

The diagnosis is made definitively with the use of nuclear scintigraphy (Meckel's scan). The test relies on the presence of ectopic gastric mucosa within the diverticulum, which has an affinity for the radionucleotide. The test has been shown to have an accuracy of up to 85%.[98] The condition is treated with surgical resection.

Ovarian torsion

Adnexal torsion is a surgical entity that must be diagnosed in a timely fashion in order to maximize salvage of the organ. Torsion may involve the fallopian tube, ovary, or both.[99] It is most likely to occur at or before menarche; however, it has been reported in premenarchal girls and even infants. It has been reported to account for up to 2.7% of all cases of pediatric abdominal pain.[100] Despite the fact that torsion is most commonly associated with adnexal conditions,[101] up to 25% of patients with torsion have normal ovaries.[102] When an adnexal mass is present, it is more likely to be benign.[103] Older patients may have torsion secondary to a corpus luteum or follicular cyst.

The diagnosis of adnexal torsion can be difficult, because the signs and symptoms associated with torsion may mimic other conditions, such as appendicitis, when the right side is involved. Symptoms of adnexal torsion and their frequency are listed in **Table 4**.

Proper diagnosis of adnexal torsion is made with the use of ultrasound imaging. Ovarian enlargement may be seen early in adnexal torsion, even before infarction has occurred. Other findings include free intraperitoneal pelvic fluid and the presence of cystic follicles along the periphery of the ovary, with thickening of the cyst wall.[104–106] The addition of Doppler imaging, which provides information regarding vascular blood flow, may also aid in the diagnosis; however, the presence of flow should not reassure the clinician of no adnexal torsion because this may be a late finding. Sensitivity has been reported to be 100%, with a specificity of 87% to 98%.[107,108] Pelvic CT may be useful in the diagnosis of adnexal torsion when the

Table 4	
Signs and symptoms of adnexal torsion	
Signs/Symptoms	**Prevalence (%)**
Abdominal pain	100
Nausea/vomiting	70–85
Fevers	18–20
Palpable mass	20–36
Leukocytosis	56

Data from Refs.[170–173]

ovaries are unable to be visualized on ultrasound or if ultrasound is unavailable. Although CT may not provide information regarding blood flow to the adnexa, it may show the presence of an enlarged ovary with peripheral follicles, similar to ultrasound.[109] The greatest fear with ovarian torsion is the loss of ovarian function secondary to loss of blood flow to the ovary. The duration of vascular interruption necessary to produce irreversible damage is unknown, and normal ovarian function has been reported after up to 72 hours of torsion.[110] Nonetheless, a high level of clinical suspicion, expeditious imaging, and familiarity with the varied clinical and imaging presentations of ovarian torsion should decrease the surgical delay and improve the likelihood of ovarian salvage.[111]

Incarcerated hernia

Indirect inguinal hernias occur in 1% to 3% of all children and are 6 times more likely to occur in males than in females.[2] Premature infants are at higher risk than those born full-term because of the timing of the final descent of the testes into the scrotum at approximately 28 to 36 weeks' gestation. It is not until this descent that closure of the peritoneal opening of the internal ring begins, which, although patent, allows for bowel contents to herniate through the inguinal canal. Most incarcerated hernias requiring surgical reduction occur during the first year of life.[112] The risk of incarceration is highest within the first 6 months of life[113,114] and rarely occurs after 8 years of age.[114]

The diagnosis of an inguinal hernia is suggested by a history of an intermittent bulge in the groin with crying, both of which usually resolve. This condition usually is brought to the parents' attention during a routine diaper change. If the clinician is able to easily reduce the hernia on examination, then the patient may be discharged with reassurance, guidance on when to return, and a referral to a pediatric surgeon on an outpatient basis. However, the persistence of this inguinal bulge, along with other symptoms such as crying, irritability, fever, refusal to eat, or vomiting, should prompt the clinician to consider the diagnosis of incarceration. On examination, a smooth, firm, sausage-shaped, mildly tender, erythematous mass may be palpated in the groin. The hernia originates proximal to the inguinal ring and can extend into the scrotum.[2]

The diagnosis of an incarcerated inguinal hernia is usually made clinically; however, if the diagnosis is uncertain, scrotal ultrasound may be helpful in distinguishing other scrotal conditions such as a hydrocele. Most incarcerated hernias can be reduced manually unless there is clear peritonitis or bowel compromise.[115] This procedure is usually performed at the bedside by either the emergency physician or a pediatric surgeon or urologist. There is a high rate of early recurrent incarceration, and therefore many surgeons recommend admission to the hospital for observation after manual reduction.

Nonsurgical

Acute gastroenteritis

AGE is characterized by acute diarrhea with or without nausea, vomiting, fever, and abdominal pain.[116] Worldwide, diarrhea is responsible for 1.4 to 2.5 million deaths per year.[117,118] In children less than 5 years of age, up to 150,000 hospitalizations (10% of hospitalizations) and 3.7 million physician visits per year in the United States are because of diarrheal illnesses.[119,120]

Because AGE is the most common reason for a child to present to the ED with gastrointestinal symptoms, it is easy for the emergency physician to become complacent with the diagnosis. However, it is important to distinguish the child with gastroenteritis from the patient with another diagnosis that may present in a similar manner, such as diabetic ketoacidosis, an inborn error of metabolism, a urinary tract infection/pyelonephritis, increased intracranial pressure, or any of the aforementioned surgical causes of abdominal pain.

The management of a patient with gastroenteritis and dehydration should be dictated by the patient's clinical picture, rather than by laboratory values. Numerous studies have attempted to identify laboratory predictors (serum bicarbonate, blood urea nitrogen) of the degree of dehydration.[121–126] However, in most patients with uncomplicated AGE, serum electrolytes are not helpful in predicting the degree of dehydration or determining appropriate management of these patients.[116] In patients with lethargy or altered mental status, it is helpful to obtain a serum glucose level and possibly serum electrolytes, a recommendation that is supported by the American Academy of Pediatrics.[127] For patients with hypoglycemia (serum glucose <60 mg/dL), treatment should include a 2.5 to 5 mL/kg bolus of 10% dextrose (D10W), or a 1 to 2 mL/kg bolus of 25% dextrose (D25W)[128,129] with the addition of dextrose-containing intravenous fluids (5%–10% dextrose 1/2 normal saline) at 1 to 1.5 times the maintenance rate[129] to maintain euglycemia.

Stool cultures are not routinely indicated in immunocompetent patients with diarrhea, because most cases of gastroenteritis are viral in nature, and identification of the exact pathogen does not influence management of the patient. However, if the patient is experiencing grossly bloody stools, the presence of a bacterial pathogen (*Escherichia coli*, *Shigella*, *Salmonella*, *Yersinia*, or *Campylobacter* species) should be suspected, and stool cultures should be sent.

Patients with gastroenteritis represent a spectrum of disease, from those with mild dehydration to those with severe dehydration, or even hypovolemic shock. The level of dehydration dictates the treatment and ultimately the disposition of such patients. **Table 5** provides an objective measure of classifying patients with dehydration as mild, moderate, or severe.

Until recently, the management of patients with gastroenteritis included intravenous therapy. However, over the last decade numerous studies have been conducted showing the success of oral rehydration therapy (ORT) as the first-line therapy for the treatment of ED patients with mild to moderate dehydration secondary to AGE.[130–132] **Table 6** lists the treatment of patients with gastroenteritis based on their degree of dehydration and takes into account both the amount of fluid that should be replaced based on losses that have occurred and those that continue to occur while in

Table 5
Signs and symptoms associated with levels of dehydration

	Mild (<5% Weight Loss)	Moderate (5%–10% Weight Loss)	Severe (>10% Weight Loss)
Heart rate	Slight increase	Increased	Significantly increased
Blood pressure	Normal	Normal	Low
Capillary refill	<2 s	2–3 s	>3 s
Mucous membranes (tongue)	Normal/dry	Dry	Dry
Mental status	Normal	Altered	Depressed
Appearance of eyes	Normal	Sunken	Sunken
Urine output	Small	Oliguric	Oliguric/anuric

Data from Shaw K. Dehydration. In: Fleisher G, Ludwig S, Henretig F, et al, editors. Textbook of pediatric emergency medicine, 4th edition. Philadelphia: Lippincott Williams & Wilkins; 2000.

Table 6		
Treatment of gastroenteritis based on the degree of dehydration		
Degree of Dehydration	Rehydration Therapy	Replacement of Losses
Mild to moderate	Oral rehydration solution, 50–100 mL/kg body weight for 3–4 h Initiate therapy with 5 mL (1 tsp) every 5 min and advance as tolerated If not improving or tolerating ORT, consider IVF	Additional 2 mL/kg body weight of ORT per emesis, and 10 mL/kg body weight per diarrheal episode
Severe	0.9 normal saline or lactated Ringer bolus 20 mL/kg until mental status and perfusion improve, followed by 5% dextrose 1/2 normal saline intravenously at twice maintenance rates	As above If unable to tolerate oral fluids, administer additional losses as above as 5% dextrose 1/2 normal saline

Abbreviation: IVF, intravenous fluids.
Data from King CK, Glass R, Bresee JS, et al. Managing acute gastroenteritis among children: oral rehydration, maintenance, and nutritional therapy. MMWR Recomm Rep 2003;52:1–16.

the ED. The World Health Organization recommends a reduced osmolarity solution for ORT, such as Pedialyte, Rehydralyte, and Infalyte. Gatorade is not recommended as a rehydrating solution in children with gastroenteritis.

Historically, antiemetics have not been recommended for use in pediatric patients. Studies involving phenothiazines specifically have shown their association with adverse reactions such as acute dystonic reactions and apnea.[133–135] In addition, many of these drugs are associated with sedation and drowsiness, which may interfere with the ability to orally rehydrate these patients. Furthermore, the US Food and Drug Administration has required a black box warning on promethazine hydrochloride,[136] which cautions against its use in children less than 2 years of age because of the potential for fatal respiratory depression. The warning also calls for caution in those older than 2 years and avoidance of coadministration of other medications with respiratory depression effects. Recently, several studies have shown the efficacy and safety of the use of ondansetron, a 5-HT$_3$ receptor antagonist, as an antiemetic in patients with vomiting attributed to gastroenteritis.[137–141] These studies concluded that the use of ondansetron reduced the rate of emesis, improved the amount of oral intake, and decreased lengths of stay in the ED.

The decision to admit the child with gastroenteritis and dehydration to the hospital should include several factors. Potential indications for admission include dehydration greater than 5% with the inability to tolerate oral fluids, intractable or bilious emesis, significant electrolyte disturbances, or suspicion for parental noncompliance with home ORT and/or follow-up.[116]

Henoch-Schönlein purpura
Henoch-Schönlein purpura (HSP) is the most common vasculitis of childhood, associated with the classic palpable purpuric rash on the lower extremities. It occurs most frequently between 5 and 15 years of age, with the mean age of about 5 to 6 years, and 90% of patients are less than 10 years old.[142–144] Gastrointestinal involvement has been reported in approximately 50% to 75% of cases, with the most

common presentation being colicky abdominal pain.[142,144,145] In addition, patients may have vomiting, and although gastrointestinal bleeding is usually occult, about 30% of patients have grossly bloody or melanotic stools.[146] Approximately 2% of patients have massive gastrointestinal hemorrhage.[147] Symptoms are caused by bowel wall edema and hemorrhage secondary to vasculitis. HSP may also present as intussusception caused by areas of edematous bowel serving as a lead point. Other extraintestinal manifestations of HSP include arthritis or arthralgia, renal disease manifesting as hematuria with or without proteinuria, and orchitis in boys. The diagnosis of HSP is usually made on clinical grounds, especially when the patient presents with the characteristic rash. There are no distinctive or diagnostic laboratory abnormalities associated with HSP.[146] HSP is usually a self-limited disease lasting an average of about 4 weeks. Treatment is largely supportive, with no specific therapy required.[146] Steroids are often used for the relief of abdominal pain, although their use is not yet considered standard of care because of the lack of sufficient evidence in the literature. The abdominal pain usually resolves within a few days with or without treatment.[147]

Constipation

Constipation is a common reason why pediatric patients present to the ED with abdominal pain and is of particular concern to many parents. Despite the fact that most constipation outside the neonatal period is functional, physicians must take care to rule out other conditions that may be causing the constipation.

There is wide variability in the normal frequency of bowel movements, which can vary with diet and age. Functional constipation is caused by painful bowel movements with resultant voluntary withholding of feces by the child.[148]

The first step in evaluating a child with suspected constipation is a thorough medical history, including what the family or child mean when they use the term constipation, the duration of symptoms, the frequency of bowel movements, consistency and size of the stools, presence of abdominal and anal pain, and the presence of blood on the stool or toilet paper. Parents may report a history of diarrhea, which may be a sign of encopresis (leakage of liquid stool around firm feces in the rectum). The practitioner should inquire about stool-withholding behavior and medications that may be a source of constipation. Signs of organic conditions[148] include fever, abdominal distension, anorexia, nausea, vomiting, weight loss, poor weight gain, or a delay in the first bowel movement after birth (>48 hours).

The physical examination should include external examination of the perineum and perianal area and a digital rectal examination to assess tone, rectal size, anal wink, volume and consistency of stool that may be present in the rectal vault, and the presence of fecal occult blood.[148] **Box 2** lists those findings on physical examination that should prompt an evaluation for an organic cause of constipation.

Organic causes of constipation that should be considered, particularly in the newborn and infant age groups, include imperforate anus, anal stenosis, meconium plug syndrome, meconium ileus (cystic fibrosis), Hirschprung disease, volvulus, infant botulism, hypocalcemia, hypercalcemia, and hypothyroidism.[2] In general, the diagnosis of functional constipation can be made based on clinical grounds alone; however, when the diagnosis is in question, or other diagnoses are being considered, an abdominal obstruction series should be obtained.

Management consists of disimpaction, if fecal impaction is present, initiation of oral medications, and parental education. Fecal impaction occurs when there is a hard mass in the lower abdomen, a dilated rectum filled with a large amount of stool, or excessive stool in the colon identified by abdominal radiograph.[149] Disimpaction may occur with oral medication such as high doses of mineral oil or polyethylene

---

Box 2
Physical examination findings suggesting organic conditions in a child with constipation

Failure to thrive

Abdominal distension

Lack of lumbosacral curve

Pilonidal dimple covered by a tuft of hair

Midline pigmentary abnormalities of the lower spine

Sacral agenesis

Flat buttocks

Anteriorly displaced anus

Patulous anus

Tight, empty rectum in presence of palpable abdominal fecal mass

Gush of liquid stool and air from rectum on withdrawal of finger

Occult blood in stool

Absent anal wink

Absent cremasteric reflex

Decreased lower extremity tone and/or strength

Absence or delay in relaxation phase of lower extremity deep-tendon reflexes

Data from Baker SS, Liptak GS, Colletti RB, et al. Constipation in infants and children: evaluation and treatment. A medical position statement of the North American Society for pediatric gastroenterology and nutrition. J Pediatr Gastroenterol Nutr 1999; 29:612–26.

---

glycol electrolyte solutions. However, these medications are poorly tolerated in the pediatric age group, are usually reserved for inpatient management of refractory patients, and may require the use of a nasogastric tube for administration. Rectal disimpaction may be performed with an array of enemas, such as saline, mineral oil, or polyethylene glycol electrolyte solution. In infants, rectal disimpaction may be performed with glycerin suppositories.[150] The next step in management is prescribing maintenance therapy. This therapy consists of dietary interventions (increased intake of fluids, fiber, and carbohydrates, particularly those found in some juices), behavioral modification (encouragement of unhurried toilet time after meals, maintenance of stool diaries), and laxatives. The choice of laxatives depends on the age of the child, consideration of side effects, and practitioner preference. Some suggested options include mineral oil (not to be used in those <1 year of age secondary to the risk of aspiration), lactulose, sorbitol, polyethylene glycol, and docusate. Stimulants, such as bisacodyl and senna, should be reserved for short-term use and may be initiated with the other medications listed until regular stooling habits are maintained.

Functional abdominal pain

Functional abdominal pain is a common childhood complaint seen in the absence of significant organic conditions.[151] Despite the lack of a true condition to explain the symptoms, up to 30% of patients are diagnosed with functional disorders,[152–154] such as irritable bowel syndrome, functional dyspepsia, and abdominal migraine. The pain can be severe and disruptive to the child's (and the family's) routine daily life. Studies have reported the prevalence to be between 0.5% and 19%.[153–158]

The diagnosis of functional abdominal pain is a diagnosis of exclusion in patients who usually present to the ED with symptoms of chronic or recurrent abdominal pain. Several definitions have been proposed to describe chronic or recurrent abdominal pain; however, most investigators agree that it represents pain lasting for a period of at least 3 months and is either chronic or episodic.[151] In evaluating the child with chronic or recurrent abdominal pain, the emergency physician must determine the likelihood of serious conditions by performing a preliminary evaluation, including a thorough history and physical examination. This strategy should point the clinician to specific red flags that require a more thorough evaluation, such as weight loss, reduced growth, significant vomiting, chronic severe diarrhea, hematochezia, hematemesis, unexplained fever, and a family history of inflammatory bowel disease.[151] The suggested initial laboratory evaluation should include a complete blood count with differential, basic metabolic panel, inflammatory markers (eg, CRP test, erythrocyte sedimentation rate), liver enzyme and function tests, pancreatic enzyme tests, and UA. Further investigations depend on the possible differential diagnosis suggested by the history and physical examination.

Most cases of chronic or recurrent abdominal pain, in the absence of the red flags and laboratory values found to be within normal limits, do not require any treatment in the ED setting, other than reassurance that there is no evidence of an underlying organic condition.[159] This observation should not minimize or deny the symptoms experienced by the child, but rather emphasize that the pain has not arisen from a harmful process. The family should be counseled on returning to the ED for a change in symptoms, including those consistent with dehydration as a result of significant output or a lack of intake. In addition, the patient should be referred to a pediatric gastroenterologist for further management as an outpatient.

Extraabdominal

Pneumonia
Although pneumonia is a known cause of pediatric abdominal pain, its diagnosis may be missed initially. Diagnostic uncertainty has resulted in the removal of normal appendices[160,161] in patients with acute abdominal pain. **Fig. 8** shows right-sided lung infiltrates in a patient who presented with severe abdominal pain in the right lower quadrant and was being evaluated for possible appendicitis. In general, intrathoracic processes may mimic an acute abdomen by referred pain.[162] The diaphragmatic pleura is innervated by the 6 or 7 lowest intercostal nerves peripherally and by the phrenic nerve centrally,[163,164] and therefore pain may be referred to the abdominal wall during the course of a basilar pneumonia. The reported prevalence of pneumonia in children with abdominal pain ranges from 2.7% to 5%.[160,165] It is difficult to rely on the classic triad of fever, cough, and rales when deciding to obtain a chest radiograph, because the positive predictive value of this constellation is 27% and the sensitivity only 35%.[166] This observation is of particular importance in young children, because these patients may offer suboptimal examinations, and it may be difficult to identify clinical signs and symptoms consistent with pneumonia. In a study of 51 patients with extraabdominal causes of acute abdominal pain, 15 patients were diagnosed with pneumonia and 10 of them were 3 years of age or younger.[167] Therefore, in the evaluation of pediatric abdominal pain, it is important to consider evaluating for pneumonia as an occult cause.

Group A beta-hemolytic streptococcal pharyngitis
Patients with group A beta-hemolytic streptococcal (GABHS) pharyngitis commonly present with sore throat, odynophagia, and fever. However, other symptoms, such

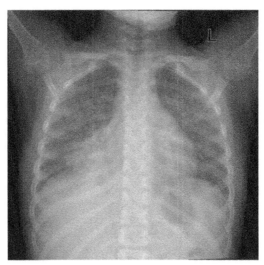

Fig. 8. Posteroanterior chest radiograph of a patient presenting with severe right lower quadrant pain and concern for appendicitis. The radiograph shows right middle and lower lobe infiltrates.

as headache, vomiting, and abdominal pain, may also be present. One study reported a 27% prevalence of abdominal pain among patients with culture-positive GABHS.[168] Another study of pediatric patients found a prevalence of either bacterial or viral pharyngitis of 16.6% in patients presenting with abdominal pain.[5] GABHS is primarily a disease of children between 5 and 15 years of age[169] and its prevalence is highest in the winter and early spring.[169] Despite attempts at developing clinical scoring systems in an effort to identify patients at low risk of infection with GABHS, and therefore to forgo rapid and culture testing for GABHS, the signs and symptoms of GABHS and non-GABHS pharyngitis overlap too broadly,[169] making an exclusively clinical diagnosis inaccurate in many cases. Therefore, pharyngitis, specifically that caused by GABHS, should be considered and tested for in patients who present to the ED with abdominal pain and signs and symptoms consistent with pharyngitis.

SUMMARY

Abdominal pain is a common chief complaint among children presenting to the ED. The emergency physician must have a high index of suspicion for surgical emergencies requiring immediate attention, nonsurgical gastrointestinal diagnoses, as well as extraabdominal conditions, which may also be a cause of abdominal pain.

REFERENCES

1. Ruddy RM. Pain–abdomen. In: Fleisher G, Ludwig S, Henretig F, et al, editors. Textbook of pediatric emergency medicine. 5th edition. Philadelphia: Lippincott Williams & Wilkins; 2006. p. 469–76.
2. McCollough M, Sharieff GQ. Abdominal surgical emergencies in infants and young children. Emerg Med Clin North Am 2003;21(4):909–35.
3. Mason JD. The evaluation of acute abdominal pain in children. Emerg Med Clin North Am 1996;14(3):629–44.

4. Reynolds SL, Jaffe DM. Diagnosing abdominal pain in a pediatric emergency department. Pediatr Emerg Care 1992;8(3):126–8.
5. Scholer SJ, Pituch K, Orr DP, et al. Clinical outcomes of children with acute abdominal pain. Pediatrics 1996;98(4 Pt 1):680–5.
6. Smink DS, Fishman SJ, Kleinman K, et al. Effects of race, insurance status, and hospital volume on perforated appendicitis in children. Pediatrics 2005;115(4):920–5.
7. Bratton SL, Haberkern CM, Waldhausen JH. Acute appendicitis risks of complications: age and Medicaid insurance. Pediatrics 2000;106(1 Pt 1):75–8.
8. Addiss DG, Shaffer N, Fowler BS, et al. The epidemiology of appendicitis and appendectomy in the United States. Am J Epidemiol 1990;132(5):910–25.
9. Horwitz JR, Gursoy M, Jaksic T, et al. Importance of diarrhea as a presenting symptom of appendicitis in very young children. Am J Surg 1997;173(2):80–2.
10. Grosfeld JL, Weinberger M, Clatworthy HW Jr. Acute appendicitis in the first two years of life. J Pediatr Surg 1973;8(2):285–93.
11. Bundy DG, Byerley JS, Liles EA, et al. Does this child have appendicitis? JAMA 2007;298(4):438–51.
12. Karaman A, Cavusoglu YH, Karaman I, et al. Seven cases of neonatal appendicitis with a review of the English language literature of the last century. Pediatr Surg Int 2003;19(11):707–9.
13. Schorlemmer GR, Herbst CA Jr. Perforated neonatal appendicitis. South Med J 1983;76(4):536–7.
14. Rothrock SG, Green SM, Dobson M, et al. Misdiagnosis of appendicitis in nonpregnant women of childbearing age. J Emerg Med 1995;13(1):1–8.
15. Williams N, Bello M. Perforation rate relates to delayed presentation in childhood acute appendicitis. J R Coll Surg Edinb 1998;43(2):101–2.
16. Saidi RF, Ghasemi M. Role of Alvarado score in diagnosis and treatment of suspected acute appendicitis. Am J Emerg Med 2000;18(2):230–1.
17. Peltola H, Ahlqvist J, Rapola J, et al. C-reactive protein compared with white blood cell count and erythrocyte sedimentation rate in the diagnosis of acute appendicitis in children. Acta Chir Scand 1986;152:55–8.
18. Paajanen H, Mansikka A, Laato M, et al. Are serum inflammatory markers age dependent in acute appendicitis? J Am Coll Surg 1997;184(3):303–8.
19. Miskowiak J, Burcharth F. The white cell count in acute appendicitis. A prospective blind study. Dan Med Bull 1982;29(4):210–1.
20. Wu HP, Chang CF, Lin CY. Predictive inflammatory parameters in the diagnosis of acute appendicitis in children. Acta Paediatr Taiwan 2003;44(4):227–31.
21. Mikaelsson C, Arnbjornsson E. The value of C-reactive protein (CRP) determinations in patients with suspected acute appendicitis. Ann Chir Gynaecol 1984;73(5):281–4.
22. Rodriguez-Sanjuan JC, Martin-Parra JI, Seco I, et al. C-reactive protein and leukocyte count in the diagnosis of acute appendicitis in children. Dis Colon Rectum 1999;42(10):1325–9.
23. Paajanen H, Somppi E. Early childhood appendicitis is still a difficult diagnosis. Acta Paediatr 1996;85(4):459–62.
24. Schneider C, Kharbanda A, Bachur R. Evaluating appendicitis scoring systems using a prospective pediatric cohort. Ann Emerg Med 2007;49(6):778–84, 784 e1.
25. Kharbanda AB, Taylor GA, Fishman SJ, et al. A clinical decision rule to identify children at low risk for appendicitis. Pediatrics 2005;116(3):709–16.

26. Dado G, Anania G, Baccarani U, et al. Application of a clinical score for the diagnosis of acute appendicitis in childhood: a retrospective analysis of 197 patients. J Pediatr Surg 2000;35(9):1320–2.

27. Macklin CP, Radcliffe GS, Merei JM, et al. A prospective evaluation of the modified Alvarado score for acute appendicitis in children. Ann R Coll Surg Engl 1997;79(3):203–5.

28. Owen TD, Williams H, Stiff G, et al. Evaluation of the Alvarado score in acute appendicitis. J R Soc Med 1992;85(2):87–8.

29. Brennan GD. Pediatric appendicitis: pathophysiology and appropriate use of diagnostic imaging. CJEM 2006;8(6):425–32.

30. Albiston E. The role of radiological imaging in the diagnosis of acute appendicitis. Can J Gastroenterol 2002;16(7):451–63.

31. Weyant MJ, Eachempati SR, Maluccio MA, et al. Is imaging necessary for the diagnosis of acute appendicitis? Adv Surg 2003;37:327–45.

32. Orr RK, Porter D, Hartman D. Ultrasonography to evaluate adults for appendicitis: decision making based on meta-analysis and probabilistic reasoning. Acad Emerg Med 1995;2(7):644–50.

33. Wong ML, Casey SO, Leonidas JC, et al. Sonographic diagnosis of acute appendicitis in children. J Pediatr Surg 1994;29(10):1356–60.

34. Ramachandran P, Sivit CJ, Newman KD, et al. Ultrasonography as an adjunct in the diagnosis of acute appendicitis: a 4-year experience. J Pediatr Surg 1996; 31(1):164–7 [discussion: 167–9].

35. Crady SK, Jones JS, Wyn T, et al. Clinical validity of ultrasound in children with suspected appendicitis. Ann Emerg Med 1993;22(7):1125–9.

36. Zaki AM, MacMahon RA, Gray AR. Acute appendicitis in children: when does ultrasound help? Aust N Z J Surg 1994;64(10):695–8.

37. Hahn HB, Hoepner FU, Kalle T, et al. Sonography of acute appendicitis in children: 7 years experience. Pediatr Radiol 1998;28(3):147–51.

38. Carrico CW, Fenton LZ, Taylor GA, et al. Impact of sonography on the diagnosis and treatment of acute lower abdominal pain in children and young adults. AJR Am J Roentgenol 1999;172(2):513–6.

39. Lessin MS, Chan M, Catallozzi M, et al. Selective use of ultrasonography for acute appendicitis in children. Am J Surg 1999;177(3):193–6.

40. Rice HE, Arbesman M, Martin DJ, et al. Does early ultrasonography affect management of pediatric appendicitis? A prospective analysis. J Pediatr Surg 1999;34(5):754–8 [discussion: 758–9].

41. Pena BM, Taylor GA, Lund DP, et al. Effect of computed tomography on patient management and costs in children with suspected appendicitis. Pediatrics 1999;104(3 Pt 1):440–6.

42. Pena BM, Taylor GA, Fishman SJ, et al. Costs and effectiveness of ultrasonography and limited computed tomography for diagnosing appendicitis in children. Pediatrics 2000;106(4):672–6.

43. Hoecker CC, Billman GF. The utility of unenhanced computed tomography in appendicitis in children. J Emerg Med 2005;28(4):415–21.

44. Brenner DJ, Hall EJ. Computed tomography–an increasing source of radiation exposure. N Engl J Med 2007;357(22):2277–84.

45. Waseem M, Rosenberg HK. Intussusception. Pediatr Emerg Care 2008;24(11): 793–800.

46. Newman J, Schuh S. Intussusception in babies under 4 months of age. CMAJ 1987;136(3):266–9.

47. Lai IR, Huang MT, Lee WJ. Mini-laparoscopic reduction of intussusception for children. J Formos Med Assoc 2000;99(6):510–2.
48. Daneman A, Alton DJ. Intussusception. Issues and controversies related to diagnosis and reduction. Radiol Clin North Am 1996;34(4):743–56.
49. Stringer MD, Pablot SM, Brereton RJ. Paediatric intussusception. Br J Surg 1992;79(9):867–76.
50. Bajaj L, Roback MG. Postreduction management of intussusception in a children's hospital emergency department. Pediatrics 2003;112(6 Pt 1):1302–7.
51. DiFiore JW. Intussusception. Semin Pediatr Surg 1999;8(4):214–20.
52. Asano Y, Yoshikawa T, Suga S, et al. Simultaneous occurrence of human herpes-virus 6 infection and intussusception in three infants. Pediatr Infect Dis J 1991; 10(4):335–7.
53. O'Ryan M, Lucero Y, Pena A, et al. Two year review of intestinal intussusception in six large public hospitals of Santiago, Chile. Pediatr Infect Dis J 2003;22(8): 717–21.
54. Reijnen JA, Festen C, Joosten HJ, et al. Atypical characteristics of a group of children with intussusception. Acta Paediatr Scand 1990;79(6–7):675–9.
55. Sato M, Ishida H, Konno K, et al. Long-standing painless intussusception in adults. Eur Radiol 2000;10(5):811–3.
56. Tenenbein M, Wiseman NE. Early coma in intussusception: endogenous opioid induced? Pediatr Emerg Care 1987;3(1):22–3.
57. d'Escrienne MM, Velin P, Filippigh P, et al. Lethargic form of acute intestinal intussusception in an infant. Arch Pediatr 1996;3(1):44–6 [in French].
58. Mackay AJ, MacKellar A, Sprague P. Intussusception in children: a review of 91 cases. Aust N Z J Surg 1987;57(1):15–7.
59. Hernandez JA, Swischuk LE, Angel CA. Validity of plain films in intussusception. Emerg Radiol 2004;10(6):323–6.
60. Harrington L, Connolly B, Hu X, et al. Ultrasonographic and clinical predictors of intussusception. J Pediatr 1998;132(5):836–9.
61. Pracros JP, Tran-Minh VA, Morin de Finfe CH, et al. Acute intestinal intussusception in children. Contribution of ultrasonography (145 cases). Ann Radiol (Paris) 1987;30(7):525–30.
62. Shanbhogue RL, Hussain SM, Meradji M, et al. Ultrasonography is accurate enough for the diagnosis of intussusception. J Pediatr Surg 1994;29(2):324–7 [discussion: 327–8].
63. Verschelden P, Filiatrault D, Garel L, et al. Intussusception in children: reliability of US in diagnosis–a prospective study. Radiology 1992;184(3):741–4.
64. del-Pozo G, Albillos JC, Tejedor D, et al. Intussusception in children: current concepts in diagnosis and enema reduction. Radiographics 1999;19(2):299–319.
65. Henrikson S, Blane CE, Koujok K, et al. The effect of screening sonography on the positive rate of enemas for intussusception. Pediatr Radiol 2003;33(3):190–3.
66. Hadidi AT, El Shal N. Childhood intussusception: a comparative study of nonsur-gical management. J Pediatr Surg 1999;34(2):304–7.
67. Lui KW, Wong HF, Cheung YC, et al. Air enema for diagnosis and reduction of intussusception in children: clinical experience and fluoroscopy time correlation. J Pediatr Surg 2001;36(3):479–81.
68. Rubi I, Vera R, Rubi SC, et al. Air reduction of intussusception. Eur J Pediatr Surg 2002;12(6):387–90.
69. Applegate KE. Intussusception in children: evidence-based diagnosis and treatment. Pediatr Radiol 2009;39(Suppl 2):S140–3.

70. Crystal P, Hertzanu Y, Farber B, et al. Sonographically guided hydrostatic reduction of intussusception in children. J Clin Ultrasound 2002;30(6):343–8.

71. Yoon CH, Kim HJ, Goo HW. Intussusception in children: US-guided pneumatic reduction–initial experience. Radiology 2001;218(1):85–8.

72. Gu L, Zhu H, Wang S, et al. Sonographic guidance of air enema for intussusception reduction in children. Pediatr Radiol 2000;30(5):339–42.

73. Sorantin E, Lindbichler F. Management of intussusception. Eur Radiol 2004; 14(Suppl 4):L146–54.

74. Kenigsberg K, Lee JC, Stein H. Recurrent acute intussusception. Pediatrics 1974;53(2):269–70.

75. Torres AM, Ziegler MM. Malrotation of the intestine. World J Surg 1993;17(3): 326–31.

76. Applegate KE, Anderson JM, Klatte EC. Intestinal malrotation in children: a problem-solving approach to the upper gastrointestinal series. Radiographics 2006;26(5):1485–500.

77. Lin JN, Lou CC, Wang KL. Intestinal malrotation and midgut volvulus: a 15-year review. J Formos Med Assoc 1995;94(4):178–81.

78. Millar AJ, Rode H, Brown RA, et al. The deadly vomit: malrotation and midgut volvulus. Pediatr Surg Int 1987;2:172–6.

79. Millar AJ, Rode H, Cywes S. Malrotation and volvulus in infancy and childhood. Semin Pediatr Surg 2003;12(4):229–36.

80. Slovis TL, Klein MD, Watts FB Jr. Incomplete rotation of the intestine with a normal cecal position. Surgery 1980;87(3):325–30.

81. Williams H. Green for danger! Intestinal malrotation and volvulus. Arch Dis Child Educ Pract Ed 2007;92(3):ep87–91.

82. Shimanuki Y, Aihara T, Takano H, et al. Clockwise whirlpool sign at color Doppler US: an objective and definite sign of midgut volvulus. Radiology 1996;199(1): 261–4.

83. Weinberger E, Winters WD, Liddell RM, et al. Sonographic diagnosis of intestinal malrotation in infants: importance of the relative positions of the superior mesenteric vein and artery. AJR Am J Roentgenol 1992;159(4):825–8.

84. Zerin JM, DiPietro MA. Superior mesenteric vascular anatomy at US in patients with surgically proved malrotation of the midgut. Radiology 1992;183(3):693–4.

85. Nichols DM, Li DK. Superior mesenteric vein rotation: a CT sign of midgut malrotation. AJR Am J Roentgenol 1983;141(4):707–8.

86. Shatzkes D, Gordon DH, Haller JO, et al. Malrotation of the bowel: malalignment of the superior mesenteric artery-vein complex shown by CT and MR. J Comput Assist Tomogr 1990;14(1):93–5.

87. Pracros JP, Sann L, Genin G, et al. Ultrasound diagnosis of midgut volvulus: the "whirlpool" sign. Pediatr Radiol 1992;22(1):18–20.

88. Leonidas JC, Magid N, Soberman N, et al. Midgut volvulus in infants: diagnosis with US. Work in progress. Radiology 1991;179(2):491–3.

89. Hayden CK Jr, Boulden TF, Swischuk LE, et al. Sonographic demonstration of duodenal obstruction with midgut volvulus. AJR Am J Roentgenol 1984; 143(1):9–10.

90. Dufour D, Delaet MH, Dassonville M, et al. Midgut malrotation, the reliability of sonographic diagnosis. Pediatr Radiol 1992;22(1):21–3.

91. Ashley LM, Allen S, Teele RL. A normal sonogram does not exclude malrotation. Pediatr Radiol 2001;31(5):354–6.

92. Sagar J, Kumar V, Shah DK. Meckel's diverticulum: a systematic review. J R Soc Med 2006;99(10):501–5.

93. Levy AD, Hobbs CM. From the archives of the AFIP. Meckel diverticulum: radiologic features with pathologic correlation. Radiographics 2004;24(2): 565–87.
94. Park JJ, Wolff BG, Tollefson MK, et al. Meckel diverticulum: the Mayo Clinic experience with 1476 patients (1950–2002). Ann Surg 2005;241(3):529–33.
95. Matsagas MI, Fatouros M, Koulouras B, et al. Incidence, complications, and management of Meckel's diverticulum. Arch Surg 1995;130(2):143–6.
96. McCollough M, Sharieff GQ. Abdominal pain in children. Pediatr Clin North Am 2006;53(1):107–37, vi.
97. Kusumoto H, Yoshida M, Takahashi I, et al. Complications and diagnosis of Meckel's diverticulum in 776 patients. Am J Surg 1992;164(4):382–3.
98. St-Vil D, Brandt ML, Panic S, et al. Meckel's diverticulum in children: a 20-year review. J Pediatr Surg 1991;26(11):1289–92.
99. Breech LL, Hillard PJ. Adnexal torsion in pediatric and adolescent girls. Curr Opin Obstet Gynecol 2005;17(5):483–9.
100. Rody A, Jackisch C, Klockenbusch W, et al. The conservative management of adnexal torsion–a case-report and review of the literature. Eur J Obstet Gynecol Reprod Biol 2002;101(1):83–6.
101. Taylor S. Torsion of the ovary in childhood. Arch Dis Child 1952;27(134): 368–70.
102. Davis AJ, Feins NR. Subsequent asynchronous torsion of normal adnexa in children. J Pediatr Surg 1990;25(6):687–9.
103. Shust NM, Hendricksen DK. Ovarian torsion: an unusual cause of abdominal pain in a young girl. Am J Emerg Med 1995;13(3):307–9.
104. Graif M, Shalev J, Strauss S, et al. Torsion of the ovary: sonographic features. AJR Am J Roentgenol 1984;143(6):1331–4.
105. Graif M, Itzchak Y. Sonographic evaluation of ovarian torsion in childhood and adolescence. AJR Am J Roentgenol 1988;150(3):647–9.
106. Helvie MA, Silver TM. Ovarian torsion: sonographic evaluation. J Clin Ultrasound 1989;17(5):327–32.
107. Ben-Ami M, Perlitz Y, Haddad S. The effectiveness of spectral and color Doppler in predicting ovarian torsion. A prospective study. Eur J Obstet Gynecol Reprod Biol 2002;104(1):64–6.
108. Quillin SP, Siegel MJ. Transabdominal color Doppler ultrasonography of the painful adolescent ovary. J Ultrasound Med 1994;13(7):549–55.
109. Gittleman AM, Price AP, Goffner L, et al. Ovarian torsion: CT findings in a child. J Pediatr Surg 2004;39(8):1270–2.
110. Chen M, Chen CD, Yang YS. Torsion of the previously normal uterine adnexa. Evaluation of the correlation between the pathological changes and the clinical characteristics. Acta Obstet Gynecol Scand 2001;80(1):58–61.
111. Puri P, Guiney EJ, O'Donnell B. Inguinal hernia in infants: the fate of the testis following incarceration. J Pediatr Surg 1984;19(1):44–6.
112. Sato TT, Oldham KT. Pediatric abdomen. In: Lazar J, editor. Surgery: scientific principles and practice. 3rd edition. Greenfield (CA): Lippincott Williams & Wilkins; 2001.
113. Stevenson RJ, Ziegler MM. Abdominal pain unrelated to trauma. Pediatr Rev 1993;14(8):302–11.
114. Singer J. Acute abdominal conditions that may require surgical intervention. In: Strange GR, Ahrens W, Lelyveld S, et al, editors. Pediatric emergency medicine: a comprehensive study guide. New York: McGraw-Hill; 1996. p. 311–9.
115. Brandt ML. Pediatric hernias. Surg Clin North Am 2008;88(1):27–43, vii–viii.

116. Colletti JE, Brown KM, Sharieff GQ, et al. The management of children with gastroenteritis and dehydration in the emergency department. J Emerg Med 2010;38:686–98.

117. Kosek M, Bern C, Guerrant RL. The global burden of diarrhoeal disease, as estimated from studies published between 1992 and 2000. Bull World Health Organ 2003;81(3):197–204.

118. Parashar UD, Bresee JS, Glass RI. The global burden of diarrhoeal disease in children. Bull World Health Organ 2003;81(4):236.

119. Malek MA, Curns AT, Holman RC, et al. Diarrhea- and rotavirus-associated hospitalizations among children less than 5 years of age: United States, 1997 and 2000. Pediatrics 2006;117(6):1887–92.

120. McConnochie KM, Conners GP, Lu E, et al. How commonly are children hospitalized for dehydration eligible for care in alternative settings? Arch Pediatr Adolesc Med 1999;153(12):1233–41.

121. Teach SJ, Yates EW, Feld LG. Laboratory predictors of fluid deficit in acutely dehydrated children. Clin Pediatr (Phila) 1997;36(7):395–400.

122. Shaoul R, Okev N, Tamir A, et al. Value of laboratory studies in assessment of dehydration in children. Ann Clin Biochem 2004;41(Pt 3):192–6.

123. Bonadio WA, Hennes HH, Machi J, et al. Efficacy of measuring BUN in assessing children with dehydration due to gastroenteritis. Ann Emerg Med 1989; 18(7):755–7.

124. Narchi H. Serum bicarbonate and dehydration severity in gastroenteritis. Arch Dis Child 1998;78(1):70–1.

125. Vega RM, Avner JR. A prospective study of the usefulness of clinical and laboratory parameters for predicting percentage of dehydration in children. Pediatr Emerg Care 1997;13(3):179–82.

126. Yilmaz K, Karabocuoglu M, Citak A, et al. Evaluation of laboratory tests in dehydrated children with acute gastroenteritis. J Paediatr Child Health 2002;38(3): 226–8.

127. Practice parameter: the management of acute gastroenteritis in young children. American Academy of Pediatrics, Provisional Committee on Quality Improvement, Subcommittee on Acute Gastroenteritis. Pediatrics 1996;97(3): 424–35.

128. Ludwig S, Lavelle J. Resuscitation–pediatric basic and advanced life support. In: Fleisher G, Ludwig S, Henretig F, et al, editors. Textbook of pediatric emergency medicine. 5th edition. Philadelphia: Lippincott Williams & Wilkins; 2006. p. 21.

129. Agus M. Endocrine emergencies. In: Fleisher G, Ludwig S, Henretig F, et al, editors. Textbook of pediatric emergency medicine. 5th edition. Philadelphia: Lippincott Williams & Wilkins; 2006. p. 770.

130. Atherly-John YC, Cunningham SJ, Crain EF. A randomized trial of oral vs intravenous rehydration in a pediatric emergency department. Arch Pediatr Adolesc Med 2002;156(12):1240–3.

131. Spandorfer PR, Alessandrini EA, Joffe MD, et al. Oral versus intravenous rehydration of moderately dehydrated children: a randomized, controlled trial. Pediatrics 2005;115(2):295–301.

132. Listernick R, Zieserl E, Davis AT. Outpatient oral rehydration in the United States. Am J Dis Child 1986;140(3):211–5.

133. Olsen JC, Keng JA, Clark JA. Frequency of adverse reactions to prochlorperazine in the ED. Am J Emerg Med 2000;18(5):609–11.

134. Kahn A, Blum D. Phenothiazines and sudden infant death syndrome. Pediatrics 1982;70(1):75–8.
135. Kahn A, Hasaerts D, Blum D. Phenothiazine-induced sleep apneas in normal infants. Pediatrics 1985;75(5):844–7.
136. Hampton T. Promethazine warning. JAMA 2005;293(8):921.
137. Cubeddu LX, Trujillo LM, Talmaciu I, et al. Antiemetic activity of ondansetron in acute gastroenteritis. Aliment Pharmacol Ther 1997;11(1):185–91.
138. Ramsook C, Sahagun-Carreon I, Kozinetz CA, et al. A randomized clinical trial comparing oral ondansetron with placebo in children with vomiting from acute gastroenteritis. Ann Emerg Med 2002;39(4):397–403.
139. Reeves JJ, Shannon MW, Fleisher GR. Ondansetron decreases vomiting associated with acute gastroenteritis: a randomized, controlled trial. Pediatrics 2002; 109(4):e62.
140. Freedman SB, Adler M, Seshadri R, et al. Oral ondansetron for gastroenteritis in a pediatric emergency department. N Engl J Med 2006;354(16):1698–705.
141. Stork CM, Brown KM, Reilly TH, et al. Emergency department treatment of viral gastritis using intravenous ondansetron or dexamethasone in children. Acad Emerg Med 2006;13(10):1027–33.
142. Saulsbury FT. Henoch-Schonlein purpura in children. Report of 100 patients and review of the literature. Medicine (Baltimore) 1999;78(6):395–409.
143. Calvino MC, Llorca J, Garcia-Porrua C, et al. Henoch-Schonlein purpura in children from northwestern Spain: a 20-year epidemiologic and clinical study. Medicine (Baltimore) 2001;80(5):279–90.
144. Trapani S, Micheli A, Grisolia F, et al. Henoch Schonlein purpura in childhood: epidemiological and clinical analysis of 150 cases over a 5-year period and review of literature. Semin Arthritis Rheum 2005;35(3):143–53.
145. Chang WL, Yang YH, Lin YT, et al. Gastrointestinal manifestations in Henoch-Schonlein purpura: a review of 261 patients. Acta Paediatr 2004;93(11): 1427–31.
146. Saulsbury FT. Clinical update: Henoch-Schonlein purpura. Lancet 2007; 369(9566):976–8.
147. Tizard EJ, Hamilton-Ayres MJ. Henoch Schonlein purpura. Arch Dis Child Educ Pract Ed 2008;93(1):1–8.
148. Baker SS, Liptak GS, Colletti RB, et al. Constipation in infants and children: evaluation and treatment. A medical position statement of the North American Society for Pediatric Gastroenterology and Nutrition. J Pediatr Gastroenterol Nutr 1999;29(5):612–26.
149. Barr RG, Levine MD, Wilkinson RH, et al. Chronic and occult stool retention: a clinical tool for its evaluation in school-aged children. Clin Pediatr (Phila) 1979;18(11):674, 676, 677–9, passim.
150. Weisman LE, Merenstein GB, Digirol M, et al. The effect of early meconium evacuation on early-onset hyperbilirubinemia. Am J Dis Child 1983;137(7):666–8.
151. American Academy of Pediatrics Subcommittee on Chronic Abdominal Pain. Chronic abdominal pain in children. Pediatrics 2005;115(3):812–5.
152. El-Matary W, Spray C, Sandhu B. Irritable bowel syndrome: the commonest cause of recurrent abdominal pain in children. Eur J Pediatr 2004;163(10): 584–8.
153. Hyams JS, Treem WR, Justinich CJ, et al. Characterization of symptoms in children with recurrent abdominal pain: resemblance to irritable bowel syndrome. J Pediatr Gastroenterol Nutr 1995;20(2):209–14.

154. Croffie JM, Fitzgerald JF, Chong SK. Recurrent abdominal pain in children–a retrospective study of outcome in a group referred to a pediatric gastroenterology practice. Clin Pediatr (Phila) 2000;39(5):267–74.

155. Ramchandani PG, Hotopf M, Sandhu B, et al. The epidemiology of recurrent abdominal pain from 2 to 6 years of age: results of a large, population-based study. Pediatrics 2005;116(1):46–50.

156. van Tilburg MA, Venepalli N, Ulshen M, et al. Parents' worries about recurrent abdominal pain in children. Gastroenterol Nurs 2006;29(1):50–5 [quiz: 56–7].

157. Rasquin-Weber A, Hyman PE, Cucchiara S, et al. Childhood functional gastrointestinal disorders. Gut 1999;45(Suppl 2):II60–8.

158. Hyman PE, Milla PJ, Benninga MA, et al. Childhood functional gastrointestinal disorders: neonate/toddler. Gastroenterology 2006;130(5):1519–26.

159. Bremner AR, Sandhu BK. Recurrent abdominal pain in childhood: the functional element. Indian Pediatr 2009;46(5):375–9.

160. Jona JZ, Belin RP. Basilar pneumonia simulating acute appendicitis in children. Arch Surg 1976;111(5):552–3.

161. Munglani R, Kenney IJ. Paediatric parapneumonic effusions: a review of 16 cases. Respir Med 1991;85(2):117–9.

162. Guyton AC. Textbook of medical physiology. 8th edition. Philadelphia: WB Saunders; 1991. p. 520–31.

163. Crafts RC. A textbook of human anatomy. 2nd edition. New York: John Wiley; 1979. p. 153–212.

164. Williams PL, Warwick R, Dyson M, et al. Gray's anatomy. 37th edition. Edinburgh: Churchill Livingstone; 1989. p. 1271.

165. Winsey HS, Jones PF. Acute abdominal pain in childhood: analysis of a year's admissions. Br Med J 1967;1(5541):653–5.

166. Leventhal JM. Clinical predictors of pneumonia as a guide to ordering chest roentgenograms. Clin Pediatr (Phila) 1982;21(12):730–4.

167. Tsalkidis A, Gardikis S, Cassimos D, et al. Acute abdomen in children due to extra-abdominal causes. Pediatr Int 2008;50(3):315–8.

168. Kreher NE, Hickner JM, Barry HC, et al. Do gastrointestinal symptoms accompanying sore throat predict streptococcal pharyngitis? An UPRNet study. Upper Peninsula Research Network. J Fam Pract 1998;46(2):159–64.

169. Gerber MA. Diagnosis and treatment of pharyngitis in children. Pediatr Clin North Am 2005;52(3):729–47, vi.

170. Shadinger LL, Andreotti RF, Kurian RL. Preoperative sonographic and clinical characteristics as predictors of ovarian torsion. J Ultrasound Med 2008;27:9.

171. Houry D, Abbott JT. Ovarian torsion: a fifteen-year review. Ann Emerg Med 2001;38:158.

172. Kokoska ER, Keller MS, Weber TR. Acute ovarian torsion in children. Am J Surg 2000;180:462.

173. Provost R. Torsion of the normal fallopian tube. Obstet Gynecol 1972;53:80.

Acute Abdominal Pain in the Older Adult

Luna Ragsdale, MD, MPH*, Lauren Southerland, MD

KEYWORDS

• Acute abdominal pain • Elderly • Emergency department

Older adults, defined as those who are 65 years and older, are the fastest growing segment of the population in the United States and the highest emergency department (ED) users of any age group.[1] By some estimates, older patients will account for one-fourth of all ED visits in the United States by 2030.[2] Abdominal pain is the most common presenting complaint to the ED,[1] and in older adults, abdominal pain is the fourth most common chief complaint.[3] Challenges to the diagnosis and management of abdominal pain in older adults are multifactorial but start with the lack of overt clinical findings and varying presentations of intra-abdominal disorders. In a survey comparing younger and older adult patients, emergency medicine physicians (EPs) consistently found older patients more complex, requiring more time and resources to diagnose and treat. Out of the surveyed diagnoses EPs found abdominal pain in older adults the most difficult to evaluate.[4] This article starts with a review of the physical changes of aging and how these changes affect both the abdominal diseases to which the older adults are susceptible and the clinical features of abdominal pathology in this group. This discussion is followed by an analysis of the management of acute abdominal pain in older adults organized by the following pathologic processes: inflammatory, obstructive, vascular, and other causes.

PATHOPHYSIOLOGIC CHANGES IN THE OLDER ADULT

Pathophysiologic changes secondary to aging cause an increased susceptibility to intra-abdominal diseases, as well as atypical clinical presentations. These changes occur from cellular to systemic levels, especially in the immune, genitourinary (GU), gastrointestinal (GI), nervous, and cardiovascular systems.

Older adults are at a higher risk for more frequent and severe infections due to immunosenescence. Aging of B cells decreases the ability to develop humoral (antibody) immunity to new infections or antigens, thereby increasing the risk for

Division of Emergency Medicine, Duke University Medical Center, DUMC 3096, 2301 Erwin Road, Duke North Suite 2600, Durham, NC 27710, USA
* Corresponding author.
E-mail address: Luna.ragsdale@duke.edu

Emerg Med Clin N Am 29 (2011) 429–448
doi:10.1016/j.emc.2011.01.012
0733-8627/11/$ – see front matter © 2011 Elsevier Inc. All rights reserved.

recurrence.[5] The T cell response also changes with aging, with decreased quantity and quality of the T cells and a decreased immune response to known antigens, possibly because of changes in the phenotype towards more immunosuppressive T cells.[6,7] These derangements have consequences for interpretation of the white blood cell count; on the one hand, a low count does not exclude an acute inflammatory condition, on the other, an elevated count does not exclude functional immunodeficiency. Aging is associated with a decreased response to pyrogens, lower basal body temperature, changes in thermal homeostasis, and a decreased production and conservation of heat. In one study, 30% of older adults who had surgical abdominal pain did not present with either a fever or leukocytosis.[8] Immunosenescence also results in decreasing immunosurveillance, the body's main defense against developing cancerous cells.

Renal changes with aging include decreased numbers of glomeruli and decreased glomerular function. These changes are caused by both long-term damage from comorbidities, such as hypertension and diabetes, and dysautoregulation of the afferent and efferent arterioles resulting in glomerular damage. Glomerular filtration rate decreases with age starting in the fourth decade and then diminishes by about 8 mL/min/decade, resulting in a reduction in the clearance of drugs and metabolites. Changes to the basement membrane and the development of small diverticula in the distal renal tubules promote urinary stasis and bacterial growth.[9] The aging kidneys also have diminished ability to concentrate urine, making older adults more prone to dehydration. Hormonally, the kidneys have reduced production of epoetin, inclining the older adult toward anemia from slow losses of blood.[9]

The effects of aging on the GI system also predispose patients to abdominal pathologic conditions. The stomach has a slightly decreased emptying time and fundal compliance. Acid secretion may increase secondary to decreased prostaglandin production. Liver mass and liver blood flow decrease with aging, resulting in decreased albumin synthesis and decreased phase 1 drug metabolism. The decrease in cytochrome P450 function and drug metabolism may be even greater in older men than in older women.[10] In the colon, the number of diverticula in the bowel increases with age. Because of physiologic anorexia of aging, there is decreased fluid and nutrient intake, predisposing the older adult to constipation.[11,12] Reduced physical activity for just 2 weeks almost doubles total colonic transit time in older adults,[13] which may contribute to the higher rate of postoperative ileus in this population.

Both the central and peripheral nervous systems are affected by aging. The prevalence of dementia and cognitive impairment increases, obscuring symptoms and obfuscating the medical history. Peripherally, pain and temperature sensation decreases as the type of pain sensing nerves slowly switches from A delta fibers (fast, sharp, prickly pain) to a reliance on slower-conducting C fibers.[14] This sensation decrease may contribute to the lack of peritoneal signs in many older adults. In a study of 212 patients with peritonitis, 55% had abdominal pain, but guarding or rigidity was observed in only 34%.[15] A review of patients with perforated ulcers found that only 21% of older adults presented with peritoneal signs.[16]

DIAGNOSTIC OBSTACLES

Among the difficulties complicating the diagnosis of intra-abdominal disorders in older adults are preexisting illnesses that alter classical manifestations; an inability to obtain an accurate history; medications that can cause, confound, or mask disease processes; and alterations in laboratory baseline and physical findings.[15,17,18] In addition, older adults may be less likely to seek timely medical care and thus may have later-stage disease or more serious illness when they present for care.[4,19,20] All these factors contribute to a higher morbidity and mortality for acute abdominal disorders in older adults.[20]

Chronic diseases accumulate with aging. Diabetes decreases peripheral nerve sensation in the abdomen as well as in the extremities. Previous abdominal surgery may diminish the perception of pain in the older adult.[21] Atherosclerotic cardiovascular disease places the patient at risk for cardiac ischemia, mimicking as abdominal pain, as well as other vascular catastrophes, including mesenteric ischemia and aortic aneurysm.

The usual clinical approach of a diagnostic workup based on a history taking and physical examination is complicated in older adults by multiple factors. Some patients downplay their symptoms or are unable to understand questions pertaining to cognitive or hearing impairment. Caregivers may be a helpful source of history taking but are not always available. At times, the presenting symptom of an underlying intra-abdominal process may itself be altered mental status.[22–24]

Patients' medications can also disguise or contribute to disease. On average, the older adult takes 4.5 prescription drugs and 2.1 over-the-counter medications. Many older adults are taking nonsteroidal antiinflammatory drugs (NSAIDs). These drugs can not only cause GI and renal diseases but also diminish the febrile response. Chronic steroid use also increases the risk of ulcer disease and blunts the immune response. β-Blockers blunt the tachycardia associated with fever, pain, or infections. Narcotic or analgesic use may blunt the patient's perception of abdominal pathologic conditions. Several other medications can themselves cause abdominal pain as is discussed later.

Laboratory values are rarely diagnostic in the evaluation of abdominal pain in any age group and should be interpreted with even greater caution in the elderly. Aging is associated with a mild elevation in alkaline phosphatase. Hyperamylasemia is nonspecific and may be seen in pancreatitis but may also occur with mesenteric ischemia. Bacteriuria is common and often represents colonization rather than infection. Lean body mass and endogenous creatinine production declines with aging. High normal and minimally elevated values of creatinine may indicate substantially reduced renal function.

With atypical and delayed presentations, pathophysiologic and pharmacologic effects, decreased ability to communicate, and higher morbidity and mortality rates, accurate diagnosis of older adults with acute abdominal pain can be extremely challenging. One approach, when presented with these patients, is to organize the differential diagnosis into categories based on underlying pathologic processes: inflammatory, obstructive, vascular, or other causes.[25]

Inflammatory Causes of Abdominal Pain

Infection and inflammation are the final common pathway of most abdominal diseases in any age group. In this section inflammatory causes of pain are reviewed from the upper to the lower GI tract.

Peptic ulcer disease

Although the incidence of peptic ulcer disease (PUD) and the related complications and mortality of PUD have decreased over the past few decades in younger adults, hospital admission rates for PUD-related complications have increased in older adults. This increase may be secondary to increased use of aspirin and NSAIDs. Nearly 40% of older adults are prescribed NSAIDs, and age is an independent risk factor for developing gastroduodenal injury with NSAID use.[26] The risk of bleeding from a peptic ulcer is higher in short-term versus long-term users of NSAIDs or aspirin.[13,27–29] Another factor contributing to PUD is the increased prevalence of *Helicobacter pylori* colonization with age.[30,31] Approximately 53% to 73% of older adults who have PUD are *H pylori* positive.[32]

In older adults, the typical presentation of epigastric pain is less common than in younger adults.[33] About 35% of older adults with endoscopically proven PUD do not experience pain.[34] In many cases, the initial presentation is with complications, the most common of which is GI bleeding. With long-term blood loss, patients may present with anemia or its consequent symptoms such as angina, decreased exercise tolerance, or congestive heart failure.

Perforation is a serious complication, more commonly seen with duodenal ulcers, and occurs in 5% to 10% of older adults with PUD. In one study, only 47% of patients with a perforated gastroduodenal ulcer had a sudden onset of pain and only 21% presented with rigidity.[16] Disturbingly, plain radiographs failed to identify free air in 39% of cases of perforation.[16] Once perforation occurs, the mortality is 30%, three times higher than in younger adults. Other less common complications of PUD include gastric outlet obstruction and penetration into adjacent organs. The overall mortality of PUD is 100 times higher in older than in younger patients.

Pancreatitis

Pancreatitis is the most common nonsurgical cause of abdominal pain in older adults.[35] The top 2 causes of pancreatitis in older adults are gallstones and idiopathic causes compared with gallstones, hyperlipidemia, and alcohol use in younger patients.[36,37] Classically, the disease presents with upper abdominal pain radiating to the back, but it can also present as diffuse abdominal, back, or chest pain, with associated nausea and vomiting. Imaging is particularly helpful in patients with atypical presentations. Recent guidelines suggest that 2 out of 3 of the following should be present for the diagnosis of pancreatitis: (1) upper abdominal pain; (2) elevated levels of pancreatic enzymes; and (3) findings suggestive of acute pancreatitis on ultrasonography (U/S), computed tomography (CT), or magnetic resonance imaging (MRI). In the acute setting, CT is the preferred confirmatory imaging modality.[38]

In one series, gallstone pancreatitis accounted for more than half the cases in older adults compared with only 36% of younger patients.[39] Endoscopic retrograde cholangiopancreatography (ERCP) is the recommended therapeutic and diagnostic test for those patients who have common bile duct dilation on CT or U/S or a recent cholecystectomy.[39] ERCP is safe in older adults with a complication rate insignificantly higher than in younger patients, even when considering the subset of older adults on anticoagulation. The complication rate for ERCP remains constant for the young-old (65–74 years), the old-old (75–84 years), and the very old (>85 years).[40] Older adults may require subsequent ERCP sessions to completely clear the duct because of a higher stone burden.[41]

The Ranson criteria and the APACHE II (Acute Physiology and Chronic Health Evaluation II) criteria are used to predict patients at risk for severe disease and complications. In patients hospitalized for acute pancreatitis, older age is an independent risk factor for progression to organ dysfunction, systemic inflammatory response syndrome, or death.[42] Although mild pancreatitis can be managed in a regular unit with fluid resuscitation, analgesia, and antiemetics, patients with severe pancreatitis should be managed in an intensive care unit (ICU) with early surgical consultation and increased attention to their comorbidities and decreased physiologic reserve. Thromboprophylaxis with low–molecular weight heparin is suggested, given the increased inflammatory state.[43] Enteral nutrition via nasogastric or nasojejunal tube feed is the preferred mode of nutrition in severe acute pancreatitis because it seems to reduce oxidative stress, stabilize the catabolic state induced by pancreatitis, and improve outcomes.[44,45]

Biliary disease

Biliary tract disorders are the most common cause of abdominal pain in the older adult and the most common indication for intra-abdominal surgery.[46] The incidence of gallstones increases with age, with the prevalence reaching 33% by the age of 70 years.[47] Changes in bile acid production, bile cholesterol saturation, and decreased gallbladder sensitivity to cholecystokinin predispose older adults to the formation of gallstones.

Gallstones become symptomatic when they obstruct the neck of the gall bladder, resulting in intermittent symptoms of pain, often with associated anorexia, nausea, and vomiting. Symptomatic cholelithiasis can be managed by elective cholecystectomy if pain is controlled, if the patients are tolerating oral intake, and if patients do not appear sick. Early surgical intervention decreases repeat ED visits and complications, including acute cholecystitis (AC), pancreatitis, cholangitis, perforation and empyema.[48] Choledocholithiasis occurs more frequently in older adults[49] and can lead to obstructive jaundice, pancreatitis, and ascending cholangitis. U/S has low sensitivity but high specificity for detecting these stones. Magnetic resonance cholangiopancreatography and endoscopic U/S can detect bile duct stones with higher sensitivity and specificity than U/S and have comparable accuracy to ERCP but are much less invasive.[49] ERCP is the first-line therapeutic intervention.

If gallbladder outlet obstruction lasts more than 12 to 24 hours, there is increasing likelihood of progression to inflammatory changes in the gallbladder walls and onset of AC. A third of older adults with AC will present with minimal abdominal pain and minimal to no peritoneal signs, and presentation may not correlate with the severity of disease.[50] In one study of older adults with AC, 40% of severely ill patients had empyema of the gallbladder, gangrenous AC, or free perforation, and 15% had concomitant subphrenic or hepatic abscess; yet, of these patients, more than one-third were afebrile and a quarter did not have abdominal tenderness.[51] Fever is also not a sensitive indicator in older adults, as in one series only 71% with nongangrenous AC and 59% with gangrenous AC were afebrile. Approximately, 32% lacked leukocytosis and 28% lacked both fever and leukocytosis. In patients with gangrenous AC, more than a quarter of the patients lacked leukocytosis, and 16% lacked both fever and leukocytosis.[52] The ED treatment of AC begins with fluid resuscitation, administration of broad-spectrum antibiotics, and surgery consultation with cholecystectomy as definitive treatment.[53]

Emphysematous cholecystitis occurs predominately in older adults, particularly in men and diabetic patients, and is less likely to be associated with gallstones. This disease accounts for only 1% of all cases of AC but carries a mortality ranging from 15% to 25%, five times greater than the operative mortality for nonemphysematous AC.[54] Gas-forming clostridial species are the most common causative agent. With the high risk of perforation, empiric broad-spectrum antibiotic administration, including anaerobic coverage and surgical intervention, are critical for survival. Diagnostic imaging considerations for biliary disease in the elderly are similar to those in other age groups.

Appendicitis

Acute appendicitis is a diagnostic challenge in patients of all ages, but more so in older adults. Appendicitis presents classically with periumbilical pain that later localizes to the right lower quadrant with associated anorexia, nausea, and vomiting. Approximately 3% to 4% of older adults presenting with acute abdominal pain will have appendicitis.[46,55] The oldest old patients, octogenarians and older, have a significantly higher risk of delayed surgery and perforation compared with even younger-old (65–79 years old) patients.[56] In a case series of 601 patients older than 65 years with acute appendicitis, patients with perforation tended to wait a day longer before presenting to the ED and to have greater delays from presentation to surgery. Age had a larger effect on perforation than comorbidities.[57] As with other age groups, no laboratory test reliably diagnoses appendicitis in the elderly. Recent efforts to use C-reactive protein for this purpose and for risk stratification show some promise, but definitive imaging or laparotomy is still required.[58,59] Diagnostic imaging considerations in the elderly are similar to those of other age groups.

Diverticulitis and colitis

Aging and lifestyle changes place the elderly at high risk for constipation and diverticulosis and thus for colitis and diverticulitis. In necropsy studies, the prevalence of diverticulosis increases from 13% in those younger than 55 years to 50% in those older than 75 years.[60] In Western nations, left-sided diverticulosis and diverticulitis are more prevalent. Uncomplicated diverticular disease (diverticulosis) is not typically associated with acute abdominal pain.[61] A prospective study following patients with bowel complaints (pain, constipation, bloating) and diverticulosis found a crossover of only 1.7% to acute diverticulitis over 5 years.[62]

Diverticulitis classically presents as left lower abdominal pain associated with cramping, change in bowel movements, nausea, or fever. Diagnosis is confirmed by contrast-enhanced CT. One study comparing CT with U/S showed similar accuracy for diagnosing diverticulitis.[63] A recent meta-analysis shows summary sensitivities of 92% for U/S versus 94% for CT and summary specificities of 90% for U/S versus 99% for CT.[64] CT, however, is the preferred test because it can rule out alternative diagnoses that may not be well visualized by other imaging modalities. Initial treatment consists of broad-spectrum antibiotics against gram-negative and anaerobic bacteria, with a typical course of 7 to 10 days.[65] Admission decisions depend on the severity of the illness as well as the presence or absence of complications. Approximately, 25% of patients have a recurrence in which complications of abscess, phlegmon, or perforation are as likely as in the initial episode.[66,67] In sick or unstable patients, ED surgical consultation should be obtained. With contraindications to surgery, CT-guided drainage of diverticular abscess is an alternative.

Colitis can have a similar presentation to diverticulitis. Causes include infectious agents, such as *Clostridium difficile*, and inflammatory bowel disorders, such as ulcerative colitis (UC) and Crohn disease. *C difficile* is the most common cause of infectious diarrhea in nursing homes in the United States with a mortality estimated at more than 17%.[68] UC and Crohn disease have bimodal age distributions, and thus a significant portion of new diagnoses is made in older adults. Older patients make up more than 20% of admissions for Crohn disease and more than 30% of admissions for UC.[69] Stool antigen analysis, CT scan, and colonoscopy may help delineate between these different causes of colonic inflammation.

Obstructive Causes of Abdominal Pain

In the elderly, bowel obstruction accounts for 10% to 12% of ED visits for abdominal pain.[20,55,70] Obstruction is 3 times more common in older adults than in younger patients.[50] After biliary disease, bowel obstruction is the second most common reason for emergency surgical intervention in this age group.[71] Presentations vary and depend on the type and location of obstruction. Complications of obstructions include dehydration, ischemia, sepsis, and perforation. The types of obstruction can be broken down into small versus large bowel and mechanical versus functional obstruction.

Small bowel obstruction

The small bowel is the most common site of obstruction. The small bowel is more mobile, smoother, and smaller in diameter, making it more prone to both adhesions and herniation than large bowel.[72] The 3 most common causes of small bowel obstruction (SBO) are adhesions (50%–74%), hernias (15%), and neoplasms (15%).[71,73] As with younger patients, older adults with SBO present with colicky abdominal pain, nausea, vomiting, abdominal distension, and constipation. Gallstone ileus is a rare disease that accounts for 1% to 4% of mechanical obstructions.[74]

Plain radiography, often the initial study of choice, have a sensitivity of 66% and specificity of 57%.[75] Flat and upright abdominal radiographs may show distended loops of bowel, collapsed loops of bowel distal to the obstruction, paucity of gas in the rectum, air fluid levels, or stack-of-coins appearance (**Fig. 1**). Plain radiography is limited in assessing the degree, location, and cause of obstruction. CT imaging should be obtained when radiographs are nondiagnostic or to discriminate between complicated (vascular involvement) and uncomplicated (bowel involvement only) obstruction and assess the location and cause of obstruction. Closed-loop obstructions have a higher risk of strangulation. When strangulation of the bowel occurs, mortality increases 10-fold.[76] The clinician should bear in mind that even CT only has a sensitivity of 92% and specificity of 93% in the diagnosis of complete SBO.[77]

The acute management of SBO includes nasogastric decompression, intravenous (IV) fluid hydration, bowel rest, and symptomatic management. Patients with signs and symptoms of complications, such as strangulation and ischemia, require aggressive resuscitation and immediate surgical involvement. When considering disposition, it is important to recognize that morbidity and mortality in older adults with SBO is approximately 26%.[78] Studies show that patients with SBO managed on a surgical service have decreased length of stay and lower incidence of postoperative complications compared with those admitted to medical services.[78–80] Thus, it is prudent to

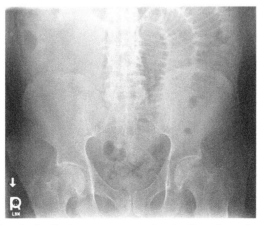

Fig. 1. SBO showing stack-of-coins appearance due to the plicae circulares that extend across the entire bowel in contrast to the haustra of the colon. (*Courtesy of* Joshua Broder, MD, Duke University, Durham, NC)

obtain early surgical consultation for almost all elderly patients with SBO. Those with uncomplicated bowel obstructions can sometimes be managed by the medical service because 30% to 50% resolve with conservative treatment.[79]

Large bowel obstruction

Most large bowel obstructions (LBOs) are caused by malignancy (60%), volvulus (10%–15%), or diverticulitis.[81,82] Across all age groups, these obstructions are much less common than SBO but are more prevalent in older adults because the prevalence of underlying causes increases with age. LBO classically presents as abdominal pain, distension, and constipation. Vomiting occurs late in the disease process, if at all. Patients with malignant obstruction may provide a history of unintentional weight loss or change in stool caliber.

In older adults, sigmoid volvulus is the most common type, accounting for 40% to 85% of all cases.[83–85] Mortality in the United States from sigmoid volvulus ranges from 12% to more than 50% depending on whether the sigmoid is viable or gangrenous.[86] Medications and diseases that alter bowel motility can predispose patients to volvulus.[87] Sigmoid volvulus tends to present with gradual onset of symptoms of left lower quadrant crampy or intermittent pain that progress to abdominal distension and obstipation. Cecal volvulus tends to have a younger age of distribution and occurs less frequently than sigmoid volvulus. Predisposing factors in the older adult include previous abdominal surgeries and adhesions. Unlike sigmoid volvulus, cecal volvulus presents with acute onset of abdominal pain similar to SBO with associated nausea and vomiting. Patients with these conditions are at high risk for perforation and require immediate surgical intervention.

Although plain radiographs are more accurate in detecting LBO than SBO, CT remains the imaging study of choice.[88,89] Other diagnostic modalities include a barium enema, although this does not allow for visualization of mural changes and extracolonic abnormalities.[88] Sigmoid volvulus presents classically on radiographs as a dilated colon with a bent inner-tube appearance with the "bend" directed to the right upper quadrant (**Fig. 2**). CT or contrast enema may be used when diagnosis is unclear. Typical findings on barium enema include the "bird's beak" deformity at the point of narrowing in the pelvis. Definitive diagnosis of a cecal volvulus is more difficult with

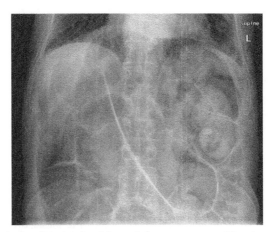

Fig. 2. Sigmoid volvulus showing bent inner-tube appearance. (*Courtesy of* Joshua Broder, MD, Duke University, Durham, NC)

plain radiographs. Radiographs may show the classic coffee bean sign, a large oval gas shadow with a line down the middle, representing the bowel bent over on itself.

Ileus and acute colonic pseudo-obstruction

Impaired intestinal transit time can be because of mechanical obstructions as discussed or because of decreased peristalsis from functional impairment of the GI system. The latter, an ileus, is seen most often postoperatively and can occur anywhere in the GI tract. Many medications can also cause ileus, including opioids, anticholinergics, and tricyclic antidepressants (TCAs).[90] Other causes of ileus include critical illness, metabolic derangements, neurologic disorders, intra-abdominal or retroperitoneal inflammation, or severe infections.[91] Patients present with mild diffuse abdominal pain and distension with hypoactive bowel sounds. Plain radiographs may show findings similar to SBO, and CT scan is necessary to rule out this condition. Treatment is mainly supportive.

Acute colonic pseudo-obstruction, also known as Ogilvie syndrome, is more common in adults older than 60 years, with a slight predisposition in men.[92,93] Ogilvie syndrome is an uncommon cause of functional obstruction that tends to occur in debilitated patients who have had prolonged hospitalizations or are institutionalized or have had recent non-GI surgery.[94,95] Anticholinergic medications, antiparkinsonism medications, phenothiazines, calcium channel blockers, and H_2 blockers are associated with this condition.[92,96] Symptoms tend to develop over days. Plain radiography and CT show massive colonic dilatation that extends to the rectum, in contrast to other forms of LBO. Barium enemas and colonoscopy are helpful in establishing the diagnosis, and colonoscopy successfully decompresses 80% of cases, but there is a 22% recurrence rate.[93] Immediate treatment is similar to that of SBO and involves IV hydration, nasogastric tube suctioning if there is evidence of small bowel involvement, and close observation. Electrolyte abnormalities should be corrected and offending medications discontinued. In stable patients, pharmacologic decompression can be achieved with the use of neostigmine with an immediate response rate of 90%.[97–99] Surgical intervention is typically reserved for patients with perforation or ischemia.

Vascular Causes of Abdominal Pain

Vascular causes of abdominal pain are typically seen only in older adults because of the high prevalence of atherosclerosis, atrial fibrillation, hypertension, and peripheral artery disease. Although the incidence of disease is relatively low, mortality is very high. Vascular diseases can be grouped into those causing end-organ ischemia, arterial aneurysms, and arterial dissections.

Acute mesenteric ischemia

Although acute mesenteric ischemia is a relatively rare cause of acute abdominal pain in older adults, it is frequently difficult to diagnose and has a high reported mortality rate of 60% to 90% depending on cause.[100–102] Mortality is directly associated with the time from presentation to surgical interventions. Mortality can range from 14%, if the time from evaluation to surgery is less than 6 hours, to 65%, if the time delay is greater than 12 hours.[103] Despite advances in imaging, mortality has not changed over the past several decades. A high index of suspicion is required to save these patients.

Mesenteric ischemia is classified by chronicity and etiology. Acute mesenteric ischemia accounts for 80% of intestinal ischemia. Acute mesenteric ischemia can be occlusive or nonocclusive, with occlusive forms more prevalent. Occlusion can occur in either the arterial or venous system. Arterial occlusions are responsible for 75% of cases, whereas occlusions in the venous system cause 8% of the cases; the remaining 17% are secondary to nonocclusive mesenteric ischemia.[104]

Arterial occlusions are caused by emboli or by intra-arterial thrombosis. Most acute emboli lodge in the superior mesenteric artery (SMA) perhaps because of its orientation almost parallel with the aorta. The usual source of emboli is the heart where thrombi can form as the result of dysrhythmias, such as atrial fibrillation, recent myocardial infarction, or chronic congestive heart failure.

Mesenteric ischemia secondary to intra-arterial thrombus occurs most commonly in the setting of atherosclerotic disease. Patients may have had prior symptoms of postprandial abdominal discomfort (intestinal angina) and weight loss. Typically, this process occurs over time, so collaterals have developed and symptoms progress subacutely. Ischemia or infarction may occur when the remaining visceral artery or collaterals become completely occluded. Occlusions typically occur in the proximal portion of the vessel and can affect a larger portion of the bowel than embolic disease. Risk factors are similar to those for cardiac ischemia.

Nonocclusive mesenteric ischemia is caused by mesenteric vasoconstriction in response to dehydration, intravascular hypovolemia, or hypotension, often in combination with a systemic low-flow state, such as heart failure. Medications that alter mesenteric vascular flow include digoxin, ergotamine, catecholamines, angiotensin II blockers, vasopressin, and β-blockers. Patients are often already in the ICU setting for other processes, obscuring the diagnosis and symptoms. Abdominal pain may gradually increase or be discontinuous and colicky in nature.

Mesenteric venous thrombosis is the least common cause of mesenteric ischemia and the least fatal. Presentations can be acute or subacute. Risk factors include hypercoagulable states, portal hypertension, portal vein thrombosis, abdominal inflammations, and a history of previous surgery or abdominal trauma.

Classically, acute mesenteric ischemia presents with pain out of proportion with abdominal examination, associated with nausea, vomiting, and diarrhea. Early on, the abdomen is often soft and nontender. As ischemia evolves into infarction, peritoneal signs emerge. Only one-third of patients present with the classic triad of abdominal pain, fever, and heme-positive stools.[105] As noted, venous occlusion can present more indolently, with more colicky symptoms lasting for more than 48 hours. Nausea, vomiting, anorexia, and diarrhea may occur. Occult blood in stools is frequent; massive hemorrhage is an ominous sign of infarction. High white blood cell counts more than 20,000; elevations in amylase, aspartate aminotransferase, lactate dehydrogenase, and creatine phosphokinase levels; and a metabolic acidosis are indicative but neither sensitive nor specific.[106,107] Elevations in phosphate and lactate levels suggest bowel necrosis.[108,109] D-Dimer levels may also be elevated.[110,111] Importantly, the absence of abnormal laboratory values does not exclude the diagnosis.

Thumbprinting or thickening of bowel loops is seen on plain radiographs in less than 40% of patients. CT is more sensitive, 82% to 100% sensitive, for venous thrombosis but may miss arterial thrombi.[112] Bowel wall thickening is most often seen in arterial occlusion, although bowel walls may be normal.[113] Bowel dilatation or wall attenuation may be present but is nonspecific. Pneumatosis is a nonspecific late finding present in only 6% to 30% of cases.[114]

Angiography is the gold standard for the diagnosis of arterial mesenteric ischemia and allows for the direct intravascular therapeutic interventions described later. However, angiography is invasive, is not readily available, is not feasible in unstable patients, and may delay surgical embolectomy. An alternative is multidetector

CT angiography. This technology is more readily available, rapidly acquired, and less invasive, with a sensitivity of 93% to 96% and a specificity of 94% to 100%.[115,116] Doppler U/S and MRI are helpful in the diagnosis of chronic mesenteric ischemia but have little role in the diagnosis of acute ischemia.

Treatment is initially supportive with fluid resuscitation, circulatory stabilization, and treatment of the underlying condition. In settings of hypotension unresponsive to fluid resuscitation, vasopressors may be required but are likely to exacerbate ischemia. Vasopressin and alpha-agonists should be avoided, except in extremis.[117] In cases of arterial emboli and nonocclusive ischemia, infusion of papaverine or other vasodilators into the SMA may be successful. If there are no contraindications, pharmacologic treatment includes the initiation of heparin and broad-spectrum antibiotics. Patients with peritoneal signs or evidence of perforation should be taken to the operating room immediately.

Ruptured abdominal aortic aneurysm

Aortic aneurysms are the 14th leading cause of death in the United States and the 10th leading cause of death in older men.[118] Ruptured abdominal aortic aneurysm (AAA) is a leading cause of sudden death, with 50% prehospital mortality. For patients who reach the hospital, mortality is still 80% to 90%. Even in a cohort of patients with rapid diagnosis who were transported to the operating room within 12 minutes of arrival, there was a 30-day mortality of 70%.[119]

Risk factors for AAA include older age (>60 years), smoking, male sex, white race, family history of AAA, occlusive atherosclerotic disease, and connective tissue disorder.[120] Aneurysm size is the most likely predictor of rupture. The yearly risk of rupture for an AAA with an initial diameter of 3 cm ranges from 0.2% to 0.4%; with a 4-cm aneurysm, the range increases to 0.8% to 1.1%, and for aneurysms measuring 4.5 cm, the yearly risk increases to 1.2% to 2.1%.[121] This risk is increased in patients with hypertension, chronic obstructive pulmonary disease, familial AAA, and tobacco abuse.[122]

The classic triad of hypotension, pulsatile mass, and abdominal or low-back pain is diagnostic but only seen in 30% to 50% of acute AAA.[123] Initially, patients may experience transient hypotension or syncope but may be stable by the time of presentation to the ED. A study of ruptured AAA showed that hypotension and tachycardia was absent in 50% of admitted patients who progressed to death within the next 2 hours. Signs and symptoms of acute AAA can be varied and nonspecific. The symptoms in 30% of patients are initially misdiagnosed or mistaken for renal colic, diverticulitis, and GI bleed.[124] Acute AAA may present with abdominal pain (83.6%) or back pain (over 50%).[125] It may mimic renal colic with unilateral flank pain radiating to the groin and microscopic hematuria. Any older adult presenting with symptoms of new-onset renal colic should be evaluated for acute AAA. Other symptoms include lower-extremity neuropathy with or without dysesthesias caused by ischemia and or compression of neural structures and intractable back pain. Aneurysms can rupture into the GI tract, leading to massive GI bleeding, or into the vena cava or left renal vein, but these are usually rapidly fatal.[123] Physical examination for the diagnosis of AAA may be impeded by increased abdominal girth.[126] Bedside U/S by ED physicians is highly accurate but does not distinguish an acute from a nonacute AAA, although this difference is usually clear from the clinical context.[127] U/S may be technically limited by habitus or bowel gas in a small proportion of patients. For stable patients, a noncontrast CT scan can evaluate the caliber of the aorta as well as identify nephrolithiasis.

Early consultation with a vascular surgeon and immediate resuscitation is imperative for suspected acute AAA. In unstable patients, a bedside ultrasonography can be obtained during ongoing resuscitation. At least 2 large-bore IV catheters should be established, and the patient should be typed and crossed for a minimum of 10 units of packed red blood cells. Expeditious transfer to the operating room may decrease mortality. Confirmatory imaging studies may be obtained in stable patients. IV contrast-enhanced CT is considered the gold standard, with a sensitivity ranging from 79% to 94% and specificity ranging from 77% to 95% for the identification of acute AAA.[120] If IV contrast is contraindicated, a noncontrast CT scan is done to visualize AAA and many cases of acute hemorrhage.

Aortic dissection

The incidence of aortic dissection is low but potentially fatal if not treated. The typical patient is a man in his seventh decade of life.[128] Risk factors include systemic hypertension, previous coronary cardiac surgeries, and atherosclerosis.[128] Patients can present with acute onset of abdominal pain, particularly, if the dissection is in the descending aorta. In patients who present with pain or symptoms above and below the diaphragm, a high index of suspicion should be maintained. Contrast-enhanced CT is the diagnostic imaging study of choice. MRI or U/S (a combination of transthoracic, transesophageal, and transabdominal approaches may be needed) can be used in cases in which IV contrast is contraindicated. This condition is managed with immediate resuscitation, blood pressure management, and either surgical or medical treatment depending on the location of the dissection.

Other Causes of Abdominal Pain

Many other intra-abdominal and extra-abdominal causes present with either vague or localized abdominal pain in the elderly.

GU

Acute urinary tract infections (UTIs) and pyelonephritis are common causes of abdominal pain in older adults. UTIs are frequent in older adults and are a consequence of previously discussed changes of aging. Caution should be exercised in ascribing abdominal pain to a UTI because asymptomatic bacteriuria is found in up to 18% of community-dwelling women who are 65 years or older and in up to 10% of all community-dwelling men older than 65 years.[129,130] The rate increases to 27% in women older than 80 years and to 16% in men older than 80 years,[131] and, approximately 58% of institutionalized older adults have been found to have asymptomatic bacteriuria.[132] Acute urinary retention usually presents with anuria, abdominal pain, and a palpable bladder but may be easily overlooked in patients unable to provide a history of this condition. Causes include medications (anticholinergics, antihistamines, and TCAs), bladder outlet obstruction, or neurogenic disease processes.

Renal causes account for 5% to 10% of abdominal pain in the older adult.[55,70] The incidence of renal stones is increasing in the older adult population.[133] Patients may present with abdominal pain and/or flank pain, often with concomitant nausea and vomiting. Noncontrast CT scan is the study of choice and can also rule out AAA. Treatment is similar to that of younger adults, with the exception that more caution should be taken in prescribing NSAIDs. Other GU causes of abdominal pain to consider in older adults are prostatitis, epididymitis, gonadal cancer, testicular torsion, and Fournier gangrene.[134]

Constipation

As discussed earlier, the older adult is at high risk for constipation. Unlike younger patients in whom constipation tends to be mainly the result of low fiber intake, in the older adult, medication effects, decreased stomach emptying time, impaired mobility, and comorbid diseases all make constipation increasingly prevalent. Constipation occurs more frequently in women than in men, possibly because of the association with pelvic floor dysfunction.[135] Symptoms of constipation include the feeling of fullness, urgency, abdominal pain, and inability to pass stool. Unlike children, radiography is still a recommended first-line diagnostic test in older adults because many serious diseases, including bowel obstruction and perforation, may present with similar symptoms.

Malignancy

Intra-abdominal malignancy may cause acute abdominal pain, as well as biliary symptoms, obstruction, peritonitis, ascites (with or without pain), and abdominal mass. A history of unexplained weight loss, anorexia, or night sweats or a lack of primary care or cancer screening tests makes newly diagnosed carcinoma more likely. In the setting of known intra-abdominal cancer, obstruction as well as cancer-specific diagnoses should be considered. Colon cancer has a propensity for GI bleeds and perforation. Prostate cancer can cause bone metastases to the pelvis and spine with pain or urinary obstruction. Gynecologic cancers may cause painful masses, peritoneal spread with peritonitis, and intermittent obstructive or urinary symptoms. Pancreatic and biliary cancers can cause upper or lower abdominal symptoms. In a study of more than 2000 patients presenting with acute abdominal pain, 2.8% were found to have an abdominal malignancy at 1-year follow-up, with almost half undiagnosed at discharge. Constipation, intestinal obstruction, and nonspecific abdominal pain were the most common diagnoses in patients whose malignancy was initially unrecognized.[136] GI and GU system cancers are also disproportionately common among older adults. At present, comprising only 12.8% of the US population,[137] this group makes up most of the new diagnoses of GI cancers (63.1%) and diagnoses of GU cancers in men (59.4%).[138] According to the American Cancer Society, 1 in 6 men and 1 in 10 women older than 60 years will develop invasive cancers.[139] With the expected population growth in this age group and increasing longevity, an increase in the number of malignancies should be expected.

Extra-abdominal causes

The many extra-abdominal and systemic diseases that are known to cause abdominal symptoms are discussed by Dean and McNamara elsewhere in this issue. Almost all such diseases occur with increasing frequency with aging and can be divided into cardiac/vascular, pulmonary, metabolic, neurologic, or other causes. Vascular causes include myocardial infarction (most notably inferior wall) that can present with epigastric pain, nausea, or vomiting. An electrocardiogram should be obtained in older adults who present with epigastric pain. Pulmonary processes, such as pneumonia, pneumothorax, and pulmonary embolus, can present as abdominal pain. Metabolic causes of abdominal pain include alcoholic or diabetic ketoacidosis, heavy metal poisoning, addisonian crisis, hemachromatosis, aspirin overdose, opioid withdrawal, and porphyria. Neuropathic pain from herpes zoster or radiculopathies can present as abdominal pain.

Older adults with processes occurring in the abdominal wall, such as ventral hernias, rectal sheath hematomas (particularly in patients who are anticoagulated), cellulitis, and abscess, may also complain of abdominal pain. As noted earlier, medications can predispose patients to abdominal diseases by a variety of mechanisms and interfere with patients' ability to recognize these diseases. In addition, several medications can also be directly responsible for abdominal symptoms. Digoxin, colchicine, and metformin and antibiotics can cause nausea, vomiting, diarrhea, and abdominal pain. Erythromycin is commonly known to cause gastric irritation and intestinal cramping. Phenothiazines, antidepressants, oral hypoglycemic agents, and diuretics may cause abdominal pain by causing liver dysfunction.[113] Although rarely overwhelming, these extra-abdominal causes should be considered when evaluating older patients with abdominal pain.

SUMMARY

Evaluation of acute abdominal pain in older adults can be challenging in the ED. Atypical or delayed presentations of abdominal diseases are much more common among older adults who are also at higher risk of complications and have higher mortality rates. Inaccurate diagnosis can lead to an increase in morbidity and mortality.[16] Given the wide range of possible acute abdominal emergencies in older adults, it is helpful to categorize the possibilities into groups based on causes, such as inflammatory, obstructive, vascular, and other causes.

REFERENCES

1. McCaig LF, Nawar EN. National hospital ambulatory medical care survey: 2004 emergency department summary. Advance data from vital and health statistics. Adv Data 2006;372:1–29.
2. Wilber ST, Gerson LW, Terrell KM, et al. Geriatric emergency medicine and the 2006 Institute of Medicine reports from the Committee on the Future of Emergency Care in the U.S. health system. Acad Emerg Med 2006;13:1345–51.
3. Wofford JL, Schwartz E, Timerding BL, et al. Emergency department utilization by the elderly: analysis of the National Hospital Ambulatory Medical Care Survey. Acad Emerg Med 1996;3:694–9.
4. McNamara RM, Rousseau E, Sanders AB. Geriatric emergency medicine: a survey of practicing emergency physicians. Ann Emerg Med 1992;21:796–801.
5. Ongradi J, Stercz B, Kovesdi V, et al. Immunosenescence and vaccination of the elderly, I. Age-related immune impairment. Acta Microbiol Immunol Hung 2009; 56(3):199–210.
6. Cusi MG, Martorelli B, DiGenova G, et al. Age related changes in T cell mediated immune response and effector memory to Respiratory Syncytial Virus (RSV) in healthy subjects. Immun Ageing 2010;7:14.
7. Grubeck-Loebenstein B. Fading immune protection in old age: vaccination in the elderly. J Comp Pathol 2010;142(Suppl 1):S116–9.
8. Potts FE, Vukov LF. Utility of fever and leukocytosis in acute surgical abdomens in octogenarians. J Gerontol A Biol Sci Med Sci 1999;54:M55–8.
9. Zhou XJ, Saxena R, Liu Z, et al. Renal senescence in 2008: progress and challenges. Int Urol Nephrol 2008;40:823–39.
10. Cotreau MM, von Moltke LL, Greenblatt DJ. The influence of age and sex on the clearance of cytochrome P450 3A substrates. Clin Pharmacokinet 2005;44: 33–60.
11. Radley S, Keighley MR, Radley SC, et al. Bowel dysfunction following hysterectomy. Br J Obstet Gynaecol 1999;106:1120–5.
12. Bhutto A, Morley JE. The clinical significance of gastrointestinal changes with aging. Curr Opin Clin Nutr Metab Care 2008;11:651–60.
13. Griffin MR, Piper JM, Daugherty JR, et al. Nonsteroidal anti-inflammatory drug use and increased risk for peptic ulcer disease in elderly persons. Ann Intern Med 1991;114:258–63.
14. Wickremaratchi MM, Llewelyn JG. Effects of ageing on touch. Postgrad Med J 2005;82:301–4.

15. Wroblewski M, Mikulowski P. Peritonitis in geriatric inpatients. Age Ageing 1991; 20:90–4.
16. Fenyo G. Acute abdominal disease in the elderly: experience from two series in Stockholm. Am J Surg 1982;143:751–4.
17. Glaspy JN, Ma OJ, Schwab RA, et al. Abdominal pain in geriatric emergency medicine. In: Meldon SW, Ma OJ, Woolard R, editors. Geriatric emergency medicine. New York: The McGraw Hill Companies, Inc; 2004. p. 173–8.
18. van Geloven AA, Biesheuvel TH, Luitse JS, et al. Hospital admission of patients aged over 80 with acute abdominal complaints. Eur J Surg 2000;166:866–71.
19. Copper GS, Shlaes DM, Salata RA. Intraabdominal infection: differences in presentation and outcome between younger patients and the elderly. Clin Infect Dis 1994;19:46–148.
20. Kizer KW, Vassar MJ. Emergency department diagnosis of abdominal disorders in the elderly. Am J Emerg Med 1998;16:357–62.
21. Watters JM, Clancey SM, Moulton SB, et al. Impaired recovery of strength in older patients after major abdominal surgery. Ann Surg 1993;218:390–3.
22. Cobden I, Lendrum R, Venables CW, et al. Gallstones presenting as mental and physical debility in the elderly. Lancet 1984;1:1062–4.
23. Rockwood K. Acute confusion in elderly medical patients. J Am Geriatr Soc 1989;37:150–4.
24. Fontanarosa PB, Kaeberlein FJ, Gerson LW, et al. Difficulty in predicting bacteremia in elderly emergency patients. Ann Emerg Med 1992;21:842–8.
25. Dang C, Aguilera P, Dang A, et al. Acute abdominal pain: four classifications can guide assessment and management. Geriatrics 2002;57:30–42.
26. Griffin MR. Epidemiology of nonsteroidal anti-inflammatory drug-associated gastrointestinal injury. Am J Med 1998;104:23S–9S.
27. Pilotto A, Franceschi M, Leandro G, et al. NSAID and aspirin use by the elderly in general practice: effect on gastrointestinal symptoms and therapies. Drugs Aging 2003;20:701–10.
28. Pilotto A, Leandro G, Di Mario F, et al. Role of Helicobacter pylori infection on upper gastrointestinal bleeding in the elderly: a case-control study. Dig Dis Sci 1997;42:586–91.
29. Laporte JR, Ibáñez L, Vidal X, et al. Upper gastrointestinal bleeding associated with the use of NSAIDs: newer versus older agents. Drug Saf 2004;27:411–20.
30. Graham DY, Malaty HM, Evans DG, et al. Epidemiology of Helicobacter pylori in an asymptomatic population in the United States. Gastroenterology 1991;100:1495–501.
31. Marshall BJ. Helicobacter pylori. Am J Gastroenterol 1994;89:S116–28.
32. Pilotto A, Salles N. Helicobacter pylori infection in geriatrics. Helicobacter 2002; 7:56–62.
33. Kemppainen H, Räihä I, Sourander L. Clinical presentation of peptic ulcer in the elderly. Gerontology 1997;43:283–8.
34. Leverat M. Peptic ulcer disease in patients over 60: experience in 287 cases. Am J Dig Dis 1966;11:279–85.
35. Martin SP, Ulrich CD. Pancreatic disease in the elderly. Clin Geriatr Med 1999; 15:579–605.
36. Rossetti B, Spizzirri A, Migliaccio C, et al. Acute pancreatitis in the elderly: our experience. BMC Geriatr 2009;9(Suppl 1):15.
37. Xin M, Chen H, Sun J. Severe acute pancreatitis in the elderly: etiology and clinical characteristics. World J Gastroenterol 2008;14:2517–21.

38. Kiriyama S, Gabata T, Takada T, et al. New diagnostic criteria of acute pancreatitis. J Hepatobiliary Pancreat Sci 2010;17(1):24–36.
39. Horakova M, Vadovicova I, Katuscak I, et al. Consideration of endoscopic retrograde cholangiopancreatography in cases of acute biliary pancreatitis. Bratisl Lek Listy 2009;110:553–8.
40. Hu KC, Chang WH, Chu CH, et al. Findings and risk factors of early mortality of endoscopic retrograde cholangiopancreatography in different cohorts of elderly patients. J Am Geriatr Soc 2009;57:1839–43.
41. Ito Y, Tsujino T, Togawa O, et al. Endoscopic papillary balloon dilation for the management of bile duct stones in patients 85 years of age and older. Gastrointest Endosc 2008;68:477–82.
42. Gardner TB, Vege SS, Chari ST, et al. The effect of age on hospital outcomes in severe acute pancreatitis. Pancreatology 2008;8:265–70.
43. Tonsi A, Bacchion M, Crippa S, et al. Acute pancreatitis at the beginning of the 21st century: the state of the art. World J Gastroenterol 2009;15:2945–59.
44. McClave SA, Chang WK, Dhaliwal R, et al. Nutrition support in acute pancreatitis: a systematic review of the literature. JPEN J Parenter Enteral Nutr 2006;30:143–56.
45. Petrov MS, Correia MI, Windsor JA. Nasogastric tube feeding in predicted severe acute pancreatitis. A systematic review of the literature to determine safety and tolerance. JOP 2008;9:440–8.
46. Laurell H, Hansson LE, Gunnarsson U. Acute abdominal pain in elderly patients. Gerontology 2006;52:336–44.
47. McSherry CK, Ferstenberg H, Calhoun WF, et al. The natural history of diagnosed gallstone disease in symptomatic and symptomatic patients. Ann Surg 1985;202:59–63.
48. Gurusamy KS, Samrai K, Fusai G, et al. Early versus delayed laparoscopic cholecystectomy for biliary colic. Cochrane Database Syst Rev 2008;4:CD007196, 1–20.
49. Attasaranya S, Fogel EL, Lehman GA. Choledocholithiasis, ascending cholangitis, and gallstone pancreatitis. Med Clin North Am 2008;92:925–60.
50. Telfer S, Fenyo G, Holt PR, et al. Acute abdominal pain in patients over 50 years of age. Scand J Gastroenterol Suppl 1998;144:47–50.
51. Morrow DJ, Thompson J, Wilson SE. Acute cholecystitis in the elderly: a surgical emergency. Arch Surg 1978;113:1129–52.
52. Gruber PJ, Silverman RA, Gottesfeld S, et al. Presence of fever and leukocytosis in acute cholecystitis. Ann Emerg Med 1996;28:273–7.
53. Elwood DR. Cholecystitis. Surg Clin North Am 2008;88:1241–52.
54. Seow VK, Lin CM. Acute emphysematous cholecystitis with initial normal radiological evaluation: a fatal diagnostic pitfall in the ED. Am J Emerg Med 2007;25:488.e3–5.
55. Bugliosi TF, Meloy TD, Vukov LF. Acute abdominal pain in the elderly. Ann Emerg Med 1990;19:1381–6.
56. Young YR, Chiu TF, Chen JC, et al. Acute appendicitis in the octogenarians and beyond: a comparison with younger geriatric patients. Am J Med Sci 2007;334:255–9.
57. Sheu BF, Chiu T, Chen JC, et al. Risk factors associated with perforated appendicitis in elderly patients presenting with signs and symptoms of acute appendicitis. ANZ J Surg 2007;77:662–6.
58. Wu H, Lin C, Chang C, et al. Predictive value of C-reactive protein at different cutoff levels in acute appendicitis. Am J Emerg Med 2005;23:449–53.

59. Sulberg D, Chromik AM, Kersting S, et al. Appendicitis in the elderly. CRP value as decision support for diagnostic laparoscopy. Chirurg 2009;80:608–14 [in German].
60. Commane DM, Arasaradnam RP, Mills S, et al. Diet, ageing and genetic factors in the pathogenesis of diverticular disease. World J Gastroenterol 2009;15: 2479–88.
61. Thompson WG, Patel DG, Tao H, et al. Does uncomplicated diverticular disease produce symptoms? Dig Dis Sci 1982;27:605–8.
62. Salem TA, Molloy RG, O'Dwyer PJ. Prospective five-year follow-up study of patients with symptomatic uncomplicated diverticular disease. Dis Colon Rectum 2007;50:1460–4.
63. Pradel JA, Adell JF, Taourel P, et al. Acute colonic diverticulitis: prospective comparative evaluation with US and CT. Radiology 1997;205:503–12.
64. Lameris W, van Randen A, Bipat S, et al. Graded compression ultrasonography and computed tomography in acute colonic diverticulitis: meta-analysis of test accuracy. Eur Radiol 2008;18:2498–511.
65. Byrnes MC, Mazuski JE. Antimicrobial therapy for acute colonic diverticulitis. Surg Infect (Larchmt) 2009;10:143–54.
66. Janes S, Meagher A, Frizelle FA. Elective surgery after acute diverticulitis. Br J Surg 2005;92:133–42.
67. Issa N, Dreznik S, Dueck DS, et al. Emergency surgery for complicated acute diverticulitis. Colorectal Dis 2009;11:198–202.
68. Crogan NL, Evans BC. Clostridium difficile: an emerging epidemic in nursing homes. Geriatr Nurs 2007;28:161–4.
69. Sonnenberg A. Demographic characteristics of hospitalized IBD patients. Dig Dis Sci 2009;54:2449–55.
70. Abi-Hanna P, Gleckman P. Acute abdominal pain: a medical emergency. Ann Emerg Med 1990;19:1383–6.
71. Hendrickson MH, Naparst TR. Abdominal surgical emergencies in the elderly. Emerg Med Clin North Am 2003;21:937–69.
72. Romano S, Bartone G, Romano L. Ischemia and infarction of the intestine related to obstruction. Radiol Clin North Am 2008;46:925–42.
73. Miller G, Voman J, Shrier I, et al. Etiology of small bowel obstruction. Am J Surg 2000;180:33–6.
74. Kauvar DR. The geriatric abdomen. Clin Geriatr Med 1993;9:547–58.
75. Maglinte DD, Balthazar EJ, Kelvin FM, et al. The role of radiology in the diagnosis of small-bowel obstruction. Am J Roentgenol 1997;168:1171–80.
76. Qalbani A, Paushter D, Dachman AH. Multidetector row CT of small bowel obstruction. Radiol Clin North Am 2007;45:499–512.
77. Mallo RD, Salem L, Flum DR. Computed tomography diagnosis of ischemia and complete obstruction in small bowel obstruction: a systematic review. J Gastrointest Surg 2005;9:690–4.
78. Schwab DP, Blackhurst DW, Sticca RP. Operative acute small bowel obstruction: admitting service impacts outcome. Am Surg 2001;67:1034–40.
79. Malangoni MA, Times ML, Kozik D, et al. Admitting service influences the outcomes of patients with small bowel obstructions. Surgery 2001;130:706–12.
80. Oyasiji T, Angelo S, Kyriakides TC, et al. Small bowel obstruction: outcome and cost implications of admitting service. Am Surg 2010;76:687–91.
81. Sufian S, Matsumoto T. Intestinal obstruction. Am J Surg 1975;130:9–14.
82. Buechter KJ, Boustany C, Caillouette R, et al. Surgical management of the acutely obstructed colon: a review of 127 cases. Am J Surg 1988;56:163–8.

83. Mulas C, Bruna M, Garcia-Armengol J, et al. Management of colonic volvulus. Experience in 75 patients. Rev Esp Enferm Dig 2010;102:239–48.
84. Ballantyne GH, Brandner MD, Beart RW, et al. Volvulus of the colon. Incidence and mortality. Ann Surg 1985;202:83–92.
85. Ballantyne GH. Volvulus of the splenic flexure. Dis Colon Rectum 1981;24: 630–2.
86. Ballantyne GH. Review of sigmoid volvulus: history and results of treatment. Dis Colon Rectum 1982;25:494–501.
87. Bak MP, Boley SJ. Sigmoid volvulus in elderly patients. Am J Surg 1986;151:71–5.
88. Stoker J, van Randen A, Lameris W, et al. Imaging patients with acute abdominal pain. Radiology 2009;253:31–46.
89. Raveenthiran V, Madiba TE, Atamanalp SS, et al. Volvulus of the sigmoid colon. Colorectal Dis 2010;12:e1–7.
90. Foxx-Orenstein AE. Ileus and pseudo-obstruction. In: Feldman M, Friedman LS, Brandt LJ, editors. Sleisenger and Fordtran's gastrointestinal and liver disease: pathophysiology/diagnosis/management. 9th edition. Philadelphia: WB Saunders; 2010.
91. Batke M, Cappell MS. Adynamic ileus and acute colonic pseudo-obstruction. Med Clin North Am 2008;92:649–70.
92. Jetmore AM, Timmcke AE, Gathright JB, et al. Ogilvie's syndrome: colonoscopic decompression and analysis of predisposing factors. Dis Colon Rectum 1992; 35:1135–42.
93. Vanek VW, Al-Salti M. Acute pseudo-obstruction of the colon (Ogilvie's syndrome): an analysis of 400 cases. Dis Colon Rectum 1986;29:203–10.
94. Villar HV, Norton LW. Massive cecal dilation: pseudoobstruction vs cecal volvulus? Am J Surg 1979;137:170–4.
95. Adams JT. Adynamic ileus of the colon. Arch Surg 1974;109:503–7.
96. Young RP, Wu H. Intestinal pseudo-obstruction caused by diltiazem in a neutropenic patient. Ann Pharmacother 2005;39:1749–51.
97. Ponec RJ, Saunder MD, Kimmey MB. Neostigmine for the treatment of acute colonic pseudo-obstruction. N Engl J Med 1999;341:137–41.
98. Abeyta BJ, Albrecht RM, Schermer CR. Retrospective study of neostigmine for the treatment of acute colonic pseudo-obstruction. Am Surg 2001;67:265–9.
99. Trevisani GT, Hyman NH, Church JM. Neostigmine: safe and effective treatment for acute colonic pseudo-obstruction. Dig Dis Sci 2000;43:599–603.
100. Kassahun WT, Schulz T, Richter O, et al. Unchanged high mortality rates from acute occlusive intestinal ischemia: a six year review. Langenbecks Arch Surg 2008;393:163–71.
101. Mamode N, Pickford I, Leiberman P. Failure to improve outcome in acute mesenteric ischaemia: seven year review. Eur J Surg 1999;165:203–8.
102. Park WM, Gloviczki P, Cherry KJ, et al. Contemporary management of acute mesenteric ischemia: factors associated with survival. J Vasc Surg 2002;35: 445–52.
103. Acosta-Merida MA, Marchena-Gomez J, Hemmersbach-Miller M, et al. Identification of risk factors for perioperative mortality in acute mesenteric ischemia. World J Surg 2006;30:1579–85.
104. Edwards MS, Cherr GS, Craven TE, et al. Acute occlusive mesenteric ischemia: surgical management and outcomes. Ann Vasc Surg 2003;17:72–9.
105. Chang RW, Chang JB, Longo WE. Update in management of mesenteric ischemia. World J Gastroenterol 2006;12:3243–7.

106. Block T, Nilsson TK, Bjorck M, et al. Diagnostic accuracy of plasma biomarkers for intestinal ischaemia. Scand J Clin Lab Invest 2008;68:242–8.
107. Sarr MG, Bulkley GB, Zuidema GD. Preoperative recognition of intestinal obstruction: prospective evaluation of diagnostic capabilities. Am J Surg 1983;145:176–82.
108. Feretis CB, Koborozos BA, Vyssoulis GP, et al. Serum phosphate levels in acute bowel ischemia. Am Surg 1985;51:242–4.
109. Murray MJ, Gonze MD, Nowak LR, et al. Serum D(–)-lactate levels as an aid to diagnosing acute intestinal ischemia. Am J Surg 1994;167:575–8.
110. Kurt Y, Akin ML, Demirbas S, et al. D-dimer in the early diagnosis of acute mesenteric ischemia secondary to arterial occlusion in rats. Eur Surg Res 2005;37:216–9.
111. Altinyollar H, Boyabatli M, Berberoğlu U. D-dimer as a marker for early diagnosis of acute mesenteric ischemia. Thromb Res 2006;117:463–7.
112. Brandt LJ, Boley SJ. AGA technical review on intestinal ischemia. Gastroenterology 2000;118:954–68.
113. Sanson TG, O'Keefe KP. Evaluation of abdominal pain in the elderly. Emerg Med Clin North Am 1996;14:615–27.
114. Horton KM, Fishman EK. Multidetector CT angiography in the diagnosis of mesenteric ischemia. Radiol Clin North Am 2007;45:275–88.
115. Kirkpatrick ID, Kroeker MA. Greenberg HM biphasic CT with mesenteric CT angiography in the evaluation of acute mesenteric ischemia: initial experience. Radiology 2003;229:91–8.
116. Aschoff AJ, Stuber G, Becker BW, et al. Evaluation of acute mesenteric ischemia: accuracy of biphasic mesenteric multidetector CT angiography. Abdom Imaging 2009;34:345–57.
117. Berland T, Oldenburg WA. Acute mesenteric ischemia. Curr Gastroenterol Rep 2008;10:341–6.
118. Silverberg E, Boring CC, Squires TS. Cancer statistics, 1990. CA Cancer J Clin 1990;40:9–26.
119. Johansen K, Kohler TR, Nicholls SC, et al. Ruptured abdominal aortic aneurysm: the Harborview experience. J Vasc Surg 1991;13:240–5.
120. Lederle FA. In the clinic: abdominal aortic aneurysm. Ann Intern Med 2009;150: ITC5-1–15.
121. Vardulaki KA, Prevost TC, Walker NM, et al. Growth rates and risk of rupture of abdominal aortic aneurysms. Br J Surg 1998;85:1674–80.
122. Van der Vliet JA, Boll AP. Abdominal aortic aneurysm. Lancet 1997;349: 863–6.
123. Banerjee A. Atypical manifestations of ruptured abdominal aortic aneurysms. Postgrad Med J 1993;69:6–11.
124. Marston WA, Ahlquist R, Johnson G, et al. Misdiagnosis of ruptured abdominal aortic aneurysms. J Vasc Surg 1992;16:17–22.
125. Fielding JWL, Black F, Ashton F, et al. Diagnosis and management of 528 abdominal aortic aneurysms. BMJ 1981;283:355–9.
126. Lederle FA, Walker JM, Reinke DM. Selective screening for abdominal aortic aneurysms with physical examination and ultrasound. Arch Intern Med 1998; 148:1753–6.
127. Kuhn M, Bonnin RL, Davey MJ, et al. Emergency department ultrasound scanning for abdominal aortic aneurysm: accessible, accurate, and advantageous. Ann Emerg Med 2000;36:219–23.

128. Hagan PG, Nienaber CA, Isselbacher EM, et al. The international registry of acute aortic dissection (IRAD): new insights into an old disease. JAMA 2000; 283:897–903.

129. Abrutyn E, Mossey J, Levinson M, et al. Epidemiology of asymptomatic bacteriuria in elderly women. J Am Geriatr Soc 1991;39:388–93.

130. Boscia JA, Kobasa WD, Knight RA, et al. Epidemiology of bacteriuria in an elderly ambulatory population. Am J Med 1986;60:208–14.

131. Rodhe N, Lofgren S, Matussek A, et al. Asymptomatic bacteriuria in the elderly: high prevalence and high turnover of strains. Scand J Infect Dis 2008;30: 804–10.

132. Lin YT, Chen LK, Lin MH, et al. Asymptomatic bacteriuria among the institutionalized elderly. J Chin Med Assoc 2006;69:213–7.

133. Usui Y, Matsuzaki S, Matsushita K, et al. Urolithiasis in geriatric patients. Tokai J Exp Clin Med 2003;28:81–7.

134. Yeh EL, McNamara R. Abdominal pain. Clin Geriatr Med 2007;23:255–70.

135. Mccrea GL, Miaskowski C, Stotts N, et al. A review of literature on gender and age differences in the prevalence and characteristics of constipation in North America. J Pain Symptom Manage 2009;37:737–45.

136. Laurell H, Hansson LE, Gunnarsson U. Why do surgeons miss malignancies in patients with acute abdominal pain? Anticancer Res 2006;26:3675–8.

137. USA QuickFacts. 2008. Available at: http://quickfacts.census.gov/qfd/states/00000.html. Accessed January 10, 2010.

138. Altekruse SF, Kosary CL, Krapcho M, et al, editors. SEER Cancer Statistics Review, 1975–2007. Bethesda (MD): National Cancer Institute. Available at: https://owa. dm.duke.edu/owa/redir.aspx?C=248fb19587764fdb896bec1b96600e13&URL= http%3a%2f%2fseer.cancer.gov%2fcsr%2f1975_2007%2f; http://seer.cancer. gov/csr/1975_2007/. Based on November 2009 SEER data submission, posted to the SEER web site, 2010. Accessed January 22, 2011.

139. American Cancer Society, Cancer facts & figures 2009. Available at: http://ww2. cancer.org/downloads/STT/500809web.pdf. Accessed January 20, 2010.

Abdominal Pain in Special Populations

Esther H. Chen, MD[a],*, Angela M. Mills, MD[b]

KEYWORDS
- Abdominal pain • Immunocompromised • Immunosuppressed
- Post-procedure

THE IMMUNOCOMPROMISED PATIENT

Patients with altered immunologic function comprise a heterogeneous population ranging from those who are mildly immunocompromised (eg, elderly, uremic, diabetic) to those who are moderately to severely immunocompromised (eg, current immuno-suppressive therapy, post transplant, acquired immunodeficiency syndrome [AIDS], active malignancy undergoing chemotherapy). Compared with immunocompetent hosts, this population suffers from the same spectrum of diseases, but because of their blunted immune response they may present with atypical symptoms such as altered mental status and tachycardia, lack the classic signs of an acute abdomen, and/or seek medical attention later in their disease course.[1] For example, transplanted organs lack native innervation, so even pain is an unreliable sign of underlying disease.[2] In addition to the surgical conditions that must be considered in any patient with acute abdominal pain, the differential diagnosis should be expanded to include nonsurgical problems and infections that may be unique to this population. These diseases include cytomegalovirus (CMV) infection, neutropenic enterocolitis (typhlitis), and intra-abdominal abscesses. Because they are so challenging to diagnose and are more likely to harbor a potentially life-threatening disease, immunosuppressed patients will often receive diagnostic imaging with abdominal-pelvic computed tomography (CT) as part of their emergency department (ED) evaluation.

Human Immunodeficiency Virus/AIDS

The introduction of highly active antiretroviral therapy (HAART) has decreased the incidence of opportunistic infections (OIs) and gastrointestinal diseases. A retrospective study of 108 human immunodeficiency virus (HIV)-positive patients (84% on

---

The authors have no financial conflict.
[a] Department of Emergency Medicine, University of San Francisco, San Francisco General Hospital, 1001 Potrero Avenue, #1E25, San Francisco, CA 94110, USA
[b] Department of Emergency Medicine, University of Pennsylvania School of Medicine, 3400 Spruce Street, Ground Ravdin, Philadelphia, PA 19104, USA
* Corresponding author.
E-mail address: esther.chen@emergency.ucsf.edu

Emerg Med Clin N Am 29 (2011) 449–458
doi:10.1016/j.emc.2011.01.006
0733-8627/11/$ – see front matter © 2011 Elsevier Inc. All rights reserved.

antiretroviral therapy or HAART, 44% with CD_4 <200 cells/mm^3) with undifferentiated abdominal pain[3] showed that only 10% of patients had an OI as compared with pre-HAART reports of 41% to 86%.[4–6] Disseminated mycobacterial disease was the most common diagnosis. Other OIs included *Candida* esophagitis, AIDS cholangiopathy, lymphoma, and intra-abdominal tuberculosis. Well-described causes of abdominal pain such as CMV colitis or peritonitis, cryptosporidiosis, and Kaposi sarcoma were not seen at all in this San Francisco population. Moreover, only 9 patients (8%) required surgical intervention, one of which was for drainage of a *Mycobacterium* abscess (the only HIV-associated OI). A more recent study of opportunistic gastrointestinal disorders in HIV patients corroborated these findings, showing that 26% of patients on HAART (vs 80% in the no-treatment group) had an OI, most commonly *Candida* esophagitis and CMV esophagitis or colitis.[7] Kaposi sarcoma and lymphoma were less common.

The primary conditions requiring acute surgical intervention in HIV patients are appendicitis, cholecystitis, bowel obstruction, and intestinal perforation.[8] These surgical conditions occur as frequently in HIV patients on HAART as in non-HIV patients,[7,9] although the underlying pathology may be different. In immunocompromised patients, CMV infection can cause vasculitis in the gastrointestinal tract leading to ulcerations in the bowel wall, particularly in the terminal ileum and colon. CMV colitis may present acutely as gastrointestinal hemorrhage, perforation, or toxic megacolon.[10] Appendicitis can also be caused by CMV infection and may present with more indolent symptoms. In addition, intestinal obstruction and intussusception may be caused by Kaposi sarcoma and lymphoma.[8,9] Finally, although gallstone cholecystitis occurs equally in non-HIV and HIV patients, acalculous cholecystitis occurs more frequently in the HIV population. Moreover, these patients can develop cholangiopathy, both as an adverse effect of antiretroviral medications and from infiltration of opportunistic pathogens into the biliary ducts causing obstruction.[9]

In addition to the conditions already mentioned, abdominal pain in HIV patients may be an adverse effect of the same antiretroviral medications that have been shown to decrease gastrointestinal diseases. Patients will often present with associated symptoms of nausea, vomiting, and diarrhea, sometimes severe enough to cause dehydration or hemodynamic instability. Some medications are associated with specific conditions. For example, didanosine (Videx) can cause acute pancreatitis and indinavir (Crixivan) can precipitate in the kidneys, leading to nephrolithiasis.[8] More often than not, the discomfort caused by these medications results in intermittent medication noncompliance and sometimes discontinuation of the treatment entirely.[11] Lapses in treatment may increase a patient's risk of developing OI.

Malignancy

Approximately 40% of the ED visits by cancer patients are for abdominal pain.[12] The differential diagnosis of abdominal pain in this patient group should include conditions directly related to the malignancy itself in addition to complications of the malignancy treatment.[13] Not surprisingly, intra-abdominal cancers increase a patient's risk of developing a small bowel or large bowel obstruction,[14] although non–intra-abdominal cancers (ie, breast, melanoma) can also cause bowel obstruction due to diffuse peritoneal carcinomatosis.[15] A diagnosis of large bowel or gastric outlet obstruction in an otherwise healthy patient or someone with a history of prior cancer should increase the suspicion of an underlying or recurrent malignancy.[13,14] Furthermore, solid tumors can become a lead point in causing intussusception, which is otherwise uncommon in healthy adults.[16] Bowel perforation may be caused by transmural erosion of gastrointestinal cancers, intestinal metastatic lesions, and atypical infections. Pneumoperitoneum can be challenging to diagnose, as patients may have difficulty localizing the infection and therefore have a delayed presentation.[1] In addition, patients with cancer can develop malignant ascites, causing abdominal distention and pain, and Budd-Chiari syndrome, a constellation of symptoms caused by hepatic venous outflow obstruction from thrombosis.[13] In evaluating these patients, Abdominal CT is more clinically useful because it can detect closed-loop or strangulation obstruction, identify a transition point, and diagnose intestinal pneumatosis or vascular thrombosis,[13] as compared with plain radiography, which has a sensitivity of only 66%[17] for detecting small bowel obstruction and an inability to identify strangulated bowel or vascular thrombosis.[18]

Gastrointestinal symptoms can also be an adverse effect of the treatment of the underlying malignancy. Chemotherapeutic agents frequently cause abdominal pain associated with nausea, vomiting, and/or diarrhea. Radiation therapy to the abdomen or pelvis can lead to a progressive occlusive vasculitis and local narrowing of the intestinal lumen. Radiation enteritis is a spectrum of disease including acute bowel ulceration, intestinal perforation, and/or massive gastrointestinal hemorrhage, and may lead to chronic fistula formation and strictures.[19]

Cancer treatment with chemotherapy can also cause profound neutropenia. In neutropenic patients, the most common cause of an acute abdomen is neutropenic enterocolitis (NEC) or typhlitis.[13] NEC is a necrotizing inflammation of the cecum and the adjacent small intestine in the setting of chemotherapy-induced neutropenia or bone marrow transplantation. Also known as necrotizing enterocolitis, it has been described in patients with aplastic anemia, AIDS, and organ transplantation. Cytotoxic agents such as the taxanes and vinorelbine (Navelbine) may also increase a patient's risk of NEC.[20]

Symptoms of NEC include fever, nausea, vomiting, abdominal distension, diarrhea, and right lower quadrant pain, which may be initially thought to be due to appendicitis. Patients may also present with hypotension and other signs of sepsis. Although the symptoms of NEC may be difficult to distinguish from the routine side effects of the chemotherapeutic agents themselves, it is more likely to be associated with bowel wall thickening on abdominal CT of more than 4 mm, with a very poor prognosis if greater than 10 mm (**Fig. 1**).[21,22] Treatment includes fluid resuscitation, broad-spectrum antibiotics effective for enteric gram-negative bacilli, *Enterococcus* spp, and anaerobes, bowel rest, and parenteral nutrition as needed.[20] Surgical intervention is reserved for bowel ischemia and perforation.[23] Mortality and morbidity rates are high so prompt recognition may be life-saving.[24]

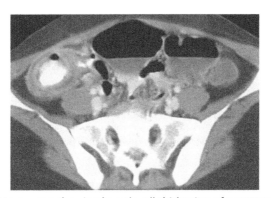

Fig. 1. Computed tomogram showing bowel wall thickening of neutropenic enterocolitis.

Solid Organ Transplant Patients

Like many postsurgical patients, the two most common reasons for solid organ transplant patients to visit the ED are abdominal pain (31%), often associated with other gastrointestinal symptoms, and infectious symptoms (17%) such as fever or wound infection.[2] In this ED study, infection (36%) and gastrointestinal or genitourinary pathology (20%) were the most common ED diagnoses, regardless of the time elapsed since transplantation. Moreover, the majority of transplant patients (61%) were hospitalized (compared with the 17% overall admission rate in the same institution during the study period), regardless of their diagnosis, presumably because a missed diagnosis may have serious consequences for both the graft and the patient. Any posttransplant patient with abdominal pain must be evaluated for organ rejection, systemic infection, and drug toxicity.

Specific conditions to consider in these patients will depend on the time elapsed since transplantation. In the early posttransplant period (<1 month), postsurgical complications and infections predominate.[2] The surgical anastomosis may constrict or leak, causing bowel obstruction or peritonitis. Graft injuries, such as bile duct ischemia, can later become a liver abscess. Viral or candidal infections may be either donor-derived or a surgical complication. *Clostridium difficile* colitis is also common during this period, as opposed to OIs, which are typically absent.[25] In addition, patients have a slightly higher risk of graft rejection within the first month than within the intermediate or late posttransplant period.[2]

During the intermediate posttransplant period (1–6 months), viral infections and graft rejection are the most common reasons for patients to develop a fever.[25] Because the full effect of immunosuppressants is now present, OIs such as CMV colitis and intra-abdominal abscesses caused by fungal (eg, *Candida*, *Cryptococcus*) and bacterial infections (eg, *Nocardia*, *Legionella*) may develop. These patients should be considered severely immunocompromised and highly susceptible to infection.

In the late posttransplant period (>6 months), the risk of infection typically declines slightly as immunosuppressive therapy is tapered down in patients with good graft function. However, patients continue to be at risk for developing chronic rejection, often as a result of chronic viral infections.[25] Acute diverticulitis is a common gastrointestinal infection seen during this period; patients may present with perforation due to a delay in diagnosis. In addition, this population may also develop posttransplantation lymphoproliferative disorder (PTLD), a lymphoproliferative disorder thought to be associated with Epstein-Barr virus infection. Patients with suspected PTLD may present with fever, a mononucleosis-like syndrome, gastrointestinal obstruction, bleeding, or perforation, and have significant hepatic or pancreatic dysfunction. Regression of PTLD may occur with a reduction in immunosuppressant therapy, although this disease often will require chemotherapy or immunotherapy.[25]

THE POSTPROCEDURE PATIENT

Percutaneous interventions are minimally invasive procedures increasingly being performed by interventional radiologists and noninterventionalists. Acute abdominal pain and other gastrointestinal symptoms are common reasons these patients seek emergency care following their procedure. The remaining sections of this article focus on the gastrointestinal complications of several common procedures.

Vena Cava Filters

Potential complications of inferior vena cava (IVC) filters include recurrent deep vein thrombosis (DVT), IVC thrombosis, migration, fracture, and infection. Thus, acute abdominal pain or flank pain in a patient with an IVC filter may be due to a device-related complication. Older permanent filters are more likely to migrate or fracture than those placed in the past 6 years (5%–30% [migration] and 2% [strut fracture] vs 0.3%–3% and 0%, respectively) (**Fig. 2**).[26–28] Filter or strut migration may be entirely asymptomatic or may cause ischemic (vessel obstruction) or hemorrhagic (vessel perforation) end-organ damage. Furthermore, limited IVC penetration by the filter has increased recently from 10% to 95% with the newer filters,[26,28] due to an anchoring improvement that may partially explain the decrease in migration rate; through-and-through caval penetration is rare. Patients with filter migration or more significant caval penetration may report tearing pain in their groin or flank followed by fever or signs of organ dysfunction (eg, small bowel obstruction, duodenal perforation, rectal bleeding). These patients require CT imaging for diagnosis and immediate interventional radiology consultation for filter removal.

Percutaneous Gastrostomy Tubes

The major gastrointestinal complications of percutaneously placed gastrostomy, gastrojejunostomy, and jejunostomy tubes include peritonitis (1.3%) from pericatheter leakage of gastric contents into the peritoneum, gastric perforation or hemorrhage (1.7%), deep stomal infection or abscess (0.8%), and inadvertent injury to adjacent organs during placement.[29,30] Patients may also present with minor complications including superficial wound infection, peristomal leakage, and tube malfunction (eg, dislodgment, blockage, balloon rupture). A case series of 400 gastrostomy procedures reported 4 cases of peritonitis in patients with significant comorbidities; one patient developed a liver abscess after inadvertent liver puncture during the procedure.[31] Major complications occur early, within a few days after the procedure, and patients may present with abdominal pain and fever or severe sepsis. These patients often require CT imaging to detect intra-abdominal abscesses or gastric perforation, followed by interventional radiology or surgical consultation for tube removal and/or abscess drainage.

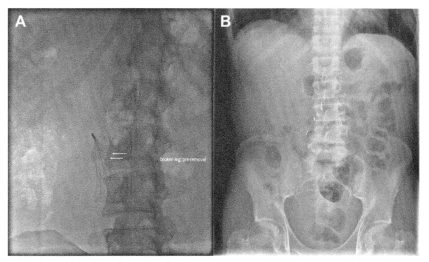

Fig. 2. (*A*) IVC filter strut fracture. The arrows point to the broken struts. (*B*) IVC filter strut fracture and migration.

Transvenous Hepatic and Renal Biopsy

Transvenous biopsies are most commonly performed on the liver and kidneys. Most transvenous liver biopsy complications require no intervention and are detected before hospital discharge.[32] However, discharged patients may return with abdominal pain radiating to the right shoulder, indicating a delayed formation of a perihepatic hematoma. Ultrasonography of the right upper quadrant may be used to confirm the diagnosis (**Fig. 3**). Acute intervention is often not required unless there is associated hemodynamic instability or a significant, life-threatening drop in the hemoglobin level. Finally, although transient pyrexia may be routinely observed up to 24 hours after the procedure,[33] persistent pyrexia with concurrent gastrointestinal symptoms suggests the presence of an intrahepatic or perihepatic abscess and requires further evaluation.

Similar to liver biopsies, complications following transjugular renal biopsy typically do not require acute intervention. Almost ubiquitous after a renal biopsy is gross hematuria from a perinephric hematoma or calyceal hemorrhage (66%); both conditions typically resolve spontaneously.[34,35] Patients with significant hematuria or symptomatic anemia due to an arteriovenous or arteriocalyceal fistula[36] may develop abdominal pain and distention from clot retention, with subsequent urethral obstruction. In this clinical scenario, the bladder must be manually irrigated through a large-bore (20 French or larger) Foley catheter. Continuous bladder irrigation is often reserved for patients without clot formation, as the clots can obstruct the smaller lumen of the catheter and cause bladder perforation. Alternatively, patients with symptomatic anemia in the absence of hematuria may have a retroperitoneal hematoma[37] also causing abdominal or flank pain. Urgent consultation for vessel embolization should be obtained for patients with intractable bleeding or retroperitoneal bleed.

Transjugular Intrahepatic Portosystemic Shunts

Transjugular intrahepatic portosystemic shunts (TIPS) are used to treat patients with complications of liver failure by diverting blood from the abnormally high-pressure portal system to the low-pressure caval system.[38] Because inadvertent puncture of the hepatic capsule (5%–30%), gallbladder (5%–10%), and right kidney (<2%) can occur during the procedure,[39] patients may develop acute abdominal pain or flank pain from a slowly expanding perihepatic hematoma, acute cholangitis, or perinephric

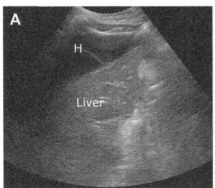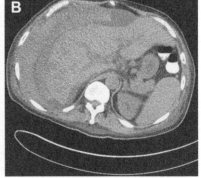

Fig. 3. (*A*) Ultrasonogram showing perihepatic hematoma (H) post transvenous liver biopsy; (*B*) Computed tomogram of the same patient, demonstrating perihepatic hematoma following transvenous liver biopsy.

hematoma, respectively. Acute ED management of TIPS-related issues requires stabilizing the patient, initiating treatment of the active issues (eg, antibiotics for infection, blood transfusion for gastrointestinal bleeding), and obtaining CT imaging to identify intra-abdominal sources of infection or bleeding.

Uterine Artery Embolization

Women who undergo uterine artery embolization (UAE) will often present to the ED with abdominal/pelvic pain and vaginal discharge or bleeding.[40–42] These symptoms, along with bloating, fever, dysuria, hot flushes, mood swings, and fibroid passage, are collectively referred to as postembolization syndrome, thought to be caused by fibroid infarction.[41] The two most clinically significant reasons for hospital readmission are severe, intractable abdominal pain and pelvic infection.[41] Even though the pain may be caused by postembolization syndrome, fibroid passage, or fibroid necrosis—all relatively benign conditions—the differential diagnosis should also include pelvic infections (eg, endometritis, myometritis, infected necrotic leiomyoma, pelvic abscess). The most reliable diagnostic study to distinguish a uterine infection or abscess from postembolization syndrome is magnetic resonance imaging with gadolinium (**Fig. 4**).[43] If this is not readily available, CT is preferred to ultrasonography.

Percutaneous Biliary Drains

There are 3 types of percutaneous biliary drains: external (sits above the obstruction and drains bile into an external drainage bag), internal (metallic or plastic stent drains into the bowel), and internal-external (external catheter enters a duct above the obstruction and crosses the obstruction into the duodenum) drainage catheters.[44] Two common causes of acute abdominal pain are intraperitoneal bile leakage and tube obstruction, which can result in ascending cholangitis and intrahepatic abscesses, especially in patients with malignant biliary obstruction.[45] CT imaging may be useful in detecting these fluid collections. Before imaging, a simple maneuver that may promptly relieve the obstruction (and the patient's pain) is to uncap the external portion of an external or internal/external catheter where the external catheter is capped.

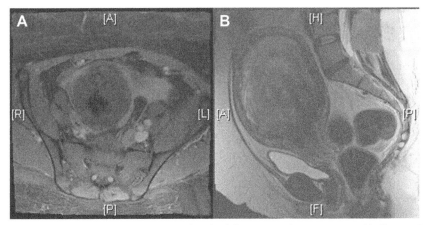

Fig. 4. (*A*) Magnetic resonance imaging (MRI) of the uterus, showing gas and inflammation within the endometrium characteristic of endometritis; (*B*) MRI of the uterus, showing extrusion of a uterine fibroid.

EMERGENCY DEPARTMENT MANAGEMENT

The ED management of patients with altered immunologic function and who are post-procedure includes immediate resuscitation, a broadened differential diagnosis with timely diagnosis, and urgent consultation as appropriate. As these patients are at high risk of abdominal emergencies, radiologic imaging such as CT or ultrasonography is often necessary to confirm a diagnosis and guide therapy. Infections, both intra-abdominal and otherwise, should be treated with the appropriate antibiotics. Patients with acute symptoms and an unclear diagnosis warrant admission until serious pathology may be reasonably excluded.

SUMMARY

Evaluation of abdominal pain in special populations includes recognition of atypical and delayed patient presentations. As classic presentations of abdominal emergencies can be altered, life-threatening conditions may be easily missed. Consideration of the underlying condition of the patient (ie, immunocompromised host, postprocedural) will enable the emergency practitioner to appropriately evaluate and manage these patients for those specific disease processes in the differential diagnosis.

REFERENCES

1. Scott-Conner CE, Fabrega AJ. Gastrointestinal problems in the immunocompromised host. A review for surgeons. Surg Endosc 1996;10(10):959–64.
2. Unterman S, Zimmerman M, Tyo C, et al. A descriptive analysis of 1251 solid organ transplant visits to the emergency department. West J Emerg Med 2009; 10(1):48–54.
3. Yoshida D, Caruso JM. Abdominal pain in the HIV infected patient. J Emerg Med 2002;23(2):111–6.
4. Barone JE, Gingold BS, Arvanitis ML, et al. Abdominal pain in patients with acquired immune deficiency syndrome. Ann Surg 1986;204(6):619–23.
5. Parente F, Cernuschi M, Antinori S, et al. Severe abdominal pain in patients with AIDS: frequency, clinical aspects, causes, and outcome. Scand J Gastroenterol 1994;29(6):511–5.
6. O'Keefe EA, Wood R, Van Zyl A, et al. Human immunodeficiency virus-related abdominal pain in South Africa. Aetiology, diagnosis and survival. Scand J Gastroenterol 1998;33(2):212–7.
7. Monkemuller KE, Lazenby AJ, Lee DH, et al. Occurrence of gastrointestinal opportunistic disorders in AIDS despite the use of highly active antiretroviral therapy. Dig Dis Sci 2005;50(2):230–4.
8. Slaven EM, Lopez F, Weintraub SL, et al. The AIDS patient with abdominal pain: a new challenge for the emergency physician. Emerg Med Clin North Am 2003; 21(4):987–1015.
9. Saltzman DJ, Williams RA, Gelfand DV, et al. The surgeon and AIDS: twenty years later. Arch Surg 2005;140(10):961–7.
10. Davidson T, Allen-Mersh TG, Miles AJ, et al. Emergency laparotomy in patients with AIDS. Br J Surg 1991;78(8):924–6.
11. Hill A, Balkin A. Risk factors for gastrointestinal adverse events in HIV treated and untreated patients. AIDS Rev 2009;11(1):30–8.

12. Swenson KK, Rose MA, Ritz L, et al. Recognition and evaluation of oncology-related symptoms in the emergency department. Ann Emerg Med 1995;26(1): 12–7.
13. Ilgen JS, Marr AL. Cancer emergencies: the acute abdomen. Emerg Med Clin North Am 2009;27(3):381–99.
14. Hirst B, Regnard C. Management of intestinal obstruction in malignant disease. Clin Med 2003;3(4):311–4.
15. Ripamonti CI, Easson AM, Gerdes H. Management of malignant bowel obstruction. Eur J Cancer 2008;44(8):1105–15.
16. Takeuchi K, Tsuzuki Y, Ando T, et al. The diagnosis and treatment of adult intussusception. J Clin Gastroenterol 2003;36(1):18–21.
17. Maglinte DD, Kelvin FM, Sandrasegaran K, et al. Radiology of small bowel obstruction: contemporary approach and controversies. Abdom Imaging 2005; 30(2):160–78.
18. Sarr MG, Bulkley GB, Zuidema GD. Preoperative recognition of intestinal strangulation obstruction. Prospective evaluation of diagnostic capability. Am J Surg 1983;145(1):176–82.
19. Yeoh E. Radiotherapy: long-term effects on gastrointestinal function. Curr Opin Support Palliat Care 2008;2(1):40–4.
20. Rolston KV. Neutropenic enterocolitis associated with docetaxel therapy in a patient with breast cancer. Clin Adv Hematol Oncol 2009;7(8):527–8.
21. Gorschluter M, Mey U, Strehl J, et al. Neutropenic enterocolitis in adults: systematic analysis of evidence quality. Eur J Haematol 2005;75(1):1–13.
22. Spencer SP, Power N, Reznek RH. Multidetector computed tomography of the acute abdomen in the immunocompromised host: a pictorial review. Curr Probl Diagn Radiol 2009;38(4):145–55.
23. Blijlevens NM. Neutropenic enterocolitis: challenges in diagnosis and treatment. Clin Adv Hematol Oncol 2009;7(8):528–30.
24. Gomez L, Martino R, Rolston KV. Neutropenic enterocolitis: spectrum of the disease and comparison of definite and possible cases. Clin Infect Dis 1998; 27(4):695–9.
25. Fishman JA. Infection in solid-organ transplant recipients. N Engl J Med 2007; 357(25):2601–14.
26. Berczi V, Bottomley JR, Thomas SM, et al. Long-term retrievability of IVC filters: should we abandon permanent devices? Cardiovasc Intervent Radiol 2007; 30(5):820–7.
27. Chung J, Owen RJ. Using inferior vena cava filters to prevent pulmonary embolism. Can Fam Physician 2008;54(1):49–55.
28. Ray CE Jr, Kaufman JA. Complications of inferior vena cava filters. Abdom Imaging 1996;21(4):368–74.
29. Given MF, Hanson JJ, Lee MJ. Interventional radiology techniques for provision of enteral feeding. Cardiovasc Intervent Radiol 2005;28(6):692–703.
30. Wollman B, D'Agostino HB, Walus-Wigle JR, et al. Radiologic, endoscopic, and surgical gastrostomy: an institutional evaluation and meta-analysis of the literature. Radiology 1995;197(3):699–704.
31. Silas AM, Pearce LF, Lestina LS, et al. Percutaneous radiologic gastrostomy versus percutaneous endoscopic gastrostomy: a comparison of indications, complications and outcomes in 370 patients. Eur J Radiol 2005;56(1):84–90.
32. Kalambokis G, Manousou P, Vibhakorn S, et al. Transjugular liver biopsy—indications, adequacy, quality of specimens, and complications—a systematic review. J Hepatol 2007;47(2):284–94.

33. Gamble P, Colapinto RF, Stronell RD, et al. Transjugular liver biopsy: a review of 461 biopsies. Radiology 1985;157(3):589–93.
34. Cluzel P, Martinez F, Bellin MF, et al. Transjugular versus percutaneous renal biopsy for the diagnosis of parenchymal disease: comparison of sampling effectiveness and complications. Radiology 2000;215(3):689–93.
35. Misra S, Gyamlani G, Swaminathan S, et al. Safety and diagnostic yield of transjugular renal biopsy. J Vasc Interv Radiol 2008;19(4):546–51.
36. See TC, Thompson BC, Howie AJ, et al. Transjugular renal biopsy: our experience and technical considerations. Cardiovasc Intervent Radiol 2008;31(5):906–18.
37. Fine DM, Arepally A, Hofmann LV, et al. Diagnostic utility and safety of transjugular kidney biopsy in the obese patient. Nephrol Dial Transplant 2004;19(7): 1798–802.
38. Haskal ZJ, Martin L, Cardella JF, et al. Quality improvement guidelines for transjugular intrahepatic portosystemic shunts. J Vasc Interv Radiol 2003;14(9 Pt 2): S265–70.
39. Freedman AM, Sanyal AJ, Tisnado J, et al. Complications of transjugular intrahepatic portosystemic shunt: a comprehensive review. Radiographics 1993;13(6): 1185–210.
40. Marshburn PB, Matthews ML, Hurst BS. Uterine artery embolization as a treatment option for uterine myomas. Obstet Gynecol Clin North Am 2006;33(1):125–44.
41. Pron G, Mocarski E, Bennett J, et al. Tolerance, hospital stay, and recovery after uterine artery embolization for fibroids: the Ontario uterine fibroid embolization trial. J Vasc Interv Radiol 2003;14(10):1243–50.
42. Ganguli S, Faintuch S, Salazar GM, et al. Postembolization syndrome: changes in white blood cell counts immediately after uterine artery embolization. J Vasc Interv Radiol 2008;19(3):443–5.
43. Kitamura Y, Ascher SM, Cooper C, et al. Imaging manifestations of complications associated with uterine artery embolization. Radiographics 2005;25(Suppl 1): S119–32.
44. Covey AM, Brown KT. Palliative percutaneous drainage in malignant biliary obstruction. Part 2: mechanisms and postprocedure management. J Support Oncol 2006;4(7):329–35.
45. Wu SM, Marchant LK, Haskal ZJ. Percutaneous interventions in the biliary tree. Semin Roentgenol 1997;32(3):228–45.

Index

Note: Page numbers of article titles are in **boldface** type.

A

Abdomen, surgery of, abdominal pain and, 163
   vascular anatomy of, 253–255
Abdominal aortic aneurysm, 264–266
Abdominal emergencies, vascular, **253–272**
Abdominal hernias. See *Hernia(s), abdominal.*
Abdominal pain, acute, analgesia in, 168
      approach to, **159–173**
      diagnostic imaging in, 176–179
      diagnostic studies in, 169–170
      imaging and laboratory testing in, **175–193**
         integration based on pain location and disease process, 179–190
      in older adult, **429–448**
      in unstable patient, 168–169
      laboratory testing in, 175–176
   assessment of patient's pain in, 160–162
   epigastric, evaluation of, 184
   extra-abdominal and systemic causes of, 196–197
   functional, in children, 418–419
   generalized, evaluation of, 179–181
   hematologic causes of, 200
   history taking in, 159–163
   imflammatory causes of, 200–202
   in children, diagnosis of, 403–420
     differential diagnosis of, 403, 404
     due to infections, 202–203
     functional, 418–419
     history taking in, 401
     physical examination in, 402–403
   in older adults. See *Adult(s), older, abdominal pain in.*
   in right upper quadrant, evaluation of, 182–183
   in special populations, **449–458**
   infectious causes of, 202–203
   left lower quadrant, evaluation of, 188–189
   left upper quadrant, evaluation of, 187–188
   metabolic/endocrine causes of, 197–199
   neurogenic causes of, 205
   right lower quadrant, evaluation of, 184–187
   suprapubic, evaluation of, 189–190
   symptoms associated with, abdominal examination in, 164–166

Emerg Med Clin N Am 29 (2011) 459–467
doi:10.1016/S0733-8627(11)00026-5
0733-8627/11/$ – see front matter © 2011 Elsevier Inc. All rights reserved.

emed.theclinics.com

Moving?

Make sure your subscription moves with you!

To notify us of your new address, find your **Clinics Account Number** (located on your mailing label above your name), and contact customer service at:

Email: journalscustomerservice-usa@elsevier.com

800-654-2452 (subscribers in the U.S. & Canada)
314-447-8871 (subscribers outside of the U.S. & Canada)

Fax number: 314-447-8029

Elsevier Health Sciences Division
Subscription Customer Service
3251 Riverport Lane
Maryland Heights, MO 63043

*To ensure uninterrupted delivery of your subscription, please notify us at least 4 weeks in advance of move.

Printed and bound by CPI Group (UK) Ltd, Croydon, CR0 4YY

03/10/2024

01040449-0009